g.uk/libra

KT-430-661

BRITISH MEDICAL ASSOCIATION
0646885

Menorrhagia

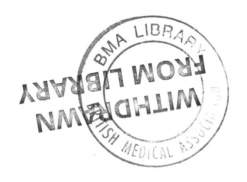
BMA LIBRARY
WITHDRAWN FROM LIBRARY
BRITISH MEDICAL ASSOCIATION

Menorrhagia

Edited by

Shirish S. Sheth MD FRCOG FACS FCPS FICS FICOG FAMS
*Hon. Professor, Obstetrician and Gynaecologist, King Edward Memorial Hospital
and Seth G. S. Medical College (until 1994) Mumbai, India
President Elect, International Federation of Gynaecology and Obstetrics (FIGO)*

and

Christopher J. G. Sutton MA (Cantab) MB BCh FRCOG
Professor of Gynaecological Surgery, University of Surrey, Guildford, UK

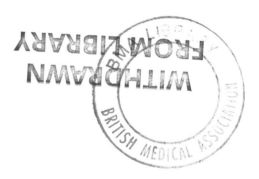
WITHDRAWN FROM LIBRARY
BMA
BRITISH MEDICAL ASSOCIATION

I S I S
MEDICAL
MEDIA

© 1999 by Isis Medical Media Ltd.
59 St. Aldates
Oxford OX1 1ST, UK

First published 1999

All rights reserved. No part of this publication
may be reproduced, stored in a retrieval system,
or transmitted in any form or by any means, electronic,
mechanical, photocopying, recording or otherwise
without the prior permission of the copyright owner.

The Authors have asserted their right under the
Copyright, Designs and Patents Act, 1988,
to be identified as the Authors of this work.

British Library Cataloguing in Publication Data.
A catalogue record for this title is available from
the British Library.

ISBN 1 899066 93 4

Sheth, S. S. (Shirish)
Menorrhagia
Shirish S. Sheth and Christopher J. G. Sutton (eds)

Always refer to the manufacturer's Prescribing
Information before prescribing drugs cited in this book.

Typeset by
Wyvern 21 Ltd, Bristol, UK

Page layout and design by
Design Online, Oxford, UK

Image reproduction by
Track Direct, London, UK

Illustration by
Oxford Designers & Illustrators

Index by
Dr Laurence Errington

Cover photography
Courtesy of Professor P.M. Motta, S. Makabe and E. Vizza/Science Photo Library

Isis Medical Media staff
Commissioning Editor: John Harrison
Senior Editorial Controller: Catherine Rickards
Production Controller: Geoff Holdsworth

Printed and bound by
KHL Printing Ltd., Singapore

Distributed in the USA by
Books International Inc., PO Box 605
Herndon VA 20172, USA

Distributed in the rest of the world by
Plymbridge Distributors Ltd., Estover Road,
Plymouth, PL6 7PY, UK

Contents

Contents

List of contributors

Gautam N. Allahbadia
Consultant in Infertility and Reproductive Medicine, Bombay Hospital and Medical Research Center, Mumbai; The Appollo Clinic, Mumbai; Rotunda — The Centre for Human Reproduction, Mumbai, India

Gunasinghe J. Arachchi
Research Fellow, Department of Obstetrics and Gynaecology, University of Sydney, Sydney NSW 2006, Australia

Sunil K. Bichile
Consultant Haematologist, Department of Haematology, T.N. Medical College, Mumbai, India

John Bonnar
Professor of Obstetrics and Gynaecology, University of Dublin Trinity College; Department of Obstetrics and Gynaecology, Trinity Centre for Health Sciences, St. James's Hospital, Dublin 8, Ireland

Stanley B. Brown
Centre for Photobiology and Photodynamic Therapy, University of Leeds, Leeds, UK

Percy M. Coats
Consultant and Trust Medical Director, Royal Surrey County Hospital Trust, Egerton Road, Guildford, Surrey, UK

Kaizad R. Damania
Nowrosjee Wadia Maternity Hospital, Mumbai, India

Richard W. Dover
Research Fellow in Gynaecological Endoscopy, Royal Surrey County Hospital, Egerton Road, Guildford, Surrey, UK

Kirsten Duckitt
Royal College of Obstetricians and Gynaecologists, 27 Sussex Place, Regent's Park, London, UK

Ian S. Fraser
Professor in Reproductive Medicine, Department of Obstetrics and Gynaecology, University of Sydney, Sydney NSW 2006, Australia

Michael J. Gannon
Consultant in Obstetrics and Gynaecology, Yorkshire Menorrhagia Research Centre, Pinderfields Hospital, Wakefield, UK

Ray Garry
Consultant Gynaecologist, South Cleveland Hospital, Marton Road, Middlesbrough, Cleveland, UK; Medical Director of the WEL Foundation, St. James's University Hospital, Leeds, UK

Mehroo D. Hansotia
Consultant Gynaecologist, Fertility Clinic & IVF Centre, 12 Spring Field, 1st Floor, 19 Vaccha Ghandi Road, Gamdevi, Mumbai, India

Jemma Johns
Gynaecology Cancer Research Unit, The Royal Hospitals NHS Trust, St. Bartholomew's Hospital, West Smithfield, London, UK

Gautam Khastgir
Subspecialty Senior Registrar in Reproductive Medicine, Academic Department of Obstetrics and Gynaecology, Chelsea and Westminster Hospital, Imperial College School of Medicine, University of London, London, UK

Bruce McLucas
U.C.L.A. School of Medicine, Los Angeles, CA, USA

John M. Monaghan
Senior Lecturer in Gynaecological Oncology, Gynaecological Cancer Centre, Queen Elizabeth Hospital, Sheriff Hill, Gateshead, Tyne & Wear NE9 6SX, UK

Nargesh D. Motashaw
Consultant Obstetrician & Gynaecologist and Professor Emeritus, King Edward Memorial Hospital and Seth G. S. Medical College; DELSTAR, 9/A Patkar Marg, Godrej Chowk (Kemp's Corner), Bombay 400 036, India

Suresh Nair
Consultant Obstetrician and Gynaecologist, Kandang Kerbau Women and Children's Hospital; Gynaecology Associates Women's Medical Centre, 3 Mt. Elizabeth #12–18, Mount Elizabeth Medical Centre, Singapore 228510

David H. Oram
Consultant Gynaecological Oncologist, Gynaecology Cancer Research Unit, The Royal Hospitals NHS Trust, St. Bartholomew's Hospital, West Smithfield, London, UK

Kurush P. Paghdiwalla
Consultant Gynaecologist, Chowpatty Medical Centre, Baig Mansion, Babulnath Road, Mumbai, India

Nicholas Panay
Chelsea and Westminster Hospital, Imperial College School of Medicine, University of London, London, UK

Sunil J. Parekh
Consultant Haematologist, Parekh House, 14 M.P. Marg, Mumbai, India

Douglas R. Phillips
Long Island Women's Health Care Associates, 2260 Merrick Road, Merrick, NY 11566, USA; Clinical Associate Professor of Obstetrics and Gynaecology, S.U.N.Y. at Stony Brook School of Medicine, Stony Brook, NY, USA

Andrew Pooley
Research Fellow, Department of Obstetrics and Gynaecology, Royal Surrey County Hospital, Guildford, Surrey, UK

Margaret C. P. Rees
Honorary Senior Clinical Lecturer, Nuffield Department of Obstetrics and Gynaecology, John Radcliffe Hospital, Oxford, UK

John J. Sciarra
Thomas J. Watkins Professor and Chairman, Department of Obstetrics and Gynecology, Northwestern University Medical School, Chicago, IL, USA

Robert W. Shaw
Department of Obstetrics and Gynaecology, University of Wales College of Medicine, Heath Park, Cardiff, UK

Shirish S. Sheth
Consultant Gynaecologist, Breach Candy and Sir Hurkisondas N. Hospitals, 2/2 Navjivan Society, Lamington Road, Mumbai 8, India

Brian L. Sheppard
Trinity College Department of Obstetrics and Gynaecology, Trinity Centre for Health Sciences, St. James's Hospital, Dublin, Ireland

Rustom P. Soonawala
Nowrosjee Wadia Maternity and Breach Candy Hospitals, Mumbai, India

Mark R. Stringer
Centre for Photobiology and Photodynamic Therapy, University of Leeds, Leeds, UK

Christopher J. G. Sutton
Professor of Gynaecological Surgery, University of Surrey, Guildford, UK; Director, Minimal Access Therapy Training Unit and Consultant Gynaecologist, Royal Surrey County Hospital, Guildford, Surrey, UK; Consultant Gynaecologist, Chelsea and Westminster Hospital, Imperial College School of Medicine, University of London, London, UK

John Studd
Consultant Gynaecologist, Academic Department of Obstetrics and Gynaecology, Chelsea and Westminster Hospital, Imperial College School of Medicine, University of London, London, UK

Rafael F. Valle
Department of Obstetrics and Gynaecology, Northwestern University Medical School, Chicago, IL, USA

Woodruff J. Walker
Director of Radiology and Consultant, Department of Diagnostic Radiology, Royal Surrey County Hospital, Egerton Road, Guildford, Surrey, UK

Introduction

In the absence of good clinical acumen and appropriate investigations, it is possible that women may be subjected to many unnecessary gynaecological procedures. A young woman with submucous myoma may be hysterectomized, a pubertal virgin with idiopathic thrombocytopenic purpura (ITP) may undergo hysteroscopy and curettage, and a young hypothyroid woman may be prescribed large amounts of hormones and probably undergo curettage by every different gynaecologist she visits. This demonstrates the importance of early diagnosis by the gynaecologist of some of the most worrisome conditions. The gynaecologist must establish strategies that ensure that pertinent diagnosis is an integral part of their clinical armamentarium. In the words of Hippocrates, 'You cannot treat a patient unless you have arrived at a diagnosis'.

The ability to diagnose menorrhagia, which is an extremely common condition, is vital. Often on clinical examination dysfunctional uterine bleeding (DUB) is diagnosed and hysteroscopy reveals the cause to be an intrauterine polyp. Similarly, endometrial hyperplasia changes the diagnosis from DUB to uterine cancer or genital tuberculosis. Laparoscopic examination or laparotomy for abdominal hysterectomy likewise may show a uterine fibroid or adnexal mass, where prior to the procedure, the diagnosis was DUB. Investigations also help to pinpoint precisely the stage or severity of existing disease.

The gynaecologist should apply common sense to the science of diagnosis. It is unwise and reprehensible to perform a diagnostic laparoscopy in a patient in whom clinically-palpable fibroids are apparent. This would be as foolish as conducting a beta-HCG study to diagnose a 20-week pregnancy and is a misuse of time, money and technology. Furthermore, it may increase patient morbidity and perhaps imbue the younger generation of gynaecologists with the wrong scientific culture. An investigative approach, particularly of hidden conditions, is required for diagnosis or to modify treatment. If a given investigation is expensive or invasive and does not guide succinctly or alter the decision-making process, the surgeon should consider whether it is really worthwhile to perform the investigation.

The zeal with which a gynaecologist undertakes investigations will depend on his or her eagerness to detect the cause of a dysfunction or illness, the patient's compliance to undergo investigation and, in the current context, pressure from 'ambulance-chasing' lawyers.

Ideally, a non-invasive investigation is preferred over an invasive one and also an economical investigation preferred over an expensive one; this applies equally to affluent countries and the third world. Sadly, many investigations are carried out to satisfy a judge or a chairman of a consumer court; often they may even be performed to please insurance and equipment companies. It seems likely that if insurance companies could be sued and litigations countersued, scientific investigations would probably be performed more judiciously.

In a climate where litigation was kept to a minimum, clinical integrity and patient compliance would be high, insurance companies would scrutinize a patient's physical rather than financial condition, and the gynaecologist would live out the Hippocratic oath; the list of investigations and management of DUB would often be entirely different. Certainly, it is reasonable to assume that clinical practices in India, neighbouring and developing countries, would not be similar to those in the affluent and litigious countries.

Appropriate treatment also requires patience on the part of the gynaecologist. Before undertaking surgery rational discrimination and understanding is needed. The surgeon should dedicate time and patience to the patient so that she finds herself able to respond thoughtfully to counselling. A patient's psyche plays an important role in her response to a suggested course of treatment. A pubertal patient may go to any length to avoid hysterectomy and preserve her uterus while a perimenopausal patient may insist on hysterectomy at all costs even though her menorrhagia does not require it.

Fortunately, recent technical advances have produced a plethora of alternatives to hysterectomy and it is hoped that this book will go a long way to providing the perplexed practitioner with a guide to plotting a course through this ever-increasing maze of options.

Once the initial complications and problems of endometrial resection or ablation are overcome, it is interesting to note that regardless of the technique used results, in terms of amenorrhoea and patient satisfaction at six months, are remarkably similar. Cynics suggest that this is merely a long-term prelude to an eventual hysterectomy, but long-term follow-up to at least six years, has shown that at the end of this time approximately 83% of patients remain satisfied with the procedure and have avoided any further surgical intervention. Clearly, a favourable outcome is to some extent age-dependent and is more likely if there is no other pathology underlying the condition, such as fibroids or adenomyosis.

Newer approaches to hysteroscopic surgery are described in this book, particularly photodynamic therapy and microwave ablation of the endometrium. Various thermal techniques involving hot water balloons or balloons heated by rows of electrodes with sensors linked to a computer to monitor the output of each individual electrode (to ensure uniform destruction of the endometrium) are also discussed. Interestingly, results of all of these ablative techniques are almost identical to those of endometrial ablation by electrosurgery or neodymium-YAG laser. Understandably, there is concern among gynaecological surgeons that such alternative therapies will allow dissemination of these techniques to radiologists, and even general practitioners or their nurses. However, the Medical Devices Agency has recently issued a warning stating that unrecognised perforation and internal injury is possible with these techniques and that their use should be restricted to trained and experienced gynaecological surgeons.

Another area in which gynaecologists are concerned that their role is gradually being replaced by the interventional radiologists, is in the treatment of fibroids by arterial embolization. This technique and the alternative techniques of myolysis and myomectomy are also discussed in this volume, which is as up-to-date as we can possibly make it at the time of going to press.

Shirish S. Sheth and Christopher J. G. Sutton

CHAPTER 1

Aetiology and investigation of menorrhagia

I.S. Fraser and G.J. Arachchi

Introduction

Women in many 20th-century societies are experiencing increasing numbers of menstrual cycles during their reproductive life span, owing to progressive and substantial changes in the structure of society and in women's reproductive expectations — including greatly delayed first pregnancy, birth spacing, breast feeding for only a very short period and a trend to use sterilization as a major family planning method. There has also been a gradual decline in average age of menarche over the past century: it has been calculated that most women in modern society will experience 400–450 menstrual cycles in a lifetime, compared with 40–50 in primitive human societies. These changes have led to an increase in medical consultations, for menstrual disorders in general and for a complaint of 'heavy periods' in particular. This is, in part, associated with decreasing tolerance of the social distress of heavy bleeding in women who are expected to compete in a demanding corporate or professional world; only to a minor extent is this associated with the debilitating effects of repeated haemorrhage or iron-deficiency anaemia.

Definition

Menorrhagia means 'excessively heavy menstruation' and has been defined from population studies[1] as a measured menstrual blood loss of more than 80 ml/month. This cutoff level was recommended because those women who were repeatedly losing more than 80 ml/month had a lower haemoglobin level and other indices of mild iron deficiency compared with women whose blood loss was in the middle of the normal range. The term 'menorrhagia' is often used synonymously with the term 'hypermenorrhoea', although in some parts of the world, notably the United States, the term 'menorrhagia' is taken to signify excessively heavy bleeding with a regular pattern.

As it is not possible to measure menstrual blood loss objectively in routine clinical practice, the research definition of menorrhagia cannot be used in the average clinical situation. In clinical practice it is necessary to refine questioning concerning a complaint of 'excessive bleeding' to ensure that the presentation is one of a 'clinically convincing history of menorrhagia'.

Assessment of menorrhagia

It is now well established that a woman's complaint of excessive bleeding does not necessarily equate with objective measurements of excessive menstrual blood loss.[1–4] Several studies have shown that only about 50% of women presenting with a clinically convincing history of menorrhagia will actually have objective measurements of blood loss that exceed 80 ml/cycle. Although issues of individual perception and tolerance appear to be important, it is clear that this particular symptom is excessively difficult for a woman to quantify. It can be said that 'the physician's interpretation of the woman's description of her perception of her bleeding' may not correlate closely with the original occurrence! Some women equate prolonged bleeding with heavy flow; others may perceive change compared with previous cycles, although objective measurements may, again, demonstrate loss that is within the normal range.

Although it is well appreciated that menorrhagia is a very difficult symptom to assess correctly, there are ways in which precision can be improved. It is possible to improve considerably the accuracy of assessment of menorrhagia by a series of detailed leading questions (Table 1.1).[5] A technique that has gained some popularity recently is a pictorial blood loss assessment chart, which scores the appearance of used sanitary pads and tampons according to their degree of saturation with blood.[6] With appropriate care and counselling of the subjects it seems that this can be made fairly precise. This is one of the few promising clinical techniques likely to be semi-quantitative for assessing this difficult symptom. It must be remembered that the clinical assessment of menorrhagia is an observation on which major management decisions are made without further possibilities of quantification.

Table 1.1 Leading questions that may assist in the historical quantification of menstrual blood loss

1. Do you use pads or tampons? Do you use the regular or super varieties?
   (Most women with objectively verifiable menorrhagia will use super pads.)
2. Do you use two pads at a time or a tampon and a pad simultaneously?
   (Many women with verifiable menorrhagia will use two pads at a time or a pad and tampon together when the bleeding is heaviest.)
3. How often do you change your sanitary towels when bleeding is excessively heavy?
   (Those women who change as frequently as once every 0.5–2 hours will probably have verifiable menorrhagia.)
4. Do you have 'accidents' with substantial soiling of your underclothes and skirts from time to time, or do you sometimes wake and find 'flooding' of the menstrual flow on the sheets? (The majority of women with verifiable menorrhagia will give a history of fairly regular accidents or flooding.)

Modified from ref. 5.

Menorrhagia is a symptom that can occur acutely as a sudden severe episode of bleeding 'out of the blue' but, much more commonly, is a recurrent problem continuing over many months or years. The natural history of most underlying causes is that the symptom will persist or increase over the long term unless treatment is instituted. It appears to be unusual for the 'chronic' type to undergo spontaneous cure. The underlying aetiology may influence substantially the clinical presentation.

Aetiology

A broad spectrum of conditions can be associated with menorrhagia, but those of the chronic type can be categorized into three main groups — namely, pelvic pathology, systemic diseases and dysfunctional uterine bleeding (DUB). These are illustrated in Figure 1.1.

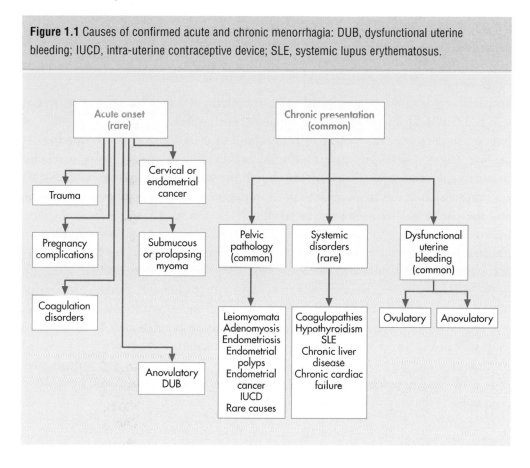

Figure 1.1 Causes of confirmed acute and chronic menorrhagia: DUB, dysfunctional uterine bleeding; IUCD, intra-uterine contraceptive device; SLE, systemic lupus erythematosus.

Menorrhagia is most frequently associated with recognizable pelvic pathology. The precise mechanisms by which these conditions cause excessive bleeding have not yet been clearly elucidated but undoubtedly include a number of complex vascular and molecular mechanisms. Systemic medical disorders are a much rarer cause of menorrhagia, and DUB is a common diagnosis of exclusion.

Acute menorrhagia

This is a relatively uncommon presentation of excessively heavy bleeding, since most women will present with a regularly recurring pattern of heavy periods. When a woman presents with excessive bleeding without a prior history, complications of an unrecognized early pregnancy should be considered as an important differential diagnosis. Other significant causes of this presentation are intra-uterine and submucous myomas (especially if prolapsing through the cervix), anovulation, coagulation disorders and trauma (Fig. 1.1).

Pelvic pathology

Uterine myomata

Uterine myomata are benign myometrial lesions and are the commonest recognizable pathological cause of menorrhagia; they can sometimes be associated with the most severe degrees of regular loss. On the other hand, it has been calculated that only 30% of myomata are actually associated with menorrhagia.

The degree of severity of menorrhagia is generally determined by the relationship of the largest myoma to the endometrium.[7] Typically, the large submucous and pedunculated intra-uterine myomatous polyps are associated with the heaviest degrees of loss. Hysteroscopy often reveals large, superficial, thin-walled and fragile vessels running across the surface of these submucous lesions.

Adenomyosis

Menorrhagia is said to occur in 40–50% of patients with adenomyosis.[8] In recent years, the association of superficial adenomyosis has been noted in up to 40% of patients undergoing endometrial resection,[9] but the relationship of this histological finding to excessive bleeding is unproven. In those women with objective menorrhagia, the distortions of the inner myometrial layer that occur with adenomyosis are probably associated with functional changes in the blood vessels, and there may be increased vascular fragility.[10]

Endometriosis

Menorrhagia is a common clinical association with endometriosis, although many women with this condition do not have this complaint. Surgical treatment of endometriosis may substantially reduce measured menstrual blood loss.[11] Again, the underlying mechanism for the menorrhagia is uncertain although, classically, it is said to be mediated through a prostaglandin-related mechanism. The actual mechanisms are almost certainly much more complex than this and will involve several molecular systems influencing vascular function and fragility and migratory leucocytes.

Endometrial polyps

Menorrhagia occurs in about 12% of women with endometrial polyps,[12] and blood loss returns to normal in most cases following removal of the polyp. The aetiology of endometrial polyps, and the mechanisms by which they cause excessive bleeding, are unknown.

Polycystic ovarian disease

The aetiology of polycystic ovarian disease (PCOD) is still uncertain, and a number of anomalies of hypothalamic pituitary and ovarian function may be involved. It is typically associated with anovulation and, in a minority of cases, may be associated with substantial anovulatory DUB at infrequent intervals.[13] Endometrial hyperplasia and occasionally even endometrial adenocarcinoma at a young age may occur in the absence of adequate progestogenic treatment of the endometrium.

Intra-uterine contraceptive devices (IUCDs)

Modern copper IUCDs are much less likely to cause menorrhagia than the outdated inert devices, but a minority of women will complain of substantial increase in blood loss.[14] In some of these cases there appears to be distortion of the IUCD within the cavity (e.g. partial rotation or twisting of the device), or embedding or partial perforation within the uterine wall. In other cases the excessive bleeding may be caused by minor movement of the device against superficial endometrial vessels. The menorrhagia may also be accompanied by disturbances of prostaglandin metabolism and fibrinolysis.

Endometrial adenocarcinoma
It has been reported that about 40% of women presenting with endometrial carcinoma prior to the menopause will present with regular and excessively heavy periods.[15] On the other hand, this is a relatively rare presenting cause for menorrhagia.

Other rare causes
A number of rare pelvic pathologies have been associated with menorrhagia: these include trauma to the genital tract,[16] myometrial hypertrophy[17] and uterine vascular malformations.[11,18]

Systemic disorders
Systemic disorders are rare causes of menorrhagia. The commonest are coagulation disorders, but hypothyroidism, severe hepatic cirrhosis, chronic renal diseases and systemic lupus erythematosus are occasional causes.[19]

Coagulation disorders
One-quarter of adolescents with excessively heavy periods and a haemoglobin of less than 100 g/l, and one-third of those who require a blood transfusion for menorrhagia, have an underlying coagulation defect.[20] The majority of patients in this category have a disorder of platelet numbers or function (such as thrombocytopenia, the thrombocytopathies, von Willebrand's disease or leukaemia.[21,22]

Dysfunctional uterine bleeding
DUB is a diagnosis of exclusion. The definition preferred by the authors is 'excessive bleeding (heavy, prolonged or frequent) of uterine origin, which is not due to organic pelvic disease, systemic diseases or complications of pregnancy'.[23] It is convenient to divide these women into those who are predominantly ovulatory and those who are predominantly anovulatory, and it is also appropriate to divide them further into those with a chronic and ongoing problem and those with a sudden acute episode of menorrhagia 'out of the blue'.

When DUB is associated with anovulation, the primary abnormality is probably at the level of the hypothalamus, although disturbances of intra-ovarian control allowing multiple follicular development may also play a role.[24] Those women with ovulatory DUB probably have a complex functional disturbance at the endometrial level, where there is disturbance of prostaglandin and prostacyclin metabolism, enhanced fibrinolytic activity, decreased endothelin production, disturbances of matrix metalloproteinases and a variety of other abnormalities (including disturbances of local blood flow, local platelet function, lysosome function, local migratory leucocyte function and, probably, disturbances of cytokines and other growth factors). All these will lead to disturbances of the control of the volume of blood lost at the time of menstruation.[25–27]

Investigations
Investigations should be geared primarily to the recognition of iron deficiency and anaemia, and to the recognition or exclusion of local pelvic pathology and systemic disease. Systemic diseases are rare causes of menorrhagia and investigations to

detect them should not be routine: their presence should usually have been highlighted by unusual features in the detailed case history or examination (Fig. 1.2).

Figure 1.2 Investigations in the patient with menorrhagia: ANA, anti-nuclear antibodies; D&C, dilatation and curettage; MRI, magnetic resonance imaging; TFTs, thyroid function tests; TSH, thyrotrophin.

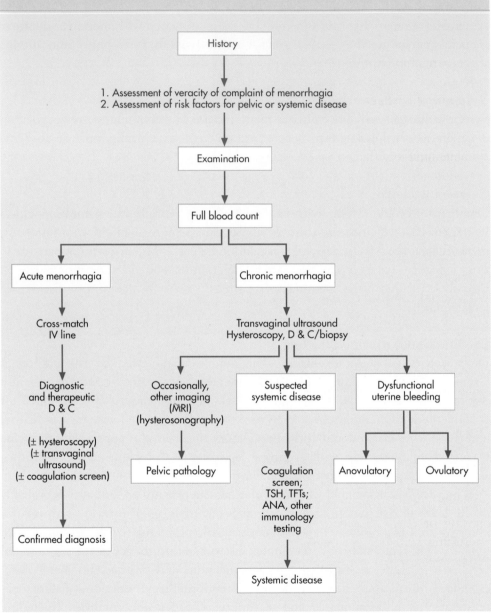

Routine investigations in most cases of menorrhagia should include the following:

1. *Full blood count, including a blood film if the haemoglobin is abnormal.* This will reveal any anaemia, and will point to the possible underlying cause (iron deficiency in the majority). It will also give information about the platelet count.
2. *Uterine imaging and endometrial sampling.* It is generally recognized that diagnostic hysteroscopy, often on an outpatient basis, with a directed biopsy or

curettage, is the most reliable means of imaging the endometrial surface and the uterine cavity, provided that the operator is experienced.[28] A much less satisfactory alternative is blind uterine curettage. The incidence of false-negative results is now known to be so high that uncritical adherence to routine use of this technique can no longer be sustained, provided that more modern methods are available.[29,30] Blind but thorough curettage is effective in detecting endometrial hyperplasia and adenocarcinoma, but it frequently misses endometrial polyps, submucous and cavitary myomas and patchy endometritis.

An alternative and increasingly widely used technique is that of high-resolution transvaginal ultrasound scanning, sometimes supplemented by contrast hysterosonography (the instillation of saline into the uterine cavity).[31] Considerable skill and experience are required to interpret the images, but in experienced hands this is a valuable technique for assessing myomata, adenomyosis, endometrial hyperplasia, intracavitary polyps, PCOD and even endometrial carcinoma. There is a great temptation for many doctors initially to order pelvic ultrasound examination because of its ease, but it should be recognized that this is a fairly expensive and highly skilled technique that has not yet been confirmed to replace adequately direct inspection by hysteroscopy, accompanied by endometrial sampling.

Additional investigations

In general, these should be carried out only if the case history is suspicious or if there is an unsatisfactory response to standard treatments. In cases of acute menorrhagia, the complications of an unsuspected pregnancy should not be overlooked. The presence of an unsuspected pregnancy can also occasionally confuse the investigation of ongoing chronic menorrhagia

Other investigations include assessment of serum ferritin, if there is doubt about iron deficiency, and other serum biochemical analyses if there is suspicion of liver or renal disease.[31] Serum thyrotrophin (TSH) and thyroid function tests (TFTs) may be necessary to exclude hypothyroidism, and appropriate immunological testing may be required if there is a suspicion of systemic lupus erythematosus (SLE). A partial coagulation screen should be considered if there is a history of easy bruising or dental bleeding. Serum levels of follicle-stimulating hormone and luteinizing hormone are rarely helpful, but may occasionally help to define a perimenopausal state or PCOD.

Very occasionally, alternative approaches to imaging may need to be considered. These may include magnetic resonance imaging (MRI), pelvic angiography, computerized tomography (CT) scanning and diagnostic laparoscopy. These techniques may be expensive and will only occasionally provide worthwhile additional information over the more simple techniques in terms of improving clinical management.

Conclusions

Menorrhagia is a common symptom that is not well understood or well assessed by the average clinician. Improvement in management will come only through an increased awareness of the problems of perception and tolerance of bleeding and of the need for improved precision in diagnosis, using techniques such as outpatient hysteroscopy with directed endometrial biopsy, and appropriate use of transvaginal ultrasound scanning in expert hands. An understanding of the underlying causes and the mechanisms of abnormal bleeding will allow a more rational approach to treatment of the individual woman.

References

1. Hallberg L, Hogdahl A M, Nilsson L, Rybo G. Menstrual blood loss — a population study. Acta Obstet Gynecol Scand 1966; 45: 320–351

2. Fraser I S, McCarron G, Markham R. A preliminary study of factors influencing perception of menstrual blood loss volume. Am J Obstet Gynecol 1984; 149: 788–793

3. Chimbira T H, Anderson A B M, Turnbull A C. Relation between measured menstrual blood loss and patient's subjective assessment of loss, duration of bleeding, number of sanitary towels used, uterine weight and endometrial surface area. Br J Obstet Gynaecol 1980; 87: 603–609

4. Barer A P, Fowler W M. The blood loss during normal menstruation. Am J Obstet Gynecol 1934; 31: 979–986

5. Fraser I S. Treatment of menorrhagia. In: Drife J O (ed) Dysfunctional uterine bleeding and menorrhagia. Bailliere's Clin Obstet Gynaecol 1989; 3: 391–402

6. Higham J M, O'Brien P M S, Shaw R W. Assessment of menstrual blood loss using a pictorial chart. Br J Obstet Gynaecol 1990; 97: 734–739

7. Fraser I S. Hysteroscopy and laparoscopy in women with menorrhagia. Am J Obstet Gynecol 1992; 162: 1264–1269

8. Azziz R. Adenomyosis: current perspectives. Obstet Gynecol Clin North Am 1989; 16(1): 221–235

9. McCausland A M, McCausland V M. Depth of endometrial penetration in adenomyosis helps determine outcome of rollerball ablation. Am J Obstet Gynecol 1996; 174: 1786–1793

10. Ota H. Evaluation of hysteroscopy in the diagnosis of adenomyosis. Jpn J Fertil Steril 1992; 37: 49–55

11. Fraser I S. Menorrhagia — a pragmatic approach to the understanding of causes and the need for investigations. Br J Obstet Gynaecol 1994; 101(suppl. 11): 3–7

12. Van Bogaert L J. Clinicopathologic findings in endometrial polyps. Obstet Gynecol 1988; 71: 771–773

13. Fraser I S, Baird D T. Endometrial cystic glandular hyperplasia in adolescent girls. J Obstet Gynaecol Br Commonw 1972; 79: 1009–1015

14. Shaw S T, Macaulay L K. Morphologic studies on IUD-induced metrorrhagia II. Surface changes of the endometrium and microscopic localization of bleeding sites. Contraception 1979; 19(1): 63–81

15. Quinn M, Neale B J, Fortune D W. Endometrial carcinoma in pre-menopausal women: a clinico-pathological study. Gynecol Oncol 1985; 20: 298–306

16. Fraser I S, Rencoret R H. Acute and severe menorrhagia due to cervical artery damage. Aust N Z J Obstet Gynaecol 1984; 24: 223–224

17. Fraser I S. Menorrhagia due to myometrial hypertrophy. Treatment with tamoxifen. Obstet Gynecol 1987; 70: 505–506

18. Fleming H, Ostor A G, Pickel H, Fortune D W. Arterio-venous malformations of the uterus. Obstet Gynecol 1989; 73: 209–214

19. Quick A J. Menstruation in hereditary bleeding disorders. Obstet Gynecol 1966; 28: 37–48

20. Claessens E A, Cowell C A. Acute adolescent menorrhagia. Am J Obstet Gynecol 1981; 139: 277–282

21. Ewenstein M B. The pathophysiology of bleeding disorders presenting as abnormal uterine bleeding. Am J Obstet Gynecol 1996; 175: 770–777

22. Van Eijkeren M A, Christiaens G C, Haspels A A, Sixma J J. Menstrual blood loss in women with a bleeding disorder or using anticoagulant therapy. Am J Obstet Gynecol 1990; 162: 1261–1263

23. Fraser I S. The dysfunctional uterus — dysmenorrhoea and dysfunctional uterine bleeding. In: Shearman R P (ed) Textbook of clinical reproductive endocrinology. Edinburgh: Churchill Livingstone, 1985: 578–598

24. Fraser I S, Baird D T. Blood production and ovarian secretion of estradiol-17β and estrone in women with dysfunctional uterine bleeding. J Clin Endocrinol Metab 1974; 39: 564–570

25. Cameron I T. Dysfunctional uterine bleeding. In: Drife J O (ed) Dysfunctional uterine bleeding and menorrhagia. Bailliere's Clin Obstet Gynaecol 1989; 3: 315–327

26. Smith S K. The pathophysiology of menorrhagia. In: Cameron I T, Fraser I S, Smith S K (eds) Clinical disorders of the endometrium and the menstrual cycle. Oxford: Oxford University Press, 1998: 105–115

27. Fraser I S, Hickey M, Song J Y. A comparison of mechanisms underlying disturbances of bleeding due to spontaneous dysfunctional uterine bleeding and to hormonal contraception. Hum Reprod 1996; 11 (suppl 2): 165–178

28. Dodson M G. Use of transvaginal ultrasound in diagnosing the aetiology of menorrhagia. J Reprod Med 1994; 39: 362–372

29. MacKenzie J Z, Bibby J G. Critical assessment of dilatation and curettage in 1029 women. Lancet 1978; ii: 566–569

30. Gimpelson R J. Panoramic hysteroscopy with directed biopsy versus dilatation and curettage for accurate diagnosis. J Reprod Med 1984; 29: 575–578

31. Parsons A K, Lense J J. Sonohysterography for endometrial abnormalities. JCU 1993; 21: 87–97

CHAPTER 2

Pathophysiology of menorrhagia

B. L. Sheppard and J. Bonnar

Introduction

Menstruation is a biological process dependent on complex hormonal and physiological changes that can be disturbed by a variety of factors. Menstrual disorders constitute a major clinical problem that affects a large number of women during their reproductive life: it is estimated that at least 25–30% will complain of excessive menstrual bleeding or menorrhagia.[1,2] Objective measurement of menstrual blood loss in representative populations has shown that the mean blood loss per period is about 30–40 ml. Menorrhagia is normally a subjective symptom based on the woman's complaint of excessive menstrual bleeding. Objective menorrhagia is defined as a total menstrual blood loss of 80 ml or more per menstruation. This was derived from the classic population study of Hallberg et al.[3] In women of reproductive years, menorrhagia is the most common cause of iron-deficiency anaemia.[4]

Menorrhagia may be the result of local pathology such as fibroids, polyps, adenomyosis, endometriosis, infection or carcinoma,[5,6] and may be associated with hypothyroidism,[7] the use of intra-uterine contraceptive devices[8] or haemostatic disorders.[9,10]

Fibroids and menorrhagia

Approximately 30% of women with fibroids have been reported to have menstrual disorders, usually in the form of menorrhagia.[11,12] Menorrhagia may occur when the uterine cavity surface area is expanded by submucous fibroids or during necrosis of the endometrium overlying the submucous fibroids.[13,14] It has also been suggested that the increased bleeding may be due to increased vascularity of the uterus. Fibroids release prostaglandins, mostly prostacyclin, in vitro,[15] but have fewer prostaglandin receptors than the surrounding myometrium.[16] The prostaglandins not only will induce vasodilatation but also may relate to a disturbance in normal myometrial contractility. Microradiographic studies have shown a marked increase in venous dilatation in association with intramural, subserous and submucosal fibroids.[17] Obstruction of these vessels by the developing fibroid may be involved in the pathogenesis of heavy menstrual bleeding.

Endometrial carcinoma and menorrhagia

Most women with endometrial cancer experience irregular bleeding rather than menorrhagia.[5,18,19] However, two studies have reported that 36–38% of premenopausal women presenting with endometrial cancer had heavy, regular menstruation.[5,20] Activators of fibrinolysis are implicated in both tumour growth and metastatic spread.[21] A local alteration in the balance of fibrinolytic enzymes has been shown in endometrial adenocarcinoma.[22] Not only may this facilitate continuous deposition of a fibrin matrix in the proliferation and invasion of epithelial cancers[23] and have a direct mitogenic effect on malignant cells[24] but also it may have an adverse effect on endometrial haemostatic control.

Intra-uterine contraceptive devices

Non-medicated and copper-releasing intra-uterine contraceptive devices (IUCDs) are associated with a striking increase in menstrual blood loss: an average increase of 148% with the Lippes Loop D and 59% with the Copper 7 have been reported.[8] Although the newer hormone-releasing devices are associated with a decrease in the amount of menstrual blood loss, they have been reported to induce an increase in the duration of menstrual bleeding and intermenstrual spotting.[25,26] Morphological studies have indicated that this may be due to focal haemorrhage from damaged, dilated vessels of atrophic endometrium in contact with the non-medicated arms of the devices.[27] All devices induce a foreign-body reaction within the endometrium, stimulating the migration of polymorphonuclear leucocytes and macrophages — which release activators of the fibrinolytic system into the uterine cavity.[28] Contractions of the uterine myometrial smooth muscle on the rigid IUCD produces damage to the superficial endometrial capillaries, stimulating the release of fibrinolytic activators and prostaglandins. These IUCD-induced changes in the uterine environment are probably the prime factors affecting the pattern of menstrual bleeding, which remains one of the main reasons for the poor continuation rate of the IUCD as a contraceptive method.

Haemostatic disorders and menorrhagia

Congenital haemostatic disorders such as the coagulation deficiencies of factors V, IX, X, XI, XII and XIII, von Willebrand's disease and severe thrombocytopenia[9,10,29] are less-common causes of menorrhagia that can present in adolescence. Von Willebrand's disease is the most common coagulopathy usually associated with heavy menstrual loss and other bleeding problems; such patients should be managed by the local haemophilia unit. Treatment with desmopressin (DDAVP) has proved to be effective for reducing menstrual loss in patients with von Willebrand's disease.

Dysfunctional uterine bleeding (DUB)

The majority of women with menorrhagia have no underlying organic disease and no hormonal abnormality, and are classified as having unexplained excessive uterine bleeding or DUB.[30,31] At the extremes of reproductive life, anovulatory cycles are more common but overall account for less than 10% of women with DUB.[32–34]

In recent years, research has focused on the possible role of local uterine factors in the control of blood loss during menstruation. Most studies have concentrated on the investigation of endometrial vasculature, the coagulation and fibrinolytic enzyme systems, platelets, prostaglandins and other vasoactive agents, both in the uterine wall and in menstrual fluid, in relation to normal and excessive menstrual bleeding.

Pathogenesis of DUB

Endometrial vasculature

The endometrium is supplied by spiral and basal arteries, which are branches of myometrial radial arteries. The basal arteries supply the basal endometrium and undergo no major changes through the menstrual cycle; in contrast, endometrial spiral arteries are influenced markedly by hormonal changes of the menstrual cycle.

Much of the present knowledge of the role of endometrial blood vessels in the physiology of menstruation stems from observations carried out over 50 years ago on endometrial explants in the anterior chamber of the eye of the rhesus monkey.[35] These studies showed the earliest changes to be endometrial regression associated with a decline in ovarian steroid levels. The coiling of endometrial spiral arterioles, intense vasoconstriction prior to menstrual bleeding from dilated spiral arterioles and a return to vasoconstriction of the vessels were described in great detail. Markee[35] estimated that at least 75% of menstrual bleeding arose from the spiral arterioles — leakage either from disrupted vessels into the endometrial stroma or from ruptured arterioles directly into the uterine cavity. The importance of Markee's findings are reflected in subsequent recent attempts to demonstrate an association between uterine vascular density and the amount of menstrual blood loss. Although arterial density is greater in the superficial myometrium adjacent to the endometrium than in basal endometrium,[36,37] there is no variation in vessel density throughout the menstrual cycle in women with normal blood loss or DUB.[36,38] Total arterial density is similar in women with normal menstrual loss to that in women with DUB; moreover, no correlation has been found between measured menstrual blood loss and arterial density in basal endometrium. Histological examination of uterine biopsies has identified increased numbers of thick-walled arterioles in the functional endometrium in women with DUB, which may represent remnant arterioles from incomplete menstrual shedding and play a role in increased menstrual bleeding in subsequent cycles. Although vascular abnormalities cannot be entirely ruled out, excessive menstrual bleeding in the absence of uterine pathology is not due to increased arterial proliferation.

Platelets and menstrual haemostasis

During normal menstruation, an active local haemostasis occurs in endometrial vasculature. Endometrial haemostasis appears to be compromised in women with DUB.[39–41] Just prior to the onset of menstruation, at a period of intense vasoconstriction, numerous vascular lesions, without haemostatic platelet plugs, appear in the uterine endometrium.[41,42] During the first 20–24 hours of normal menstrual bleeding, platelets and fibrin form intravascular plugs, which are subsequently shed with endometrial tissue.[42] Fibrin and platelets, either singularly or as small aggregates (Fig. 2.1), are consistently found in menstrual fluid during the first 48 hours of bleeding.[43,44] The consumption of platelets during the haemostatic process of menstruation leads to only small numbers being found in menstrual fluid.[45] The platelets appear to be devoid of granules and are probably spent, having already been exposed to aggregating stimuli.[44]

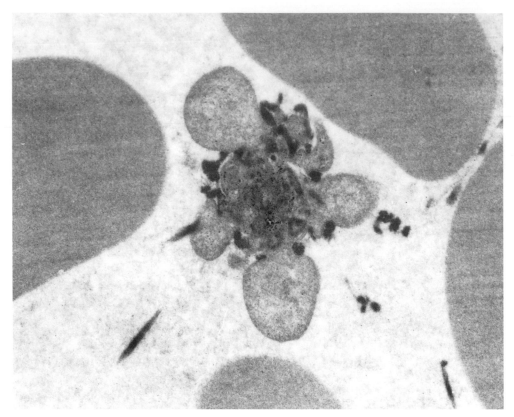

Figure 2.1 Electron micrograph of a menstrual platelet that has undergone shape change and granule release during the process of aggregation and appears to be spent. (x 15,000.)

Endometrial fibrinolysis

Local activation of the coagulation and fibrinolytic enzyme systems occurs within the uterus during the physiological process of menstruation. Blood coagulation factors are severely depleted in menstrual fluid, consistent with consumption of these components during menstruation.[46] No significant differences have been reported in coagulation factors in menstrual fluid from women with menorrhagia compared with those in women with normal menstruation;[47,48] however, a striking difference is seen in the concentrations of enzymes of the fibrinolytic system in menstrual blood from women with DUB.[49]

Fibrinolysis is dependent on the balance in production and release of activators and inhibitors of plasminogen. Early studies of plasminogen activators found high concentrations in both the uterus and menstrual fluid.[50,51] Astrup[52] suggested that tissue activators of plasminogen may interfere with uterine haemostatic mechanisms by increasing local fibrinolysis, and that increased production of these activators may play an important role in the pathology of excessive menstrual bleeding.[50] Menstrual blood contains no fibrinogen but has very high levels of fibrin degradation products (Fig. 2.2). This was thought to be the result of direct digestion of fibrin to breakdown products,[53] but subsequent electron microscopy studies identified fibrin in menstrual clots of women with normal menstruation and women with DUB.[44]

Potent fibrinolytic activity is the major mechanism responsible for maintaining the fluidity of menstrual blood. Compared with peripheral plasma, menstrual fluid contains far higher levels of tissue plasminogen activator (tPA) but significantly

Figure 2.2 Comparison of the levels of fibrinogen and fibrin degradation products (FDPs) in peripheral (☐) and menstrual (☐) blood. Menstrual blood contains no fibrinogen but very high levels of fibrin degradation products.

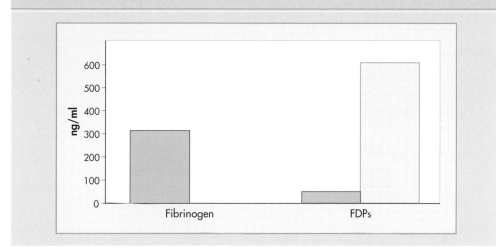

lower levels of plasminogen activator inhibitor (PAI) (Fig. 2.3).[54] The important role of increased local fibrinolytic activity in the pathogenesis of DUB is further enhanced by the finding of even higher levels of plasminogen activator in menstrual fluid of women with excessive menstrual loss.[44,55] However, throughout the menstrual cycle, women with DUB have levels of tPA in peripheral blood similar to those in women with normal menstrual loss, suggesting that the endometrium (and, perhaps, the myometrium) are the probable sources of the high levels found in menstrual fluid. Higher levels of tPA are found in the myometrium than the endometrium during the normal menstrual cycle. Indeed, not only does the activity vary from region to region in the uterine wall but also changes are seen through the menstrual cycle.[56] Several studies have reported a significant increase in endometrial tPA levels in the late secretory phase of the normal menstrual

Figure 2.3 Comparison of the levels of tissue plasminogen activator antigen (tPAag) and plasminogen inhibitor (PAI-1) in menstrual (☐) and peripheral (☐) plasma. Menstrual plasma contains higher levels of activator and lower levels of inhibitor than peripheral plasma.

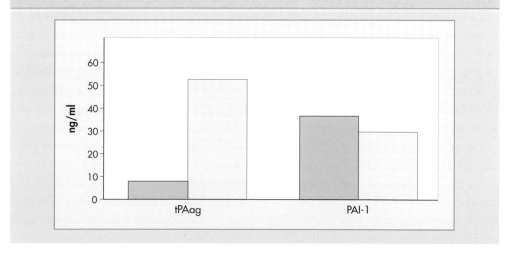

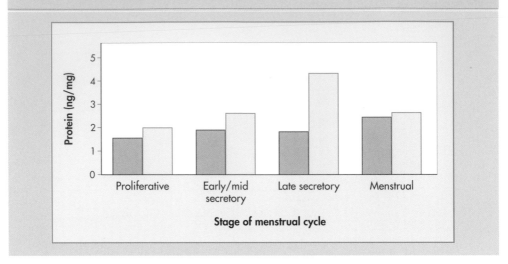

Figure 2.4 Tissue plasminogen activator antigen (tPAag) levels in extracts of endometrium from uteri removed at hysterectomy during the proliferative, early secretory, late secretory and menstrual phases of the cycle in women with normal menstrual blood loss (■; < 80 ml menstrual blood loss) and dysfunctional uterine bleeding (□; > 80 ml loss).

cycle.[56–58] The tPA has been immunocytochemically localized, predominantly in endothelial cells of small blood vessels of the myometrium throughout the cycle but more specifically in endothelial cells of capillaries and spiral arterioles of the endometrium in the late secretory phase of the cycle.[59]

Over 30 years ago, increased endometrial fibrinolytic activity was correlated with increased menstrual blood loss.[57] Significantly higher levels of plasminogen activator have been reported in extracts of late secretory endometrium from women with DUB than in those from women with normal menstrual loss (Fig. 2.4).[54,59] In this latter study a strong correlation was evident between tissue plasminogen levels in the late secretory endometrium and menstrual blood loss,[54] indicating a key role for increased local release of fibrinolytic activators in the aetiology of excessive menstrual bleeding.

Prostaglandins
Prostaglandins have been implicated in the physiological process of menstruation since Pickles et al.[60] found high concentrations of prostaglandin (PG)E_2 and PGF_2 in endometrium and menstrual fluid. Endometrium mainly produces prostaglandins PGF_2 and PGE_2, with lesser amounts of prostacyclin (PGI_2) and thromboxane A_2 (TXA_2). The myometrium principally produces PGI_2. The individual prostaglandins have differing effects on haemostasis: whereas PGE_2 and PGI_2 cause vasodilatation, PGF_2 and TXA_2 produce vasoconstriction. In addition, TXA_2 promotes platelet aggregation whereas PGI_2 inhibits the aggregatory properties of platelets.[61]

Glandular epithelium is the principal site of prostaglandin synthesis in the uterine endometrium;[62,63] production is influenced by the levels of oestrogen and progesterone. Endometrial synthesis of PGE_2 and PGF_2 increases through the secretory phase of the cycle to reach a maximum level at menstruation.[64] Elevated levels of endometrial PGE_2 and PGF_2 have been described in women complaining of excessive menstrual bleeding,[65] whereas other studies have suggested a

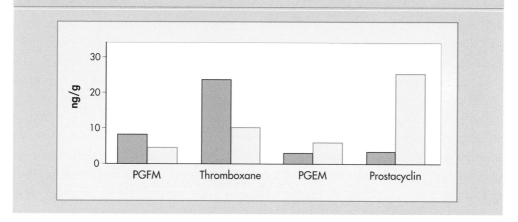

Figure 2.5 Levels of the metabolites of prostaglandins PGE$_2$ (PGEM) and PGF$_2$ (PGFM) and of 6-keto-PGF$_1$ (prostacyclin) and thromboxane B$_2$ (TXB$_2$) in menstrual endometrium from women with normal menstrual blood loss (■; < 80 ml/cycle) and women with dysfunctional uterine bleeding (DUB; □; > 80 ml/cycle). The vasodilators (PGEM and 6-keto-PGF$_1$) are higher and the vasoconstrictors (PGFM and TXB$_2$) lower in women with DUB than in women with normal menstrual blood loss.

relationship between the total prostaglandin content of the endometrium and menstrual blood loss.[66] An imbalance of prostaglandin synthesis in women with excessive menstrual bleeding has been shown in several studies: the endometrium has a greater capacity to synthesize PGE$_2$ and 6-keto-PGF$_1$ than PGF$_2$.[67–69] There is now strong evidence to support the suggestion that menorrhagia is associated with a shift within the uterine wall towards the production of increased levels of vasodilatory prostaglandins and away from prostaglandins that stimulate vasoconstriction and platelet aggregation. Studies have shown higher levels of prostacyclin, in the form of 6-keto-PGF$_1$ and the metabolite of PGE$_2$, and lower levels of thromboxane B$_2$ and the metabolite of PGF$_2$ (Fig. 2.5) in menstrual endometrium of women with DUB than in women with normal menstrual blood loss.[70,71] An interaction between prostaglandins synthesized in the endometrium and myometrium appears to be a major factor in the control of blood loss from the uterus during menstruation.

Vasoactive agents

Apart from prostaglandins, other vasoactive agents may play a role in the control of blood loss during menstruation. For example, histamine and heparin are metabolic products of mast cells that are irregularly distributed throughout the uterine endometrium and myometrium, often in close proximity to blood capillaries or venules. Studies have shown that, although mast cells predominate in the myometrium, degranulation usually occurs in the endometrium in the premenstrual phase of the cycle.[72,73] Histamine- and heparin-like activity have been identified in menstrual fluid, suggesting that these products released from mast cells are involved in the mechanism of menstrual bleeding.[74,75] Histamine may mediate contraction of endothelial cells, allowing erythrocytes to leak into the surrounding stroma through gaps in blood vessel walls; heparin-like activity may be important in maintaining menstrual blood in a fluid state. Histamine has also been shown to stimulate the release of factor VIII, tPA and PAI from cultured endothelial cells.[76,77]

Platelet-activating factor (PAF), a potent activator of platelets[78] and vasoconstrictor,[79] may be an important local mediator of vascular control in the uterine endometrium during menstruation. It is synthesized in stromal cells of the endometrium[80] and released by stimulated endothelial cells[81] and polymorphonuclear leucocytes.[82] Tissue culture studies have shown that PAF stimulates the release of PGE_2 from glandular epithelium in secretory-phase endometrium,[83,84] but inhibits the release of PGF_2 from glandular epithelial cells of proliferative endometrium.[85] The action of PAF in the endometrium may have a possible role in the altered ratio of $PGE_2:PGF_2$ synthesis found in women with DUB.

Endothelins are important vasoactive products of epithelial and endothelial cells that have been identified in uterine endometrium. Endothelin-1 is a potent constrictor of small blood vessels in the uterine wall.[86–88] This may be the vasoconstrictor described by Markee[35] and released from vascular endothelium at the time of premenstrual endometrial regression.[89] During menstruation, vasoconstriction of spiral arterioles may be further enhanced by the release of endothelins from the disruption of glandular epithelium. Although endothelin activity in the endometrium is believed to be under ovarian steroid control,[90] it is not known whether an imbalance in endothelin production is involved in the pathophysiology of DUB.

Conclusions

Extensive research during recent years suggests that most excessive uterine bleeding is due to local endometrial or myometrial dysfunction. Increased fibrinolysis, coupled with an impaired haemostasis and an imbalance in synthesis of prostaglandins towards a greater production of vasodilators, have been shown to be the major uterine factors intimately involved in the pathophysiology of menorrhagia. This laboratory research is clinically substantiated by many years of successful medical treatment of excessive menstrual bleeding with fibrinolytic inhibitors and prostaglandin synthetase inhibitors. In a recent study, the fibrinolytic inhibitor tranexamic acid reduced objectively measured menstrual blood loss by 58%, and the prostaglandin synthetase inhibitor mefenamic acid reduced menstrual loss by 20% in women with DUB.[91]

Acknowledgements

The authors are grateful to the Health Research Board and the Royal City of Dublin Hospital for support in research reported in this chapter.

References

1. Fraser I S. The 'dysfunctional' uterus: dysmenorrhoea and dysfunctional uterine bleeding. In: Shearman R P (ed) Clinical reproductive endocrinology. Edinburgh: Churchill Livingstone, 1985: 579–598

2. Coulter A. Prevalence and epidemiology of dysfunctional uterine bleeding. In: Smith S K (ed) Dysfunctional uterine bleeding. London: Royal Society of Medicine Press, 1994: 2–5

3. Hallberg L, Hogdahl A M, Nilsson L, Rybo G. Menstrual blood loss — a population study. Acta Obstet Gynecol Scand 1966; 45: 320–335

4. Cohen B J B, Gibor J. Anemia and menstrual blood loss. Obstet Gynecol Surv 1980; 35: 597–602

5. Quinn M A, Kneale B J, Fortune D W. Endometrial carcinoma in pre-menopausal women: a clinico-pathological study. Gynecol Oncol 1985; 20: 298–306

6. Fraser I S. Hysteroscopy and laparoscopy in women with menorrhagia. Am J Obstet Gynecol 1992; 162: 1264–1269

7. Scott J C, Mussey E. Menstrual patterns of myxedema. Am J Obstet Gynecol 1964; 90: 161–165

8. Guillebaud J, Bonnar J, Morehead J, Matthews A. Menstrual blood loss with intrauterine devices. Lancet 1976; 1: 387

9. Fraser I S, McCarron G, Markham R. Objective measurement of menstrual blood loss in women with a complaint of menorrhagia associated with pelvic disease or coagulation disorder. Obstet Gynecol 1986; 68: 630–633

10. Greer I A, Lowe G D O, Walker J J, Forbes C D. Congenital coagulopathies in obstetrics and gynaecology. In: Greer I A, Turpie A G G, Forbes E D (eds) Haemostasis and thrombosis in obstetrics and gynaecology. London: Chapman and Hall Medical, 1992: 459–486

11. Buttram V C, Reiter R C. Uterine leiomyomata: etiology, symptomatology and management. Fertil Steril 1981; 36: 433–445

12. Carlson K J, Nichols D H, Schiff I. Indications for hysterectomy. N Engl J Med 1993; 328: 856–860

13. West C P, Lumsden M A. Fibroids and menorrhagia. Baillieres Clin Obstet Gynaecol 1989; 3: 357–374

14. Vollenhoven B J, Lawrence A S, Healy D L. Uterine fibroids: a clinical review. Br J Obstet Gynaecol 1990; 97: 285–298

15. Rees M C P, Turnbull A. Leiomyomas release prostaglandins. Prostaglandins Leukot Med 1985; 18; 65–68

16. Hofmann G E, Rao V, Barrows G H et al. Binding sites for epidermal growth factors in human uterine tissues and leiomyomas. J Clin Endocrinol Metab 1984; 58: 880–884

17. Farrer-Brown G, Beilby J O W, Tarbit M H. Venous changes in the endometrium of myomatous uteri. Obstet Gynecol 1971; 38: 743–751

18. Peterson E P. Endometrial carcinoma in young women. A clinical profile. Obstet Gynecol 1968; 31: 702–707

19. Crissman J D, Azoury R S, Barnes A E, Schellhas H F. Endometrial carcinoma in women 40 years of age or younger. Obstet Gynecol 1981; 57: 699–704

20. Jeffrey J D, Taylor R, Robertson D I, Stuart G C. Endometrial carcinoma occurring in patients under the age of 45 years. Am J Obstet Gynecol 1987; 156: 366–370

21. Duffy M J, O'Grady P. Plasminogen activator and cancer. Eur J Cancer Clin Oncol 1984; 20: 557–582

22. Gleeson N, Gonsalves R, McGuinness E, Bonnar J. Plasminogen activators in endometrial adenocarcinoma. Int J Gynaecol Cancer 1991; 1: 223–226

23. Dvorak H F. Tumors: wounds that do not heal. N Engl J Med 1986; 315: 1650–1659

24. Kirchheimer J C, Wojta J, Christ G, Binder B R. Proliferation of an epidermal tumour cell line stimulated by urokinase. FASEB J 1987; 1: 125–128

25. Nilsson C G. Comparative quantification of menstrual blood loss with d-norgestrel-releasing IUD and Nova-T copper device. Contraception 1977; 15: 379–387

26. Rybo G. The IUD and endometrial bleeding. J Reprod Med 1978; 20: 175–182

27. Sheppard B L, Bonnar J. The effects of intrauterine contraceptive devices on the ultrastructure of the endometrium in relation to bleeding complications. Am J Obstet Gynecol 1983; 146: 829–839

28. Sheppard B L. The intrauterine contraceptive device. Clin Mater 1988; 3: 1–13

29. Van Eijkeren M, Christiaens G, Haspels A, Sixma J. Measured menstrual blood loss in women with a bleeding disorder or using oral anticoagulant therapy. Am J Obstet Gynecol 1990; 162: 1261–1263

30. Haynes P J, Anderson A B M, Turnbull A C. Patterns of menstrual blood loss in menorrhagia. Res Clin Forums 1979; 1: 73–78

31. Cameron I T. Dysfunctional uterine bleeding. Baillieres Clin Obstet Gynaecol 1989; 3: 315–326

32. Fraser I S, Michie E A, Wide L, Baird D T. Pituitary gonadotrophins and ovarian function in adolescent dysfunctional uterine bleeding. J Clin Endocrinol Metab 1973; 37: 407–414

33. Van Look P F A, Lothian H, Hunter W M et al. Hypothalamic–pituitary–ovarian function in perimenopausal women. Clin Endocrinol 1977; 7: 13–31

34. Coupey S M, Ahlstom P. Common menstrual disorders. Pediatr Clin North Am 1989; 36: 551–571

35. Markee J E. Menstruation in intraocular endometrial transplants in the rhesus monkey. Contributions to embryology. Publ no. 518. Washington: Carnegie Institute, 1940; 28: 219–308

36. Rees M C P, Dunnill M S, Anderson A B M, Turnbull A C. Quantitative uterine histology during the menstrual cycle in relation to measured menstrual blood loss. Br J Obstet Gynaecol 1984; 91: 662–666

37. Hourihan H, Sheppard B L, Bonnar J. A morphometric study of the effect of oral norethisterone and levonorgestrel in endometrial blood vessels. Contraception 1986; 34: 603–612

38. McKone E, Sheppard B L, Bonnar J. Uterine histology and menstrual blood loss. Irish J Med Sci 1991; 160: 359–360

39. Sheppard B L. The pathology of dysfunctional uterine bleeding. Clin Obstet Gynecol 1984; 11: 227–238

40. Sheppard B L. Coagulation and electron microscopy studies in menorrhagia. In: Shaw R W (ed) Reproductive endocrine disorders, Vol. 2. Lancs: Parthenon, 1990: 25–42

41. Hourihan H M, Sheppard B L, Bonnar J. The morphologic characteristics of menstrual haemostasis in patients with unexplained menorrhagia. Int J Gynecol Pathol 1989; 8: 221–229

42. Christiaens G C M L, Sixma J J, Haspels A A. Morphology of haemostasis in menstrual endometrium. Br J Obstet Gynaecol 1980; 87: 425–430

43. Christiaens G C M L, Sixma J J, Haspels A A. Fibrin and platelets in menstrual discharge before and after the insertion of an intra-uterine contraceptive device. Am J Obstet Gynecol 1981; 140: 793–798

44. Sheppard B L, Dockeray C J, Bonnar J. An ultrastructural study of menstrual blood in normal menstruation and dysfunctional uterine bleeding. Br J Obstet Gynaecol 1983; 90: 259–265

45. De Merre L J, Moss J D, Pattison D S. The haematological study of menstrual discharge. Obstet Gynecol 1967; 30: 830–833

46. Hahn L. Composition of menstrual blood. In: Diczfalusy E, Fraser I S, Webb F T G (eds) Endometrial bleeding and steroidal contraception. Bath: Pitman Press, 1980: 107–137

47. Hahn L, Cederblad G, Rybo G et al. Blood coagulation, fibrinolysis and plasma protein in women with normal and excessive menstrual blood loss. Br J Obstet Gynaecol 1976; 83: 974–980

48. Rees M C P, Cederholm-Williams S A, Turnbull A C. Coagulation factors and fibrinolytic proteins in menstrual fluid collected from normal and menorrhagic women. Br J Obstet Gynaecol 1985; 92: 1164–1168

49. Bonnar J, Sheppard B L, Dockeray C J. Coagulation, fibrinolysis and dysfunctional uterine bleeding. Res Clin Forums 1982; 4: 93–101

50. Albrechtsen O K. The fibrinolytic activity of the uterine endometrium. Acta Endocrinol 1956; 23: 207–218

51. Albrechtsen O K. The fibrinolytic activity of the human tissue. Br J Haematol 1956; 3: 284–291

52. Astrup T. The haemostatic balance. Thromb Diath Haem 1958; 2: 347–357

53. Beller F K. Observations on the clotting of menstrual blood and clot formation. Am J Obstet Gynecol 1971; 11: 535–546

54. Sheppard B L, Stack M, Jordan M, Bonnar J. Plasminogen activator in the human uterus in normal menstruation and dysfunctional uterine bleeding. Irish J Med Sci 1990; 159: 151

55. Bonnar J, Sheppard B L, Dockeray C J. The haemostatic system and dysfunctional uterine bleeding. Res Clin Forum 1983; 5: 27–36

56. Shaw S T, Macaulay L K, Tanaka M S et al. Plasminogen activator in human uterine tissue — relationship to location of sampling and time of ovarian cycle. Biochem Med 1980; 24: 170–178

57. Rybo G. Plasminogen activators in the endometrium. II. Clinical aspects. Acta Obstet Gynecol Scand 1966; 45: 97–118

58. Hourihan H M, Sheppard B L, Brosens I. Endometrial haemostasis. In: D'Arcangues C, Fraser I S, Newton J R, Odlind V (eds) Contraception and mechanisms of endometrial bleeding. Cambridge: Cambridge University Press, 1990: 95–116

59. Sheppard B L. Pathophysiology of dysfunctional uterine bleeding. In: Lowe D, Fox H (eds) Advances in gynaecological pathology. Edinburgh: Churchill Livingstone, 1992: 191–204

60. Pickles V R, Hall W J, Best F A, Smith G N. Prostaglandins in endometrium and menstrual fluid from normal and dysmenorrhoeic subjects. J Obstet Gynaecol Br Commonw 1965; 72: 185 192

61. Smith B J. The prostanoids in hemostasis and thrombosis. Am J Pathol 1980; 99: 743–803

62. Casey M L, Hemsell D L, MacDonald P C, Johnston J M. NAD⁺ dependent 15-hydroxy-prostaglandin dehydrogenase activity in human endometrium. Prostaglandins 1980; 19: 115–122

63. Rees M C P, Parry D M, Anderson A B M, Turnbull A C. Immunohistochemical localization of cyclooxygenase in the human uterus. Prostaglandins 1982; 23: 207–214

64. Downie J, Poyser N L, Wunderlich M. Levels of prostaglandins in human endometrium during the normal menstrual cycle. J Physiol 1974; 236: 465–472

65. Willman E A, Collins W P, Clayton S G. Studies on the involvement of prostaglandins in uterine symptomatology and pathology. Br J Obstet Gynaecol 1976; 83:337

66. Cameron I T, Leask R, Kelly R W, Baird D T. Endometrial prostaglandins in women with abnormal uterine bleeding. Prostaglandins, Leukot Med 1987; 29: 249–258

67. Smith S K, Abel M H, Kelly R W, Baird D T. Prostaglandin synthesis in the endometrium of women with ovular dysfunctional uterine bleeding. Br J Obstet Gynaecol 1981; 88: 434

68. Smith S K, Kelly R W, Abel M H, Baird D T. A role for prostacyclin (PGI2) in excessive menstrual bleeding. Lancet 1981; i: 522

69. Makarainen L, Ylikorkala O. Primary and myoma associated menorrhagia; role of prostaglandin and ibuprofen. Br J Obstet Gynaecol 1986; 93: 974–978

70. Sharma S C, Sheppard B L, Bonnar J. Relationship of menstrual blood loss with uterine 6-keto-PGF1 and TXB2 levels in women with normal and dysfunctional uterine bleeding. Irish J Med Sci 1990; 159: 57

71. Sharma S C, Sheppard B L, Bonnar J. Endometrial tissue levels of PGE2 and PGF2 metabolites in women with normal menstruation and dysfunctional uterine bleeding. Irish J Med Sci 1990; 159: 152

72. Drudy L, Sheppard B L, Bonnar J. Mast cells in the normal uterus and in dysfunctional uterine bleeding. Eur J Obstet Gynecol Reprod Biol 1991; 39: 193–201

73. Drudy L, Sheppard B L, Bonnar J. The ultrastructure of mast cells in the uterus throughout the normal menstrual cycle and in the menopause. J Anat 1991; 175: 51–63

74. Foley M E, Griffin B D, Zugel M et al. Heparin-like activity in uterine blood. Br Med J 1978; 2: 322–324

75. Drudy L, Sheppard B L, Bonnar J. Histamine concentration in plasma of menstrual and peripheral blood in patients with normal menstrual blood loss and in dysfunctional uterine bleeding. J Obstet Gynecol 1994; 14: 435–437

76. Hamilton K K, Sims P J. Changes in cytosolic Ca associated with von Willebrand factor release in human endothelial cells exposed to histamine. J Clin Invest 1987; 78: 600–608

77. Hanss M, Collen D. Secretion of tissue-type plasminogen activator and plasminogen activator inhibitor by cultured human endothelial cells: modulation by thrombin, endotoxin and histamine. J Lab Clin Med 1987; 109: 97–104

78. Vargraftig B B, Fouque F, Beneniste J. Adrenaline and PAF-acether synergise to trigger cyclooxygenase-independent activation of plasma free human platelets. Thromb Res 1982; 28: 557–573

79. Bjork J, Smedegard G. Acute microvascular effects of PAF-acether, as studied by intravital microscopy. Eur J Pharmacol 1983; 96: 87–94

80. Alecozay A A, Delon F D, Harper M J K et al. Platelet-activating factor (PAF) in human endometrium. Bio Reprod 1988; 38 (suppl. 1): 78

81. Camussi G, Aglietta M, Malavas F. The release of platelet-activating factor from human endothelial cells in culture. J Immunol 1983; 131: 2397–2403

82. Ludwig J C, Hoppens C L, McManus L M. Modulation of platelet-activating factor (PAF) synthesis and release from human polymorphonuclear leukocytes (PMN): role of extracellular albumin. Arch Biochem Biophys 1985; 241: 337–347

83. Smith S K, Kelly R W. Effect of platelet-activating factor on the release of PGF2 and PGE2 by separated cells of human endometrium. J Reprod Fertil 1988; 82: 271–276

84. Ahmed A, Smith S K. Platelet-activating factor stimulates phospholipase C activity in human endometrium. J Cell Physiol 1992; 152: 207–214

85. Alecozay A A, Harper M J K, Schenken R S, Hanahan D J. Paracrine interactions between platelet-activating factor and prostaglandins in hormonally-treated luteal phase endometrium. J Reprod Fertil 1991; 91: 301–312

86. Ekstrom P, Alm P, Akerlund M. Differences in vasomotor responses between main stem and smaller branches of the human uterine artery. Acta Obstet Gynecol Scand 1991; 70: 429–433

87. Fried G, Samuelson U. Endothelin and neuropeptide Y are vasoconstrictors in human uterine blood vessels. Am J Obstet Gynecol 1991; 164: 1330–1336

88. Svane D, Larson B, Andersson K E, Forman A. Endothelin-1: immunocytochemistry, localisation of binding sites, and contractile effects in human uteroplacental smooth muscle. Am J Obstet Gynecol 1993; 168: 233–241

89. Cameron I T, Irvine G, Norman J E. Menstruation. In: Hillier S G, Kitchener H C, Neilson J P. (eds) Scientific essentials of reproductive medicine. London: Saunders, 1996: 208–218

90. Casey M L, Smith J W, Nagai K et al. Progesterone-regulated cyclic modulation of membrane metalloendopeptidase (enkephalinase) in human endometrium. J Biol Chem 1991; 266: 23041–23047

91. Bonnar J, Sheppard B L. Treatment of menorrhagia during menstruation: randomized controlled trial of ethamsylate, mefenamic acid and tranexamic acid. Br Med J 1996; 313: 579–582

CHAPTER 3

Diagnosis of dysfunctional uterine bleeding

S. S. Sheth and G. N. Allahbadia

Introduction

Menorrhagia is a symptom denoting excessive menstrual bleeding. Menorrhagia can be technically defined as menses lasting longer than 7 days or a blood loss volume in excess of 80 ml. It is a complaint that is difficult to verify objectively in many cases, even with a detailed case history. Issues of perception and tolerance of symptoms are important in whether a patient presents to a doctor, and this varies considerably from one society to another.

Menorrhagia is regarded by most patients as a disease but to gynaecologists it is a symptom — an expression of pathology in the reproductive organs, the endocrine system or elsewhere in the body. Just as polyuria signals an abnormality in the renal or other systems, as manifested through the kidney, menorrhagia expresses a disorder of the uterine or other systems via the uterus.

Menorrhagia has been documented at all reproductive ages. Any woman who menstruates may develop excessive bleeding. The chances of menorrhagia increase with the number of menstrual cycles. Women with small families are especially vulnerable, owing to long spells of menstruation and short spells of amenorrhoea. The modern woman probably experiences nine times more menstrual cycles than did her ancestors.[1] The earliest reference to menorrhagia is found in Hindu texts dating back to 1400 BC, exhorting women to refrain from housework during menses, probably with the intention of giving them a well-earned rest. Hippocrates suggested cupping the breast as a cure for menorrhagia, but it was not until 1938 that the first effective treatment for the condition was described by Albright, whose use of progesterone is followed to this day.[2]

Among women with excessive bleeding, in a few the cause is immediately apparent on examination; in some, the cause reveals itself after detailed investigation; however, in the majority the cause eludes the most exhaustive search, when the condition is labelled 'dysfunctional uterine bleeding' (DUB).

In the past, definitive treatment for abnormal uterine bleeding has been either abdominal or vaginal hysterectomy although Studd finds a paucity of literature concerning the role of hysterectomy in the treatment of menorrhagia.[3] Alternatives to hysterectomy are now proposed in view of the fact that nearly 50% of uterine specimens obtained during hysterectomies for menorrhagia are disease free on pathological examination.[4] Diagnosis is essential in menorrhagia because bleeding, being a debilitating condition, interferes with a woman's normal lifestyle; occasionally, it is an early warning sign of a hidden but ominous problem. Patients vary in their subjective assessment of their condition, and objective diagnosis is often difficult in the absence of convincing or clinching clues. Therefore, pinpointing the diagnosis of menorrhagia will remain one of the challenges in gynaecological practice, even after crossing into the 21st century.

Definitions, terminology, nomenclature and classification

Definitions

Various definitions of menorrhagia exist in the literature. Definitions are useful for categorization, but not necessarily for clarity. The authors suggest that the acronym DUB be used as a working diagnosis for abnormal bleeding from the uterus for which no pelvic pathology or cause has been detected by clinical examination and routine investigations. The American College of Obstetricians and Gynecologists describes it as menstrual bleeding lasting for 7 days from a normal secretory endometrium after normal ovulation.[5] In the most widely used definition, 'menorrhagia' refers to blood loss of 80 ml or more per menstrual period.

Terminology and nomenclature

The Greek words *mene* and *rhegnymi* mean 'moon' and 'to burst', respectively. The combination 'menorrhagia', therefore, literally means 'bursting forth every month.' The term is used loosely to refer to various forms of abnormal uterine bleeding (Fig. 3.1).

Classification

In general medicine, 'pyrexia of unknown origin' (PUO) is diagnosed after excluding all causes of pyrexia. Similarly, in gynaecology, 'menorrhagia of unknown origin' (MUO) would be a more accurate description of unexplained menorrhagia than 'dysfunctional uterine bleeding' until a diagnosis is established (Table 3.1).

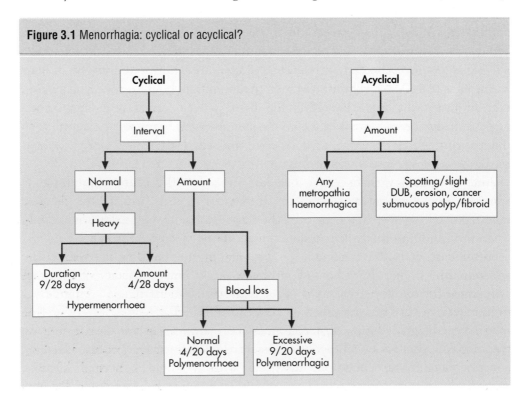

Figure 3.1 Menorrhagia: cyclical or acyclical?

Table 3.1 Classifications: menorrhagia viewed from several angles

Type	• Essential or primary (without organic cause) • Secondary (due to organic cause)
Cause	• Clinically detectable • Detectable on investigation • Detectable on HP microscopy of uterus and/or ovaries
Age group	• Pubertal • Reproductive • Perimenopausal
Blood loss	• Reduce percentage Hb • Normal percentage Hb, low serum ferritin levels
Menorrhagia of unknown origin (MUO)*	No cause on clinical examination and routine investigations → DUB

* After clinical examination and routine investigations, if no cause for MUO, working diagnosis of dysfunctional uterine bleeding (DUB).

The authors suggest that the label of DUB be reserved for those cases in which the entire gamut of studies — clinical, imaging, laboratory and (at times) histopathology — fails to identify an organic cause for abnormal bleeding.

Diagnosis

Approximately 40–70% of women who complain of excessive bleeding do not lose more than 80 ml of blood per month,[6] the cutoff point for diagnosis; conversely, about 40% of women who bleed in excess of 80 ml do not consider their blood loss to be heavy.[6] Contradictions such as these make clinical practice fascinating. However, with volumes greater than 80 ml, the risk of anaemia becomes quite high.[7] Women living in traditional societies usually show a greater tolerance towards heavy bleeding than their sisters in the industrialized world. In many uncomplaining women, menorrhagia has been diagnosed on the finding of a low haemoglobin level, often less than 60–70 g/L. At the other extreme, sometimes women with normal haemoglobin levels persist in seeking medical help for alleged excessive bleeding; such women generally need psychological support and counselling.

As always, delineation of any medical disorder involves a thorough history and physical examination. At the minimum, a focused history should address the quantity and quality of bleeding, the presence of hirsutism, galactorrhoea, symptoms of thyroid dysfunction, systemic illness (including hepatic or renal failure or diabetes mellitus) and a history of excessive bruising and prolonged bleeding after skin cuts or dental extractions. In addition, enquiry should be made with regard to sexual activity, contraceptive use, symptoms and signs of pregnancy, pelvic pain and pathology, results of previous gynaecological examinations and/or surgical procedures and details of any medication used. The woman should be asked about the pattern of menses from menarche to the present time, premenstrual molimen (suggesting ovulation), and previous therapeutic and medical evaluations. After the history is taken, a thorough physical examination should be performed. The examination should attempt to establish a differential diagnosis suggested by the patient's chief complaint following a detailed history. Laboratory evaluation is often very useful and can be critical for assessing abnormal uterine bleeding, as the aetiology can be uncertain even after a thorough history and physical examination. Laboratory evaluation may include a full blood count, serum pregnancy test, examination of cervical specimens for gonorrhoea and chlamydia, and cervical smear. The following ancillary tests can be requested according to the physician's suspicion and discretion: thyroid function tests; levels of serum transaminases, luteinizing hormone (LH), follicle-stimulating hormone (FSH) and oestradiol; prothrombin time, activated partial thromboplastin time and bleeding time; assessment of serum prolactin, quantitative beta human chorionic gonadotrophin (β-hCG), blood urea nitrogen (BUN) and serum creatinine; and adrenal function tests.

In a nutshell, the diagnosis of dysfunctional uterine bleeding is arrived at in two stages — namely (1) confirming the occurrence of menorrhagia and (2) confirming the absence of conditions that could cause menorrhagia.

Confirmation of menorrhagia

Determining whether blood loss during menses exceeds the normal limit is difficult, as the amount of bleeding cannot be easily measured. The definition of menorrhagia as bleeding in excess of 80 ml derives from population surveys[6–9] and from studies that have shown that two-thirds of women who lose more than 80 ml every month have iron-deficiency anaemia.[10–12] However, the figure of 80 ml can be misleading, as blood volume forms only a part of the menstrual discharge, ranging from 2 to 82% of the menstrual fluid;[13] moreover, it is proportional neither to the duration of bleeding nor to the number of sanitary pads and tampons.[14] Hence, it is not uncommon to encounter women who report prolonged heavy menses but have a haemoglobin of 130 g/L, and others with a haemoglobin of 60 g/L who complain of general weakness without even a mention of heavy periods.

The alkaline haematin technique, devised in 1964 by Hallberg and Nilsson,[15] has been described by O'Brien[16] as the gold standard for assessing menstrual blood loss. Although it represents an improvement over methods involving counting sanitary pads and days of bleeding, or measuring haemoglobin, the alkaline haematin method is cumbersome, offensive and time consuming. In addition, there is the risk involved in dealing with caustic reagents, as well as that of possible infection by hepatitis and AIDS virus from menstrual blood. O'Brien therefore went on to develop pictorial blood-loss assessment charts (PBAC), which make it easier to diagnose and monitor treatment by assessing the extent of soiling in standard sanitary pads.[16] A lightly soiled pad scores 1 whereas a saturated pad is assigned 20 points; for tampons the range is 1–10 points. A PBAC score of 100 translates into 80 ml of menstrual blood.[17,18] Although this method is a useful research and documentation tool, it involves a considerable expenditure of time and effort, which may be in short supply at a busy clinic. Erythrocyte ratio labelling is complicated and cannot be generally recommended. Estimation of uterine size or endometrial thickening contributes little to diagnosis. In day-to-day practice, diagnosis of menorrhagia is aided by a continuous fall in haemoglobin level in women who are not taking iron supplements. Once abnormal bleeding has been confirmed and menorrhagia diagnosed, the next step towards diagnosis of DUB is clinical examination followed by investigations.

A prospective, observational study was recently developed and validated as a method for measuring menstrual blood loss in a routine setting. Sanitary material was washed with a non-ionic detergent in a known volume of water; the haemoglobin in a sample of the resultant solution was then measured by mixing with sodium carbonate for spectrophotometric analysis. The menstrual blood loss result was revealed to each of 372 women who had been offered endometrial ablation for menorrhagia; 36 women (10%) with normal menstrual blood loss who had declined surgery continued to avoid surgery after a mean of 27 months. The authors concluded that objective diagnosis of menorrhagia can be undertaken in a routine setting and may give some women, who have a normal menstrual blood loss, sufficient reassurance to refrain from surgery.[19]

Diagnosis of DUB

In more than 50% of cases of menorrhagia of unknown origin, clinical examination and routine investigations are normal. The working diagnosis of DUB is then applied until a cause is found or the absence of a cause is confirmed.

Probing the cause of DUB begins with a detailed history and goes on to clinical examination and simple investigations. Elaborate investigations are usually deferred, except in countries where litigation is common. DUB is so widespread and the investigations so varied and numerous that they may not always be cost effective, especially in the less affluent economies.

Menorrhagia can result from a variety of conditions. In making a diagnosis of DUB, therefore, the gynaecologist must confirm the absence of all the likely causes, ranging from such obvious conditions as fibroids, retained intra-uterine contraceptive device (IUCD) or adnexal mass to subtle disruption of the endocrine system that can be detected only by special tests. It is important to remember that a lesion associated with heavy bleeding is not always obvious. Coagulation disorders such as von Willebrand's disease, deficiencies of prothrombin or of factors II, V, VII or IX, and idiopathic thrombocytopenic purpura must always be kept in mind.

History

The history makes an important contribution to diagnosis (Tables 3.2–3.4). The patient's menstrual history, from menarche to presentation, should be investigated, as should the duration and frequency of the menorrhagia. The timing of the menorrhagia is also significant: menarche and perimenopausal menorrhagia may indicate physiological dysfunction; a gradual onset of menorrhagia over months or years without other symptoms of endocrine disease is consistent with fibroids or DUB; a sudden onset, especially if bleeding continues between menstrual cycles, may indicate involution of submucosal fibroids or cancer. Cyclical weight changes, an increase in weight, or chronic obesity may suggest other causes of menorrhagia or polycystic ovarian disease.

Table 3.2 Menstrual history

Family history: Heavy bleeding, tuberculosis, uterine or ovarian malignancy in close relatives

Medications that can cause menorrhagia: Oestrogen, progesterone, anticoagulants, propranolol, phenothiazines, butyrophenones, tricyclic antidepressants, MAO inhibitors, tranquillizers, corticosteroids and digoxin

Contraception: IUCD

Other diseases: Bleeding tendency, hypertension, liver disease, or hypothyroidism

Previous surgery: Splenectomy, thyroidectomy, myomectomy, polypectomy, hysteroscopy, D&C

D&C, dilatation and curettage; IUCD, intra-uterine contraceptive device; MAO, monoamine oxidase.

Table 3.3 Associated symptoms

Symptoms	Probable cause of haemorrhage
Blood-tinged discharge	Cancer, submucous polyp, fibroid, IUCD
Painful menses	Endometriosis
Post-coital bleeding	Cervical erosion, malignancy, severe vaginitis
Intermenstrual spotting/bleeding	Surface lesion on cervix or endometrium, endometriosis, oligo-ovulation
Dyspareunia	Pelvic endometriosis, pelvic inflammatory disease (PID)
Dysuria, pain during defecation, blood in urine or stool	Pelvic endometriosis
Lower abdominal pain	Fibroid, endometriosis, adenomyosis (necrobiosis), PID, ovarian tumours, pregnancy-related conditions
General weakness, leucorrhoea, backache, pain or cramps in the leg	Anaemia, tuberculosis, malignancy
Infertility	Anovulation, fibroid, endometriosis, PID, tuberculosis
Bad obstetric history	Uterine malformation, fibroid
Post-abortion or postpartum bleeding	Retained products of conception, placental polyps

Table 3.4 Onset of menorrhagia related to diagnosis

Diagnosis	Historical clues
Physiological	Immediately after menarche, or in late 40s or 50s
Medication	Since onset of medication or soon after medication
Thyroid	Gradual onset, over months or years
Fibroid	Either gradual increase over months, or sudden or cyclic
Cancer (endometrial or cervical)	Rapid increase over few months or sudden, persistent and non-cyclic
DUB	Irregular or increasing over months
Chronic disease	Occurring with increasing disability from disease

Clinical examination

Clinical examination in patients with menorrhagia may be unremarkable or may reveal signs of severe illness, particularly when menorrhagia is due to unsuspected cancer or tuberculosis.

General examination usually reveals anaemia and gradually increasing pallor, and this could be the only physical manifestation of excessive blood loss. In a woman without overt anaemia, who is not taking haematinics, the serum ferritin level is a helpful indicator. In the absence of bleeding from any other source, frequent occurrence of anaemia despite iron supplementation confirms the presence of menorrhagia even if the woman herself makes no complaint.

Hypertension, findings indicating cardiac or liver problems causing congestion, generalized oedema, and the presence of tremors and eyeball prominence can lead the clinician to the root cause of menorrhagia. A positive history of bleeding at multiple sites and multiple times points to haematological disorders such as von Willebrand's disease.

Systemic examination may reveal no abnormality or may provide findings suggestive of liver disease or tuberculosis.

Findings on abdominal palpation may vary from normal to an extremely obvious, palpable mass encountered by the fingers. At speculum examination, the cervix may be normal or show a vascular erosion, polyp, myoma, suspicious ulcer or frank, cauliflower-like growth. Vaginal ulceration or growth, as well as neglected foreign bodies, are easily visualized. Bimanual examination, again, may be normal or reveal frank abnormalities. The uterus may be of normal or large size, or small and atrophic, with consistency ranging from normal to hard, smooth to nodular. A uterus that is tender on bimanual examination should alert the doctor to the possibility of adenomyoma. The adnexal region may be clear or covered with bilateral masses, with the abnormality felt through one or more of the fornices.

Retraction of the posterior vaginal mucosa of the pouch of Douglas can form a 'dimple'.[20] When present, the 'dimple sign' suggests infiltrating endometriosis in the rectovaginal septum or an adherent endometrial cyst of the ovary, subsequently confirmed at surgery or laparoscopy by the outpouring of chocolate-brown fluid.[20]

Table 3.5 Conditions causing menorrhagia the exclusion of which leads to diagnosis of DUB

Type	Condition
General	Hypertension
	Congestive cardiac failure
	Chronic passive venous congestion
	Purpura
	Prothrombin deficiency
	von Willebrand's disease
	Platelet disorder (number or function)
	Thrombocytopenia or thrombocytopathies
	Leukaemia
	Systemic lupus erythematosus
	Aplastic anaemia
Uterus related	Fibroid
	Adenomyosis
	IUCD
	Endometritis
	Endometrial hyperplasia
	Endometrial carcinoma
	Choriocarcinoma
	Endometrial polyp
	Tuberculosis
	Double uterus
	Symmetrical enlargement (myohyperplasia)
	Haemangioma
Cervix related	Vascular erosion
	Fibroid
	Polyp
	Malignancy
Tube related	Salpingitis
	Ectopic pregnancy
	Malignancy
Ovary related	Infection (tubovarian mass)
	Tumour (large)
	Oestrogen-secreting tumour
Vagina related	Severe vaginitis
	Ulcer
	Malignancy
	Foreign body
Vulva related	Ulcer
	Malignancy

Table 3.5 Continued

Psychogenic	Anxiety
	Overwork
	Environmental changes
	Unsatisfactory sex life
Endocrine	Hypothyroidism
Iatrogenic	Medication
	Forgotten IUCD
Pregnancy related	Incomplete, threatened or missed abortion
	Ectopic pregnancy
	Placental polyp
	Trophoblastic disease
Bleeding from lower genital tract, misleading the diagnosis	Haematuria
	Bleeding per rectum or per vulva

All detectable causes of menorrhagia should be sought and excluded before menorrhagia is attributed to DUB (Table 3.5).

Uterus size

The uterus may be enlarged in the following conditions:

- DUB
- Fibroids
- Adenomyosis
- Uterine or cervical polyps
- Endometrial hyperplasia or malignancy
- Hypertrophic tuberculosis
- Generalized myohyperplasia
- Trophoblastic disease
- Malformation
- Pyometra
- Pregnancy.

The size of the uterus may be normal in DUB, in cases of tiny fibroids, adenomyosis, small polyps, endometrial hyperplasia, malignancy or tuberculosis, trophoblastic disease and minimal pyometra. In DUB uterine size may be normal or enlarged to the size of a 10–12 weeks pregnancy, but it never exceeds that of a 14-week pregnancy. In adenomyosis the uterus usually is of 8–10 weeks' size, although in severe cases the size has been known to increase to that of 10–14 weeks but never of more than 16 weeks. Symmetrical enlargement indicates severe adenomyosis and reduces uterus-free pelvic space.[21] In endometrial carcinoma the size of the uterus usually ranges from normal to 12 weeks, but can readily increase to that of 20 weeks. A larger uterus is uncommon as, by then, heavy or irregular bleeding with or without secondaries would have demanded attention. In tuberculosis the size of the uterus rarely exceeds that of 12–14 weeks; it can, in fact, be smaller than normal. A much larger size is usually associated with pyometra with or without tubovarian pathology, including development of a mass and (uncommonly) encysted ascites.

Fibroids

Fibroids may be asymptomatic or may give rise to progressive menorrhagia which is particularly heavy on the second and third day of regular menses. A large fibroid, with increased ovarian blood supply, is associated with frequent menstrual periods, whereas submucous fibroids may lead to continuous or irregular bleeding, varying in intensity from spotting to heavy menstrual episodes, metrorrhagia or even menometrorrhagia. Fibroids may be easily felt on bimanual examination or seen on speculum examination; in some cases, however, they elude all attempts at detection until exposed by hysteroscopy. About two-thirds of women with fibroids experience no pain. Fibroids that feel soft are degenerating, whereas those that feel hard may be calcifying. A fibroid can be mistaken for adenomyoma or a bicornuate uterus. The latter is associated with menorrhagia, dysmenorrhoea and, in some cases, associated with a poor obstetric history. A uterus enlarged with fibroids has no limit in size, varying from normal to mammoth (equivalent to 28–32 weeks' pregnancy) in size. A size of over 20 weeks, particularly with marked vascularity or rapid growth, should arouse strong suspicion of malignancy — sarcomatous degeneration is found in 0.4% of fibroids removed surgically (personal series).

Adenomyosis

Adenomyosis is a common finding at histopathological examination following hysterectomy for DUB. Although dysmenorrhoea accompanies adenomyosis in some cases, in more than 70% it may be absent: hence, absence of dysmenorrhoea does not exclude adenomyosis. The uterus in adenomyosis may be enlarged, and such enlargement may be generalized or localized. Generalized enlargement may be mild, moderate or severe, depending on the endometrial extension into the myometrium. The uterus is firm and may be tender during menses in some cases. Importantly, the pouch of Douglas is free.

Brosens et al.[21] evaluated the role of endovaginal ultrasonography in the diagnosis of adenomyosis and to identify predictive characteristics: it demonstrated a sensitivity of 86%, a specificity of 50%, a positive predictive value of 86% and a negative predictive value of 77%. Adenomyosis was best predicted on the basis of ill-defined myometrial heterogeneity. The authors concluded that endovaginal sonography in symptomatic patients can be a sensitive, but not a specific, procedure for the diagnosis of adenomyosis.[21] When differentiation between adenomyosis and fibroids, with a whorled appearance, is difficult, diagnosis can be clinched by magnetic resonance imaging (MRI) or by surgery. It is important to distinguish between the two conditions, especially when the patient has infertility problems or desires future pregnancies. Absence of the capsule and of the typical whorled appearance, and the presence of coarse trabecular interlacing of fibrous and myometrial tissue, are diagnostic of adenomyosis, ruling out fibroids. When adenomyoma is severe, localized in the wall and encapsulated, only the cut surface differentiates it from fibroids. It can behave like submucous fibroids, by projecting into the uterine cavity. If the uterus removed for DUB was always painstakingly examined by an experienced pathologist, the incidence of adenomyosis would be much higher than reported at present.

Investigations

Investigations into menorrhagia of unknown origin or DUB depend on the gynaecologist's diligence in ascertaining the cause of bleeding, the patient's willingness to undergo tests, and the legal situation. Generally, non-invasive investigations are preferred to invasive tests, and economical techniques to expensive ones. The aim of the investigations is to locate or rule out the causes of bleeding. This involves (1) the diagnosis of iron-deficiency anaemia, (2) the exclusion of systemic disease causing abnormal bleeding, and (3) the exclusion of pelvic pathology. Some investigations must be initiated immediately, whereas others can be done later, when convenient or when medically needed. It is necessary to be practical, in the best interests of the patient's physical condition and economic scenario, and not to be forced into overinvestigation by the presence of a litigious environment.

The search for the cause of bleeding begins with a complete blood cell count and haemoglobin assessment, including blood film examination; hysteroscopy with endometrial curettage could be revealing, except in puberty menorrhagia, where this should be the last resort. Failure to subject the patient to hysteroscopy could result in missing such obvious causes of excessive bleeding as polyps, fibroids, and forgotten IUCDs and, occasionally, tuberculosis or pregnancy-related conditions in pubertal women.

Although the diagnostic accuracy of hysteroscopy is high, it should be considered as a diagnostic technique and used together with endometrial curettage or directed biopsy. Hysteroscopy is also useful for excluding those patients with abnormal uterine bleeding without evidence of signs of intra-uterine pathology. After a fair amount of practice, it is possible to use hysteroscopy for the identification of patients with either benign or malignant endometrial lesions, with about 20% false positives and no false negatives.[22] The combined use of hysteroscopy and biopsy leads to near-100% accuracy in the diagnosis of endometrial neoplasia and its precursors.[22]

The less-urgent tests include the following:

1. *Estimation of haemoglobin and, if required, serum ferritin levels.* Serum ferritin estimation is particularly useful in populations with a high prevalence of thalassaemia and haemoglobinopathies.[23]
2. *Haematological profile*, to exclude thrombocytopenic purpura, SLE, leukaemia, von Willebrand's disease, and aplastic anaemia. It is particularly helpful in ovulatory DUB with no anatomical uterine abnormality. After clinical assessment, relevant history and family history, the clinician often has a good idea concerning the cause of a patient's bleeding and the most appropriate laboratory tests can then be ordered, including those for prothrombin time and activated partial thromboplastin time.
3. *Thyroid function tests* — thyrotrophin (TSH), 3,5,3'-tri-iodothyronine (T3) and thyroxine (T4) to exclude myxoedema or subclinical hypothyroidism.[24]
4. *Serum tests for liver or renal disease.*

5. *Tests for antinuclear antibody, DNA binding and lupus inhibitor* to exclude SLE in difficult or refractory cases.
6. *SH and LH* to define the perimenopausal state and polycystic ovarian disease (POD) in younger women. An endocrine disorder commonly linked to menorrhagia is polycystic ovarian syndrome (PCO), characterized by hirsutism, obesity and irregular menstrual bleeding.
7. *Sonography* takes the place of invasive examination in adolescents and young girls, particularly those with an intact hymen. In the remaining patients, it has a limited role, although high-resolution transvaginal sonography is sometimes helpful. The need is to detect uterine fibroids, to differentiate fibroids from adenomyosis and uterine swelling from an adnexal mass, and to search for signs of malignancy. However, pathology or otherwise of the endometrial cavity can best be established with hysteroscopy, which is therefore preferred to transvaginal sonography. A recent study compared office hysteroscopy with transvaginal ultrasonography for diagnosing intra-uterine pathological disorders in patients with excessive uterine bleeding, with specimens obtained from either hysterectomy or operative hysteroscopy used to represent the true diagnosis.[25] Hysteroscopy was 79% sensitive and 93% specific in diagnosing intracavitary pathological disorders, whereas transvaginal ultrasonography was only 54% sensitive and 90% specific.[25] The use of contrast techniques will increase the accuracy of ultrasound in detecting intra-uterine pathology. An experienced sonologist is a critical requirement; otherwise, existing polyps will be missed and non-existing ovarian cysts will be diagnosed. Scores of misleading reports have led to unnecessary treatment and hence the results of sonography should be reviewed carefully and critically.

   Transvaginal sonography is particularly helpful in looking at endometrial thickness in postmenopausal women. In menopausal patients, endometrial thickness of more than 4 mm in the absence of oestrogen or tamoxifen therapy requires investigation.[26] Any postmenopausal woman, or a woman on oestrogen or tamoxifen with endometrial thickness of 8–10 mm or more, needs a histopathological study. A thickness less than 4 mm suggests the absence of cancer or hyperplasia. Measurement of total uterine volume may give a clue to the underlying pathology; generally, the greater the volume, the greater are the chances of failure of medical treatment.

   Ultrasonography is more accurate, more economical, more convenient and, probably, better accepted than MRI. However, it is not always able to distinguish benign from malignant conditions.[27,28]

   Transvaginal colour Doppler sonography (TVCDS) shows absence of colour in non-malignant endometrial disease, in contrast to the presence of feeder artery and venous flow in endometrial cancer.[29,30]

   Overall, endovaginal sonography is superior to MRI for evaluation of clinically suspected pelvic masses.[31–34]
8. *MRI* is significantly superior to transvaginal sonography and hysterosalpingo-graphy in the diagnosis of adenomyosis,[35–40] and this could be a valuable asset in counselling infertile women prior to surgery. Togashi et al. could distinguish adenomyosis from leiomyoma in 92 of 93 women with an enlarged uterus, using MRI.[37] However, MRI is not always efficient in differentiating small fibroids (less than 2–3 cm in diameter) from adenomyoma.[36]

In detecting adnexal mass, MRI is more specific than either sonography or CT.[41–46] Availability of MRI can be an asset, as it helps to clarify the origin of a mass, whether uterine or ovarian. MRI easily identifies ovaries in premenopausal women but is less efficient in the case of postmenopausal women with an enlarged uterus.[45] MRI is superior to both CT and ultrasound in accurately diagnosing endometriosis in the ovary and rectovaginal septum.

MRI is fast emerging as a powerful tool to aid clinical diagnosis and management. However, its high cost restricts availability, especially in the developing world. In the authors' opinion, only if MRI or CT can change the management and help preoperative counselling — such as eliminating the need for laparotomy or clinching the diagnosis of ovarian pathology — will they have a major impact on gynaecological practice.

9. *Sonohysterosalpingography*, carried out after introduction of fluid through a paediatric Foley's catheter or an infant-feeding tube, improves visualization through the 'acoustic window'.[47–49] Sonohysterography and scanning, after instillation of saline, can be helpful in the diagnosis of polyps as well as of submucous fibroids.[48,50]

10. A *Papanicolaou ('Pap') cervical smear* reflects the state of the cervix, and is of little use in assessing the endometrium. Nevertheless, it should be done in all women with menorrhagia, for its negative value in ruling out cancer. In a woman scheduled to undergo hysterectomy, a negative 'Pap' test could be very useful if histopathology indicated otherwise.

As a supplement to the 'Pap' smear, the endocervical brush or cytobrush is an efficient technique for collecting endocervical cells for early detection of neoplasms, especially from an unhealthy-looking endocervix or for repeat smears. A combination of cytobrush and spatula increases yield from the transformation zone and increases the positive cytology rate and the number of adequate smears.[51]

Occasionally, a patient may decline hysteroscopy and dilatation and curettage (D&C), preferring instead a simpler office procedure for studying the endometrium. Stovall has shown that Pipelle endometrial sampling is a viable alternative to D&C for detecting endometrial carcinoma.[52] Kaunitz et al.[53] have reported that the Pipelle method results in a larger collection of tissue than Vabra aspiration, is less painful and therefore is more acceptable to women. Moreover, it is inexpensive, which is a special advantage in developing countries, particularly when serial or mass outdoor sampling are required. However, the Pipelle method is not without drawbacks: it does not sample the entire endometrium and, like D&C, can miss an occult lesion.

11. *D&C* is mandatory in all peri- and postmenopausal women with menorrhagia, particularly when hysteroscopy is not available. Patients need to understand that this is mainly a diagnostic tool and not a therapeutic procedure, as otherwise those expecting a cure after D&C will be disappointed; at the same time, it must be pointed out that, in 30–40% of menorrhagic women, D&C provides temporary relief.[54] Between 50 and 80% of endometrial histopathological studies in menorrhagia of unknown origin will not show abnormalities, and this is reassuring to the patient.[55] Curettage is often incomplete, failing to detect polyps, fibroids, IUCD and malignancy. Sometimes, curettage is carried out when spontaneous remission is round the

corner; it then coincides with the spontaneous remission and is credited with it. Histopathology can exclude cancer, hyperplasia and, occasionally, tuberculosis, besides providing a clue to hormonal therapy through the endometrial pattern.

Grimes[56] compared 13,598 patients who underwent D&C with 5851 who underwent the Vabra procedure, and found the latter technique to be more effective in detecting fibroids, tuberculosis and malignancy, especially in women under 40 years of age. Thus, hysteroscopy and curettage are indicated in all elderly women and those with cancer predisposition, postmenopausal spotting or bleeding and abnormal endometrial thickness seen on sonography.

12. *Culture of endometrium*: it may be worth culturing endometrial tissue for acid-fast bacilli when suspecting tuberculosis, especially in endemic countries and in those patients with infertility.

13. *Laparoscopy* helps in the diagnosis of silent endometriosis, small fibroids or ovarian cyst, tuberculosis and vascularity of the broad ligament. It should be used judiciously, in selected cases most likely to benefit, such as young patients, patients in whom diagnosis is proving difficult or in whom DUB is becoming refractory — in short, very infrequently.

14. *Hysterosalpingogram*: this simple, relatively non-invasive test can detect intra-uterine polyps, uterine malformation, small fibroids and genital tuberculosis. It is particularly useful in parts of the developing world where the hysteroscope and hysteroscopist are not available. The younger the woman, the greater the need for the test.

15. *β-hCG*: pregnancy-related conditions, such as ectopic pregnancy or tropho-blastic disease, can be easily excluded by testing the blood for β-hCG. It can prove particularly useful in metromenorrhagia or intermenstrual bleeding, provided that pregnancy — either ectopic or threatened — is considered as a possible source of bleeding.

16. *Uterine biopsy*: although uterine biopsy, carried out transcervically or with the help of an imaging technique, cannot be practised routinely, it is useful in detecting uterine adenomyosis. In a recent study by Vercellini et al.,[57] myometrial needle biopsy using a 14-gauge core needle was performed on a series of women undergoing laparoscopy for suspected adenomyosis. In a small study of ten patients from Australia, Wood[58] used ultrasound to identify suspicious areas in the myometrium and to direct transabdominal needle biopsy under local anaesthesia. This may be a helpful technique for selected young women with dysmenorrhoea.

17. *Angiography* is rarely performed in cases of menorrhagia unless enforced by repeated haemorrhage and a pressing need to preserve the uterus. When combined with embolization it can be curative in refractory menorrhagia that is due to arterio-venous malformation. In patients with deep-vein thrombosis, angiography–venography is helpful in diagnosing haemangioma. Venography detects increased vascularity of the uterus when collateral circulation is established through the uterus to the veins on the opposite side.

Confirming the diagnosis of DUB

Making a diagnosis of DUB implies excluding the gamut of conditions, from the common to the rare, that could produce menorrhagia. The working diagnosis of

DUB, arrived at after ruling out organic causes by history taking and clinical examination, is firmly established as DUB only after a thorough search for the cause fails to yield a positive result.

Diagnosis in the operating room If all investigations prove to be negative, examination under anaesthesia is mandatory in women scheduled to undergo surgical procedures such as hysteroscopy and curettage, as it can provide accurate information for confirming or refuting the working diagnosis of DUB.[59] It is not unusual for the diagnosis of DUB to change on the operating table after the finding of a fibroid or adnexal mass, transforming essential or primary into secondary menorrhagia.

Examination under anaesthesia is particularly helpful to younger gynaecologists in selecting the route of hysterectomy — abdominal or vaginal, with or without laparoscopic assistance.

If the endometrium or adnexa is suspect, a frozen-section study can help to settle the issue. This facility should be available at all centres performing hysterectomy in such cases, or should be requested when there is suspicion.

Frozen-section examination Examination of frozen sections is necessary in the following circumstances:

1. When hysterectomy is undertaken without hysteroscopy and curettage, i.e. without endometrial histopathology. This is not an uncommon occurrence, as in some parts of the world the frequency of endometrial carcinoma is exceptionally low when compared with cervical cancer (1:10).[60]
2. When hysterectomy is carried out in a high-risk patient for endometrial cancer, in the absence of endometrial histopathology or with normal histopathology as assessed a year or more previously or with complex hyperplasia (atypia) detected a few months earlier.
3. When the cut-open uterus reveals suspicious or malignant-looking endometrium (every uterus removed must be opened and examined for macroscopic lesions).
4. When adnexal pathology arouses the suspicion of malignancy. The result will help to decide whether further procedures are necessary, such as salpingo-oöphorectomy or, in the case of vaginal hysterectomy, opening the abdomen for staging and omentectomy.

Diagnosis in retrospect In pubertal patients, as well as in patients of childbearing age, return of normal cycles confirms the diagnosis retrospectively;[61] however, in some perimenopausal women the final diagnosis of DUB may be arrived at after the fullest possible treatment of menorrhagia, including hysterectomy followed by histopathological examination of the uterus and adnexa. Occasionally it is realized, several months after removal of a normal-looking uterus, that the patient had hypothyroidism with delayed or masked symptoms!

Postmenopausal DUB

In 10% of cases of postmenopausal bleeding, this belongs to the DUB category and may be due to revival of ovarian function. Every single episode of postmenopausal bleeding or spotting should be thoroughly investigated.

Recurrence

Often a chronic condition, menorrhagia can recur on stopping therapy. Recurrence is defined as reappearance of menorrhagia after normal menstrual cycles for 6 months or longer, with the patient not taking treatment.

Refractory DUB

A woman should be diagnosed as having refractory DUB when she fails to respond to often-repeated medical therapies with normal or hormone-related changes in the endometrium over a period of 6 months, with a drop in haemoglobin levels.

Often, gynaecologists become so focused on looking for obstetric and gynaecological causes for menorrhagia that they forget the obscure causes or conditions from the other disciplines. Refractory DUB provides an opportunity to identify and pick up lesions that many would have missed. Submucous polyps and adenomyosis are the commonest culprits involved in DUB, and are unresponsive to therapy.

When DUB is not relieved by medical treatment, or if bleeding recurs, surgery becomes the final option and this may not be desirable if the patient is young, is reluctant to undergo surgery, or may have a haematological disorder or even a misplaced IUCD! The following conditions must always be borne in mind before resorting to surgery: haematological disorders; misplaced IUCD; hypothyroidism; ectopic pregnancy; oestrogen-secreting tumour; haemangiomas; genital tuberculosis; submucous polyp, and systemic lupus erythematosus (SLE).

It is not uncommon for menorrhagia to persist, despite all tests being negative. If, in such cases, a trial with medical treatment does not succeed, surgery is necessary.

Common errors in diagnosis

The following are common errors in diagnosis:

1. Not suspecting malignancy in perimenopausal women.
2. Not suspecting haematological disorders.
3. Not suspecting tuberculosis, particularly in a country where it is endemic.
4. Not suspecting the presence of a tiny, feminizing ovarian tumour.
5. Failure to test for hypothyroidism.
6. Failure to look for pregnancy-related conditions, such as ectopic pregnancy or trophoblastic disease.
7. When the family physician undertakes treatment on the basis of normal sonography without a gynaecological examination (this should be strongly condemned).
8. Failure to assess endometrial thickness while performing pelvic sonography.

Complications of MUO/DUB

Menorrhagia will lead to iron-deficiency anaemia and its symptoms, including general weakness and, occasionally, even cardiac failure. Missed pathology exacerbates the condition; if cancer is missed, the spread of malignancy could make surgery hazardous and change the prognosis drastically.

In gynaecological practice

During the last 30 years, the senior author has encountered more than 800 patients annually with menorrhagia in one form or another. It is not uncommon for the

Table 3.6 Final diagnosis in 1000 women with menorrhagia

Diagnosis	N
Adenomyosis	440
Fibroids	251
Dysfunctional uterine bleeding	138
Endometriosis — ovarian +	76
Tubovarian mass	25
Polyp (uterine/cervical)	18
Hypothyroidism	12
Cancer of the cervix	10
Endometrial cancer	10
Thrombocytopenic purpura	7
Oestrogen-secreting tumour	4
Tuberculosis	8
von Willebrand's disease	1

authors to see at least one patient per week with a haemoglobin level of less than 70 g/L, due to menorrhagia. Although detailed statistical analysis is not available, the breakdown of the last consecutive 1000 cases in a private clinic is instructional. The final diagnoses in this group of women were as shown in Table 3.6. Further analysis revealed that, for every 100 cases of menorrhagia, after clinical examination, menorrhagia of unknown origin or DUB was diagnosed in 60 and menorrhagia occurring secondarily to an organic cause was diagnosed in 40. In 360 cases diagnosed preoperatively as DUB, histopathological examination revealed adenomyosis in 236 (65.5%); this is in contrast to 48 (21.4%) proved to be DUB out of 224 diagnosed preoperatively as adenomyosis (personal data).

Summary

Menorrhagia gives an opportunity to look for a wide variety of causes and sharpens clinical acumen. Detection of von Willebrand's disease or of a tiny granulosa cell tumour is as gratifying to one as frustrating to the other who misses it! Diagnosis of DUB is easy to make but, the more easily it is made, the more likely it is to change to an organic cause. It should always be remembered that the diagnosis should not be reached easily but should be the outcome of thorough scrutiny. The patient's compliance, her gynaecologist's diligence and a litigious environment can play an important role in the diagnosis and management of this condition. In the words of Hippocrates, 'You cannot treat unless you have made a diagnosis'; this is particularly true for menorrhagia.

References

1. Short R V. The evolution of human reproduction. Proc R Soc Lond 1976; 195: 3–24
2. Albright A D, Weeks S R, Duffy M J. Abnormal uterine bleeding: diagnosis and medical management. Prog Obst Gynaecol 1938; 12: 309–326
3. Studd J W W. Hysterectomy and menorrhagia. Baillieres Clin Obstet Gynaecol 1989; 3: 415–424

4. Brill A L. What is the role of hysteroscopy in the management of abnormal uterine bleeding? Clin Obstet Gynecol 1995; 38: 19–34

5. American College of Obstetricians and Gynecologists. Dysfunctional uterine bleeding. Tech Bull 1982; 66: 5–6

6. Hallberg L, Hogdahl A, Nilsson L, Rybo G. Menstrual blood loss: a population study. Acta Obstet Gynecol Scand 1966; 45: 320–351

7. Cohen M A. Anaemia and menstrual loss. Obstet Gynecol Surv 1980; 35: 597–601

8. Cameron I T, Haining R, Lumbsden A J et al. The effects of mefenamic acid and norethisterone on measured menstrual blood loss. Obstet Gynecol 1990; 96: 85–88

9. Preston J T, Cameron I T, Adams E J, Smith S K. Comparative study of tranexamic acid and norethisterone in the treatment of ovulatory menorrhagia. Br J Obstet Gynaecol 1995; 102: 401–406

10. Fraser I S, McCarron G, Markham R A. Preliminary study of the factors influencing perception of menstrual blood loss volume. Am J Obstet Gynecol 1984; 149: 788–793

11. Cohen-Gibar B J B. Anaemia and menstrual blood loss. Obstet Gynecol Surv 1980; 35: 597–618

12. Cole S K, Billewicz W Z, Thomson A M. Sources of variation in menstrual blood loss. J Obstet Gynaecol Br Commonw 1971; 78: 933–939

13. Fraser J S, McCarron G, Markham R, Resta T. Blood and total fluid content of menstrual discharge. Obstet Gynecol 1985; 65: 194–198

14. Chimbira T H, Anderson A B M, Turnbull A C. Relation between measured loss and the patient's subjective assessment of loss, duration of bleeding, number of sanitary towels used, uterine weight and endometrial surface area. Br J Obstet Gynaecol 1980; 87: 603–609

15. Hallberg L, Nilsson L. Determination of menstrual blood loss. Scand J Clin Lab Invest 1964; 16: 244–248

16. O'Brien P M S. Expert perspectives in menorrhagia. Worthing, W. Sussex: Cambridge Medical 1992: 5

17. Higham J M, O'Brien P M S, Shaw R W. Assessment of menstrual blood loss using a pictorial chart. Br J Obstet Gynaecol 1990; 97: 734–739

18. Rankin G L S, Veall N, Huntsman R G, Lidell J. Measurement with Cr of red cell loss in menorrhagia. Lancet 1962; 1: 567–569

19. Gannon M J, Day P, Hammadieh N, Johnson N. A new method for measuring menstrual blood loss and its use in screening women before endometrial ablation. Br J Obstet Gynaecol 1996; 103(10): 1029–1033

20. Sheth S S. Vaginal dimple: a sign to diagnose endometriosis. J Obstet Gynecol 1991; 2: 292

21. Brosens J J, de Souza N M, Barker F G et al. Endovaginal ultrasonography in the diagnosis of adenomyosis uteri: identifying the predictive characteristics. Br J Obstet Gynaecol 1995; 102(6): 471–474

22. Mencaglia L. Hysteroscopy and adenocarcinoma. Obstet Gynecol Clin North Am 1995; 22(3): 573–579

23. Fraser I. Menorrhagia — a prognostic approach to the understanding of causes and the need for investigations. Br J Obstet Gynaecol 1994; 101: 3–7

24. Scott J C, Mussey E. Menstrual patterns of myxedema. Am J Obstet Gynecol 1981; 139: 277–280

25. Towbin N A, Gviazda I M, March C M. Office hysteroscopy versus transvaginal ultrasonography in the evaluation of patients with excessive uterine bleeding. Am J Obstet Gynecol 1996; 174(6): 1678–1682

26. Goldstein S R, Nachtigall M, Synder J R, Nachtigall L. Endometrial assessment by vaginal ultrasonography before endometrial sampling in patients with postmenopausal bleeding. Am J Obstet Gynecol 1990: 163: 119–123

27. Jain K A, Friedman D L, Jeffrey R B Jr, Sommer F G. Sonography of the pelvis. Radiology 1993; 186: 697–704

28. Bourne T. Transvaginal colour Doppler in gynaecology. In: Desai S K, Allahbadia G N (eds) Progress in infertility and transvaginal sonography. New Delhi: CBS, 1996: 100–114

29. Hota K. New pelvic sonography for detection of endometrial carcinoma. Gynecol Oncol 1992; 95: 179–184

30. Allahbadia G N. Doppler in reproductive medicine. In: Desai S K, Allahbadia G N (eds) Progress in infertility and transvaginal sonography. New Delhi: CBS 1996; 92–99

31. Baruah S. Transvaginal sonography in the diagnosis of pelvic inflammatory disease. In: Desai S K, Allahbadia G N (eds) Progress in infertility and transvaginal sonography. New Delhi: CBS, 1996; 83–86

32. Baltarowich O H, Kurtz A B, Pennell R G et al. Pitfalls in the sonographic diagnosis of uterine fibroids. J Radiol 1988; 151: 725–728

33. Hricak H, Tscholakoff D, Heinrichs L et al. Uterine leiomyomas: correlation of MR, histopathologic findings, and symptoms. Radiology 1986; 158: 385–391

34. Sumpaico W W. Ultrasound in gynaecologic oncology. In: Teodora L R (ed) Obstetric and Gynecologic Ultrasound. Makati City, Philippines: CRS Publishers, 1996; 203–210

35. Togashi K, Nishimura K, Itoh K et al. Adenomyosis: diagnosis with MR imaging: Radiology 1988; 166: 111

36. Mark A S, Hricak H, Heinrichs L W et al. Adenomyosis and leiomyoma — differential diagnosis with MR imaging. Radiology 1987; 163: 527

37. Togashi K, Ozasa H, Konishi I et al. Enlarged uterus: differentiation between adenomyosis and leiomyomas with MR imaging. Radiology 1989; 171: 531

38. Moss A A, Gamsu G et al. Abdomen and pelvis. In: Scoutt L M et al. (eds) Computed tomography of the body with magnetic resonance imaging, 2nd edn. 1992: 1181–1265

39. Togashi K, Nishimura K, Itoh K et al. Adenomyosis — diagnosis with MR imaging. Radiology 1988; 166: 111

40. Dooms G C, Hricak H, Tscholakoff D et al. Adnexal structures — MR imaging. Radiology 1986: 158: 839

41. Scoutt L M, McCarthy S M, Flynn S D et al. Evaluation of ovarian masses on MRI with ultrasound correlation. Radiology: in press

42. Mitchell D G, Mintz M C, Spritzer C E et al. Adnexal masses: MR imaging observations at 1.5T with US and CT correlation. Radiology 1987; 162: 319

43. Goldhirsch A, Triller J K, Graner R et al. Computed tomography prior to second-look operation in advanced ovarian cancer. Obstet Gynecol 1983; 62: 630–633

44. Zawin M, McCarthy S. High-field MRI and US evaluation of the pelvis in women with leiomyomas. Magn Reson Imaging 1990; 8: 371

45. Weinreb J C, Barkoff N D, Megibow A, Demopoulos R. The value of MR imaging in distinguishing leiomyomas from other solid pelvic masses when sonography is indeterminate. AJR 1990; 154: 295

46. Kawagoe H, Kataoka A, Sugiyama T et al. Leiomyosarcoma of the small intestine presenting as a pelvic mass. Eur J Obstet Gynecol Reprod Biol 1996 66(2): 187–191

47. Weigel M, Friese K, Strittmatter H J, Melchert F. Measuring the thickness — is that all we have to do for sonographic assessment of endometrium in postmenopausal women? J Ultrasound Obstet Gynecol 1995; 6: 97–102

48. Dalal A, Allahbadia G, Desai S. Hydrohysterosonography. In: Desai S, Allahbadia G (eds) Infertility and transvaginal sonography: current concepts. Delhi: Jaypee Brothers, 1995: 219–221

49. Fried A. Transvaginal sonography of the uterus. In: Desai S, Allahbadia G (eds) Infertility and transvaginal sonography: current concepts, New Delhi: Jaypee Brothers, 1995: 208–211

50. Syrop C H, Shakia V. Transvaginal sonographic detection of endometrial polyps with fluid contrast augmentation. Obstet Gynecol 1992; 79: 1041–1043

51. Taylor P T Jr, Andersen W A, Barber S R et al. The screening Papanicolaou smear contribution at the endocervical brush. Obstet Gynecol 1987; 70: 734–738

52. Stovall T G, Photopulos G J, Poston W M et al. Pipelle endometrial sampling. Obstet Gynecol 1988; 71: 54–57

53. Kaunitz A M, Masciello A, Ostrowksi. Endometrial sampling. J Reprod Med 1988; 38(5): 954–956

54. Smith S K. Physiological and pharmacological aspects of prostaglandins in the female reproductive tract. MD thesis; University of London; 1982: 59

55. Goldhaber M K, Armstrong M A, Golditch I M et al. Role of endometrial histopathology in menorrhagia of unknown origin. Am J Epidemiol 1993; 138: 508–521

56. Grimes D A. Diagnostic dilation and curettage — a reappraisal. Am J Obstet Gynecol 1982; 142: 1–6

57. Vercellini P, Trespidi L, Panazza S et al. Laparoscopic uterine biopsy for diagnosing diffuse adenomyosis. J Reprod Med 1996; 41: 220–224

58. Wood C. Direct transabdominal needle biopsy under USG guidance. Med J Aust 1996; 158: 458–461

59. Sheth S S, Shinde L. Vaginal hysterectomy for myomatous polyp. Obstet Gynecol Surv 1993; 9: 101–103

60. The incidence of genital cancers in India: an epidemiological study, 1972–1978. Indian Cancer Soc Bull 1979; 33 (No.12) Bombay, India: ICS

61. Claessens E A, Cowell C A. Acute adolescent menorrhagias. Am J Obstet Gynecol 1981; 39: 277–280

CHAPTER 4

Role of hysteroscopy in the evaluation of menorrhagia

R. F. Valle and J. J. Sciarra

Introduction

Menorrhagia is defined as excessive or prolonged uterine bleeding that exceeds 80 ml of blood loss per menstruation that occurs in the presence of a normal secretory endometrium after normal ovulation. This type of abnormal uterine bleeding occurs in about 15% of adult premenopausal women and is a frequent reason for gynaecological consultation. There are at least four known causes of menorrhagia: these are (1) organic, such as polyps and leiomyomas, (2) foreign bodies, such as intra-uterine devices (IUDs), (3) bleeding disorders, particularly from defects in the coagulation cascade, and (4) systemic disorders such as hypothyroidism.[1] Menorrhagia is termed 'essential' when its aetiology is unexplained. Haemostasis in the menstrual endometrium may be partially inhibited by changes in clotting factors, fibrinolysis and prostaglandin interaction.

Although the definition of menorrhagia is based on objective measurements of blood loss that usually results in anaemia, in clinical practice the actual perception of heavy uterine bleeding by the patient usually warrants an evaluation. There are different forms of abnormal uterine bleeding: many adolescents have dysfunctional bleeding due to the immaturity of the hypothalamic–pituitary–ovarian axis; in adult women, when the heavy bleeding is cyclic or accompanied by dysmenorrhoea, an organic aetiology is often suspected; in the perimenopausal woman, hormonal dysfunction, due to ovarian waning, mimics that of the adolescent. In this latter group a thorough evaluation of the uterine cavity is mandatory as this symptomatology may imply a malignant or premalignant endometrial lesion.[2]

Uterine evaluation

In the past, the uterine cavity has been evaluated by indirect methods to sample the endometrium. Curettage, either mechanically with metallic curettes or by suction aspiration devices, is useful in obtaining tissue samples for histological evaluation. The blind inherent approach of these methods has proved to be inadequate for accurate evaluation of intra-uterine pathology, especially malignancy. This is particularly true when the uterine cavity is evaluated in the presence of other conditions that may cause abnormal uterine bleeding. Pathology such as myomas, endometrial polyps and focal endometrial lesions located in the cornual regions or even in the lower uterine segment, may not be sampled adequately by blind techniques. For these reasons, hysteroscopy is a welcome addition to the evaluation of the uterus, both for visualization and for targeted biopsies.[3–5] Additionally, the introduction of sonography — particularly vaginal sonography — has added a new dimension in evaluating the uterine cavity. Sonography not only displays a topographic view but also allows for the evaluation of the intramural component of a myoma or other uterine lesions and the surrounding adnexal areas.[6,7]

A common method of evaluating the uterine cavity is hysterosalpingography. This determines the symmetry and contours of the uterine cavity, giving additional information about the fallopian tubes, such as symmetry, regularity of the ampullary folds and tubal patency. However, the sensitivity and specificity of this method are markedly reduced by transient uterine cavity distortion. This distortion may be caused by blood clots, mucus, debris and air bubbles, which sometimes cause difficulty in interpretation. However, when the hysterosalpingogram indicates a normal uterine cavity, usually an endoscopic evaluation will not discover a structural abnormality.[8–11]

It should be stressed that the endometrium cannot be properly evaluated unless sampled. The mechanical curette, although helpful in denuding the endometrium, can miss large portions of the lining, leaving it unsampled (Table 4.1). However, modified suction devices increase the yield of endometrial tissue and provide an adequacy of 95–99%, as reviewed by Grimes.[12] It is, none the less, well known that focal lesions can be missed when using modified suction devices, as demonstrated by Bibbo et al.[13–18] (Table 4.2). Endometrial biopsy is paramount in the evaluation of abnormal uterine bleeding. This is particularly true in adult, perimenopausal and postmenopausal women. Therefore, the physician may consider utilizing suction devices that yield more adequate tissue than mechanical curettes. However, to avoid missing focal lesions and other structural abnormalities, additional visual evaluation is necessary. Structural abnormalities, such as myomas and polyps, need to be ruled out or, when present, treated. Although sonography may outline these lesions, particularly if enhanced by intra-uterine injection of fluid, the direct view provided by hysteroscopy refines the diagnosis and conclusively diagnoses a polyp or a myoma. Additionally, hysteroscopy provides a direct method of treatment.[19]

Hysteroscopy as a method to evaluate the uterine cavity

Modern technology has provided the opportunity to use slender hysteroscopes with excellent resolution. These smaller hysteroscopes can be used in an office setting in

Table 4.1 Adequacy of dilatation and curettage (D&C)

Ref. no.	Procedure	No. of patients	Adequate curettage	Incomplete curettage
13	D&C/hysteroscopy	124	44 (35%)	80 (65%)
14	D&C/hysteroscopy	58	9 (15.5%)	49 (84.6%)
15	D&C/hysterectomy	50	<1/2 of cavity in 30 (60%)	2/3 of cavity in 42 (84%)
16	D&C/hysterectomy	512	10% of lesions missed by curettage	

Table 4.2 Adequacy of dilatation and curettage (D&C) (polyps)

Ref. no.	Procedure	No. of patients	Percentage diagnosed	Percentage missed
17	Vakutage/D&C or hysterectomy	840	83	17
18	D&C/hysterectomy	1298 specimens (121 [9.3%] had polyps)	53	47
12	Vabra: review	111	80–83	17–20
3	Hysteroscopy/D&C	553 (179 [32.4%] had polyps)	100/10	0/90

a simple and expeditious manner. Cervical dilatation is not required and the undisturbed uterine cervical canal and uterine cavity can be observed utilizing CO_2 gas as a distending medium with endoscopes of outer diameter (OD) 3–4 mm. Alternatively, low-viscosity fluids can be utilized with endoscopes of 5.5–6 mm OD with continuous-flow systems. New microhysteroscopes (2–5.5 mm OD) permit the use of both methods of uterine distention — CO_2 gas and low-viscosity fluid. Additionally, some microhysteroscopes have a collapsible plastic outer sheath that permits instrumentation with 7 Fr instruments for biopsies or minor surgical procedures.

Patients affected with coagulopathies may suggest that the abnormal uterine bleeding is due to their condition. Such patients may include those with idiopathic thrombocytopenic purpura, patients on continuous anticoagulant treatment due to thrombophlebitis, heart prosthesis patients, those patients with blood neoplasias or leukaemias, and those afflicted with von Willebrand's disease. However, even patients with such conditions should be screened for an organic aetiology of the menorrhagia.

Ultrasound provides a good delineation of the uterus, uterine walls and uterine cavity. Ultrasonic evaluation of the endometrial lining is best indicated for postmenopausal women. This method allows the thickness of the endometrial lining to be measured. If the sonographic thickness is no greater than 4 mm, and the patient experiences only sporadic bleeding, a biopsy may be necessary as the likelihood of a uterine malignancy is extremely small. However, patients with thin endometrial linings that continue to bleed abnormally should have hysteroscopy and an endometrial biopsy performed. The specificity of ultrasound in premenopausal patients is low and is best used to evaluate the uterine walls for thickness and myomas. Despite the difficulty in assessing the uterine wall penetration of submucous myomas, owing to the isoechogenicity of myometrial and myoma tissue that may interfere with their delineation, ultrasound is the best non-invasive diagnostic tool for their evaluation. When sonography demonstrates abnormal intra-uterine lesions, hysteroscopy can confirm the diagnosis, permitting also biopsy and treatment of the lesions. The adnexa can also be evaluated with ultrasound, adding more detail and precision to the bimanual pelvic examination of these areas. Sonohysterography, or fluid-enhanced sonography, is best used to delineate intra-uterine lesions and to determine their penetration of the uterine wall. This is particularly true in the case of uterine submucous myomas, in order to determine their feasibility for hysteroscopic removal. Hysteroscopy is especially useful in evaluating those patients with uterine polyps or on tamoxifen therapy and that have abnormal ultrasounds.

Because hysteroscopy can be performed safely and expeditiously in the office setting, it can be used routinely as an ambulatory procedure to evaluate the uterine cavity (Figs. 4.1–4.7).

Technique of office hysteroscopy

Hysteroscopy has been simplified with the use of small-calibre endoscopes that do not require cervical dilatation. Office hysteroscopy should be performed following menstruation in those patients who are menstruating; this is to avoid mucus, debris and bleeding in the uterine cavity that may impair visualization. A hysteroscope of less than 4 mm OD using CO_2 gas specifically delivered from an insufflator should be utilized. The CO_2 should be calibrated at a flow of 30–60 ml/min and the pressure should be maintained at less than 100 mmHg. The patient is placed on the examining table and a pelvic examination is performed to outline the uterine size and position. A vaginal speculum is introduced and the cervix is cleansed with an antiseptic solution. A paracervical block may be administered, utilizing an ester type of local anaesthetic such as chloroprocaine hydrochloride (Nesacaine 1%): 3–4 ml of the solution should be superficially injected just below the mucosa at the base of each uterosacral ligament. If a tenaculum is utilized, a small amount of anaesthetic (0.5 ml) is also injected in the anterior cervical lip. The hysteroscope is attached to a light source, distending medium and microcamera. The microcamera should be focused and the colours adjusted on a white surface. The CO_2 gas is then insufflated and the examination begins under video monitoring. The endoscope is introduced at the external cervical os. The gas slowly and gently distends the endocervical canal to create a microcavity. The endoscope is advanced gently and the endocervical canal systematically evaluated. Once the internal os is reached, a panoramic view of the uterine cavity is obtained and the uterine cavity can be explored systematically. The fore–oblique view of the endoscope is used to observe the uterotubal cones and tubal openings. Once the examination is complete, the endoscope is withdrawn under direct vision. This allows a second evaluation to be performed while the endoscope is removed. Should a non-targeted biopsy be required, a 4 mm plastic cannula is inserted and a suction endometrial aspiration performed. When targeted biopsies are required, a larger endoscope (5–6 mm OD) is needed to permit introduction of the biopsy forceps; however, with the use of new microhysteroscopes, such as the MicroSpan, this additional exchange of hysteroscopes is not required. Owing to its 3.2 mm OD, the MicroSpan permits introduction without cervical dilatation; also, owing to its special configuration, low-viscosity fluids with continuous flow can be used should distention with gas not be adequate. Additionally, because of its outer plastic sheath that is collapsed during introduction into the uterine cavity, 7 Fr instruments can be introduced to perform adequate targeted endometrial biopsies or minor surgical procedures. The versatility of these instruments adds to their use in an office setting (Fig. 4.8).

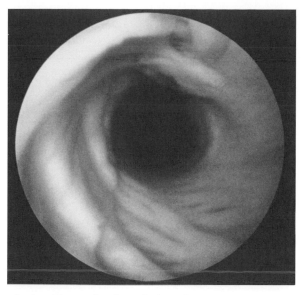

Figure 4.1 A hysteroscopic view of normal endocervical canal.

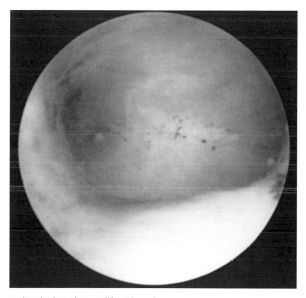

Figure 4.2 The uterine cavity during the proliferative phase.

Discussion

Menorrhagia is a frequent problem that afflicts women from menarche to menopause, as well as in the postmenopausal period. Whereas the workup of an adolescent patient is mainly hormonal following a detailed medical history, in the adult premenopausal woman — and especially those in the perimenopause — meticulous evaluation of the uterus and uterine cavity is required. In a post-menopausal woman with abnormal uterine bleeding, histological endometrial evaluation is paramount in arriving at the final diagnosis. Although endometrial suction aspiration biopsies provide evaluation of the endometrium in the majority of patients, the addition of a visual evaluation of the uterine cavity will not only facilitate the detection of structural abnormalities (such as endometrial polyps and submucous myomas) that often are the reason for the abnormal bleeding but also will offer an excellent method of evaluating the entire endometrial lining,

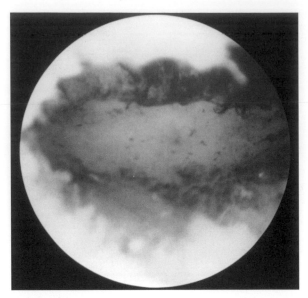

Figure 4.3 The uterine cavity in the secretory phase.

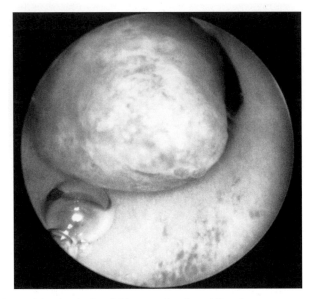

Figure 4.4 An endometrial polyp in the right cornual region of the uterus.

including the uterotubal cornual regions. Targeted biopsies of suspicious areas can be performed under direct visual guidance.

The addition of ultrasonography, particularly vaginal sonography, adds to the overall evaluation of the uterus. Ultrasound will determine the muscular thickness of the uterus and the presence of intramural or subserous leiomyomas, and will allow for evaluation of the adnexa. Additionally, when fluid is injected into the uterine cavity, submucous leiomyomas may be outlined to determine the intramural component of the myoma. In selected situations, magnetic resonance imaging (MRI) will add to the evaluation by determining the presence of adenomyosis, uterine anomalies or other uterine and adnexal lesions. MRI evaluation is particularly useful in obese patients or in those in whom sonography may not provide adequate and complete evaluation. The rational integration of these various methods of evaluation (endoscopy, ultrasound and MRI), coupled with

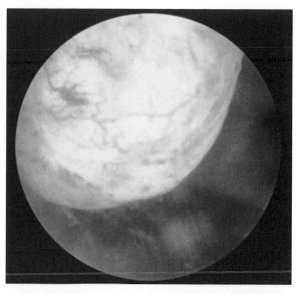

Figure 4.5 A submucous leiomyoma (note the typical peripheral vascularization).

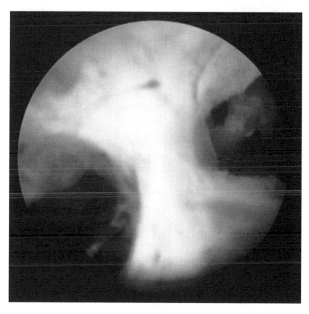

Figure 4.6 An intra-uterine adhesion connecting the uterine walls.

appropriate endometrial biopsies for histological evaluation, will provide the best uterine evaluation in order to determine the specific aetiology of abnormal uterine bleeding.

An endometrial biopsy is not routinely required in young adolescent females complaining of abnormal uterine bleeding, particularly those who respond to hormonal therapy. However, in the adult woman, especially those aged 35 years or older, endometrial sampling must be performed routinely before any hormonal treatment is undertaken. This is especially necessary as the patient approaches menopause. However, even in the younger patient who does not respond to appropriate hormonal therapy, particularly those with prolonged periods of amenorrhoea who bleed excessively, endometrial sampling should be performed to rule out any form of endometrial hyperplasia.

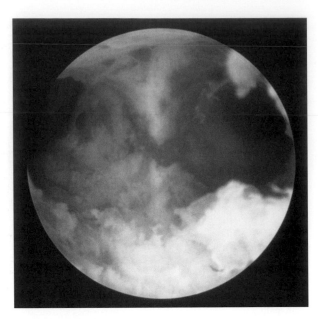

Figure 4.7 The uterine cavity divided by a wide septum.

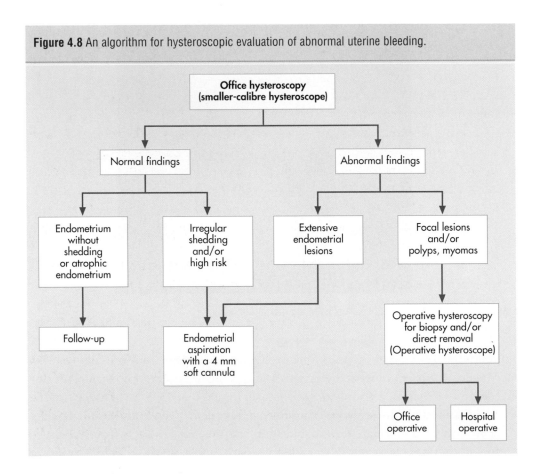

Figure 4.8 An algorithm for hysteroscopic evaluation of abnormal uterine bleeding.

Summary and conclusions

Hysteroscopy has earned a rightful place in the evaluation of abnormal uterine bleeding. Dysfunctional uterine bleeding is a diagnosis of exclusion. It is, therefore, of the utmost importance to use the most precise and accurate methods to evaluate the uterine cavity to rule out organic conditions that may cause abnormal uterine bleeding. The history and symptomatology of the patient will determine the extent and type of evaluation required. However, biopsies and evaluation of the uterine cavity should be included in practically all patients, especially adult premenopausal, perimenopausal and postmenopausal patients with persistent abnormal uterine bleeding. In selected young and adolescent women who continue to bleed despite appropriate hormonal treatment, hysteroscopic evaluation should also be considered. Ultrasound, if available, may also be helpful to outline pathology in the uterine walls and adnexa. Ultrasound, used in conjunction with hysteroscopy, provides meaningful help to the patient suffering from abnormal uterine bleeding. An MRI study may be useful if adenomyosis or a uterine anomaly is suspected.

Early definition of the problem will help outline and plan adequate treatment for these patients without unnecessary or inappropriate procedures. Furthermore, early intervention puts the patient at ease by defining the problem and indicating how it can be treated. Endoscopic follow-up is also important when endometrial lesions have been treated and symptomatology recurs.

References

1. Van Eijkeren M A, Christiaens G C M, Sixma J J, Hospels A A. Menorrhagia: a review. Obstet Gynecol Surv 1989; 44: 421–429

2. Bayer S R, DeCherney A H. Clinical manifestations and treatment of dysfunctional uterine bleeding. JAMA 1993; 269: 1823–1828

3. Valle R F. Hysteroscopic evaluation of patients with abnormal uterine bleeding. Surg Gynecol Obstet 1981; 153: 521–526

4. Gimpelson R J, Rappold H O. A comparative study between panoramic hysteroscopy with directed biopsies and dilatation and curettage. Am J Obstet Gynecol 1988; 158: 489–492

5. Loffer F D. Hysteroscopy with selected endometrial sampling compared with D&C for abnormal uterine bleeding: the value of a negative hysteroscopic view. Obstet Gynecol 1989; 73: 383–384

6. Karlsson B, Gronberg S, Wikland M et al. Transvaginal ultrasonography of the endometrium in women with postmenopausal bleeding: a Nordic multicenter study. Am J Obstet Gynecol 1995; 172: 1488–1494

7. Lerner J P, Timor-Tritsch I E, Monteagudo A. Use of transvaginal sonography in the evaluation of endometrial hyperplasia and carcinoma. Obstet Gynecol Surv 1996; 51: 718–725

8. Siegler A M. Hysterosalpingography. Fertil Steril 1983; 40: 139–158

9. Valle R F. Hysteroscopy in the evaluation of female infertility. Am J Obstet Gynecol 1980; 137: 425–431

10. Valle R F, Sciarra J J. Current status of hysteroscopy in gynecologic practice. Fertil Steril 1979; 32: 619–632

11. Fayez J A, Mutie G, Schneider P J. The diagnostic value of hysterosalpingography and hysteroscopy in infertility investigation. Am J Obstet Gynecol 1987; 156: 558–560

12. Grimes D A. Diagnostic dilatation and curettage: a reappraisal. Am J Obstet Gynecol 1982; 142: 1–6

13. Englund S E, Ingelman-Sundberg A, Westin B. Hysteroscopy in diagnosis and treatment of uterine bleeding. Gynaecologia 1957; 143: 217–222

14. Gribb J J. Hysteroscopy. An aid in gynecologic diagnosis. Obstet Gynecol 1960; 15: 593–601

15. Stock R J, Kanbour A. Prehysterectomy curettage. Obstet Gynecol 1975; 45: 537–541

16. Word B, Gravlee L C, Wideman G L. The fallacy of simple uterine curettage. Obstet Gynecol 1958; 12: 642–648

17. Bibbo M, Kluskens L, Azizi F et al. Accuracy of three sampling techniques for the diagnosis of endometrial cancer and hyperplasias. J Reprod Med 1982; 27: 622–626

18. Burnett J E. Hysteroscopy-controlled curettage for endometrial polyps. Obstet Gynecol 1964; 24: 621–625

19. Towbin N A, Gviezda I M, March C M. Office hysteroscopy versus transvaginal ultrasonography in the evaluation of patients with excessive uterine bleeding. Am J Obstet Gynecol 1996; 174: 1678–1682

CHAPTER 5

Role of imaging techniques in the diagnosis of menorrhagia

W. J. Walker

Imaging modalities

Ultrasound

Although ultrasound was initially developed at the end of the Second World War from radar, for decades images remained of poor quality and, until the mid to late 1970s, static scanners only were available. These suffered from relatively poor resolution and excessive interference due to the presence of bowel gas, etc. The development and dissemination of real-time scanning in the late 1970s and early 1980s brought about an improvement in accuracy but gynaecological scanning was still restricted to transvesical imaging. Because of the depth of penetration required, lower-frequency waves only could be used, with a consequent reduction in image resolution. In the mid 1980s and 1990s, the development of high-frequency transvaginal scanners markedly improved the accuracy of gynaecological ultrasound. Fine detail of the uterus, endometrium, adnexae, and adnexal and uterine vasculature transformed ultrasound into a highly accurate diagnostic tool in the hands of the trained and experienced.

Resolution is the critical factor in gynaecological scanning. Axial resolution, which relates to the accuracy of imaging points in the longitudinal direction of the sound beam, improves with increasing frequency, although, of course, at the expense of reduced penetration. Lateral resolution, however, is related to the diameter of the sound beam: the smaller the beam, the better the lateral resolution. Lateral resolution is mainly dependent on focusing ability. Because transvaginal scanning places the target closer to the transducer, higher frequencies can be used and, in modern scanners, frequencies of 7–10 MHz are now the norm.

Technique of transvaginal scanning

The first prerequisite is an empty bladder: even small amounts of urine in the bladder will tend to displace target organs away from the probe and beyond the penetration of the sound beam. The patient should be placed in the lithotomy position with a slight Trendelenburg tilt to displace the pelvic organs inferiorly and also to cause any fluid within the pelvis to gravitate inferiorly, improving visualization. In the author's opinion, it is better to place the legs abducted on two stools, rather than utilize stirrups which can be uncomfortable for the patient. The patient's legs and pelvic area should be covered by a blanket. The operator's free hand can be used to compress the pelvic organs while scanning and bring them more into the field of view; the diagnosis of pelvic adhesions can be aided by pushing and pulling the transducer and thereby examining the ability of the pelvic organs to slide in relation to each other. However, it should be noted that because the penetrating capacity of transvaginal scanners is reduced owing to the high frequencies employed, large masses situated just beyond the resolving capability of the sound beam may be missed and therefore a transabdominal scan may be needed in some cases. This does not mean that a full bladder has to be obtained and, if the operator is skilled in general ultrasound techniques, even without a full bladder, a mass can be differentiated from bowel. Many sonographers and gynaecologists prefer to display the ultrasound image with the apex at the top of the screen; however, radiologists tend to prefer the apex at the bottom of the screen, with the patient's right to the radiologist's left, as this perspective is the normal way in which radiologists view cross-sectional images.

Colour duplex scanning

Doppler ultrasound relies on the fact that, if an ultrasound beam is passed into a moving target such as red blood cells, reflection of the sound waves causes a frequency shift that is proportional to the velocity of the blood. In colour duplex imaging, Doppler information is provided at the same time as real-time imaging. In colour Doppler systems, the shifted Doppler frequency can be encoded in colour and incorporated into the real-time image. A colour may be assigned to a particular direction, e.g. blue for frequency shifts away from the ultrasound beam and red for shifts towards the beam. The Doppler signal can be gated to sample a specific volume of blood. Changes in colour intensity usually relate to the velocity of the blood flow.

The shift in Doppler frequency is dependent not only on the flow velocity but also on the angle of insonation. This makes direct assessment of flow velocity difficult in the case of the tortuous vessels found in the pelvis, where it is very difficult to measure a Doppler angle accurately. However, if, instead, a ratio is used, such as the resistance index, then this is independent of angle.[1] The resistance index (or resistivity index) is defined as $RI = (S - D)/S$, where S is the peak systolic and D the end diastolic frequency. A number of other ratios are available, including the pulsatility index. Vessels within the uterine myometrium and within the ovary tend to have low pulsatility and resistivity indices. The uterine arteries, however, are easy to identify using colour Doppler as they are high-resistance vessels with an early dichrotic notch.

CT scanning

Although computed tomography (CT) scanning initially held promise as an effective imaging modality in the pelvis, it has, in fact, been shown to have a limited application in the diagnosis of uterine and adnexal disorders, suffering, in particular, from a lack of specificity.[2]

Hysterosalpingography

Hysterosalpingography, although useful for the assessment of tubal status, again suffers from a lack of specificity with regard to the assessment of the uterine cavity and a susceptibility to artefacts.[3]

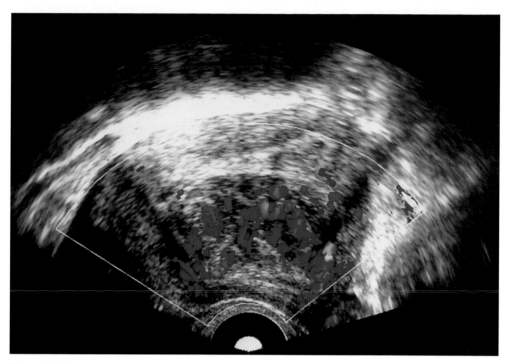

Figure 5.1 A colour Doppler ultrasonic scan of a hypervascular submucous fibroid distorting the endometrium.

Magnetic resonance imaging

Magnetic resonance imaging (MRI), developed over the last two decades and greatly improved in the 1990s, has been shown to be a very powerful diagnostic tool in the detection of gynaecological lesions. The technique utilizes the effect of powerful magnetic forces on a spinning hydrogen proton which, when knocked off its axis by pulse audio waves, produces images mainly based on chemical composition (i.e. the amount and distribution of hydrogen protons). This is unlike CT, which is reliant on density variation, or ultrasound, which is based on tissue interface reflection. Thus, MRI provides a significant improvement in tissue characterization. Scans can be performed in practically any plane and different sequences obtained — for example, fat suppression (short tau inversion recovery [STIR]) sequences — to select for different types of tissue. Although expensive, it is the single most accurate technique for gynaecological imaging; it is particularly useful for the visualization and mapping of fibroids and differentiation of fibroids from adenomyosis and adenomyomas, and for the assessment of endometrial invasion, the diagnosis of endometriomas and the characterization of ovarian lesions (particularly dermoids).

Summary

In the past, a lack of accuracy in radiological imaging techniques, together with a high operator dependency, impeded adequate confidence in diagnosis on the part of the gynaecologist and resulted in little reduction in the high level of invasive diagnostic procedures such as laparotomy and laparoscopy. The recent exponential improvement in radiological imaging techniques should make a huge impact in this area, markedly refine the pretreatment diagnosis of menorrhagia and other gynaecological conditions, and significantly reduce the necessity for surgical diagnostic procedures.

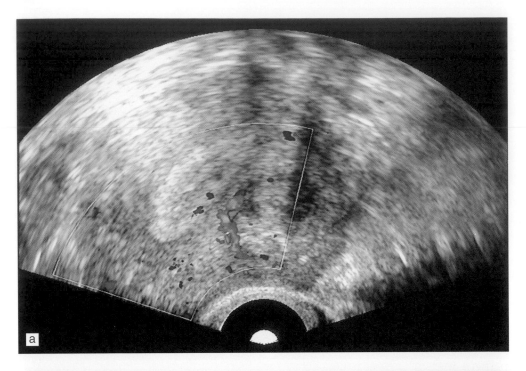

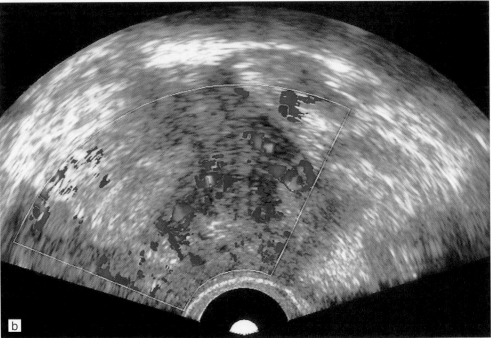

Figure 5.2 An interstitial fibroid with hypervascular pseudocapsule and extending to the endometrial border but not distorting the endometrium: (a) transvaginal scan showing anterior submucous–interstitial fibroid; (b) colour flow image demonstrating hypervascular pseudocapsule extending to the endometrial border.

Fibroids

Fibroids are conventionally described as submucous, interstitial, subserous or pedunculated. They invariably possess a peripheral pseudocapsule of hypervascularity. Internally, their vascularity is very variable but often reduced. Occasionally they may be diffusely hypervascular, arousing suspicion of sarcoma. In the case of menorrhagia, submucous myomas or interstitial myomas extending to, or affecting, the endometrium, appear to be the most important fibroids to diagnose as these can cause menorrhagia. A small submucous fibroid, with its circumferential hypervascular leash of peripheral vessels, may be associated with severe menorrhagia (Fig. 5.1), whereas a large, totally interstitial or mainly subserous fibroid may produce no alteration in the severity of menstruation.

The description of fibroids as either submucous or interstitial is rather glib. Strictly speaking, a submucous fibroid should be diagnosed only if the subendometrial layer is the fibroid itself. In reality, large fibroids arising in the interstitium and distorting the mucosa would theoretically be buffered by a normal layer of myometrium. However, fibroids are surrounded by a pseudocapsule consisting of a hypervascular ring and frequently this extends to the endometrium (Fig. 5.2). The incidence of submucous myomas is difficult to ascertain but, in a series of 1202 hysteroscopies for menorrhagia, a prevalence of 14.7% was found for submucous myoma.[4]

The cause of menorrhagia in patients with fibroids is uncertain. Pressure on the endometrium, peripheral hypervascularity affecting the endometrium, and increased endometrial surface area have all been postulated. However, most patients with peripheral hypervascularity extending to the endometrium are likely to be menorrhagic.

Ultrasound diagnosis of fibroids

Ultrasound is the most frequently used modality for demonstrating fibroids. Scans may be performed transabdominally through a full bladder or transvaginally with the bladder empty. Transabdominally performed scans are less accurate,[5] owing to the resolution factors previously described; however, Goldstein[6] has cautioned against over-reaction to normal physiological conditions that escaped detection in the past because they were not previously imaged.

In order to plan modern treatment, the gynaecologist requires from the radiologist an accurate description of uterine fibroids. A report simply stating 'fibroids are present' or 'fibroid change' is inadequate by today's standards. Radiologists should state the overall uterine dimensions and volume, the number of ultrasonically detectable fibroids, their position within the uterus (subserous, interstitial or submucous), the length of the endometrial cavity and any distortion of that cavity. A diagram drawn by the radiologist is particularly useful. It is very important that the site and prevalence of any submucous fibroids should be accurately described for the above reasons. Three-dimensional scanning (still in its infancy) holds promise for the precise mapping of fibroids so that appropriate therapy can be instituted.

The ovaries should be scanned for adnexal pathology and evidence of pressure on surrounding structures — bladder, rectum or ureter — documented. Demonstration of fibroids can be aided by overall measurement of uterine dimensions. Measurement of the uterus is more difficult with transvaginal scanning: this is because, in transvaginal scanning, the presence of a full bladder straightens out the uterus and makes longitudinal measurement easier to obtain, whereas when the uterus assumes its normal position, i.e. anteflexed or retroflexed as in transvaginal scanning, the curvature has to be allowed for in the longitudinal measurement. Measurements should be taken from the external os to the uterine fundus longitudinally and in the same plane the anteroposterior (AP) diameter should also be obtained. In the axial plane, the transverse measurement should also be obtained. In the nulliparous postpubertal woman the size of the uterus is approximately 7 cm in longitudinal dimension, fundus to exocervix, and 3–4 cm in AP and transverse diameter. After pregnancy there is an increase of about 1 cm and it is not uncommon to find normal uteri with dimensions of $8 \times 5 \times 5$ cm. Uteri over this size are usually pathologically enlarged.

The endometrium is an echogenic layer that varies in width with the cycle. The myometrium is more sonolucent, but three zones can be detected: these are the innermost layer, which is the most hypoechoic and probably the more vascular area; the middle layer, which is more echogenic; and the outer layer, which is characterized by the presence of blood vessels. Myometrial contractions may be observed.[7]

Uterine volume can be calculated on the basis of the formula for a prolate ellipse, $0.5 \times D1 \times D2 \times D3$, where D1, D2 and D3 represent the maximum length, AP diameter and width, respectively. However, although this formula is accurate for normal uteri, it becomes inaccurate for uterine volume where multiple fibroids cause a complex structure.

The ultrasonic appearance of fibroids is variable. Most have a rather heterogeneous echotexture with a tendency to be hyperechoic. They are also characterized by oval areas of acoustic shadowing. Once the position of fibroids has been documented, the adnexae should be scanned for any ovarian pathology and the kidneys to exclude hydronephrosis.

On occasion it may be difficult to differentiate between a pedunculated fibroid and a solid ovarian tumour. Colour Doppler may be useful in this regard (Fig. 5.3) but, if the stalk of the fibroid cannot be accurately visualized (which occurs in a small number of cases), differentiation may be extremely difficult. The best method of resolving this problem is to carry out a transvaginal ultrasound-guided biopsy of the lesion in question. In this procedure, under ultrasound guidance an 18 gauge Tru-cut needle is passed through the vaginal wall using a needle guide and fired through the lesion using a spring-loaded device. This procedure causes little pain and gives a rapid histological diagnosis. A similar technique can be used for the differentiation of intraligamentous fibroids from ovarian masses. Although the procedure is very effective it is much under-utilized.

Leiomyosarcoma

The true incidence of leiomyosarcoma is difficult to ascertain. In relation to asymptomatic myomas it is very small indeed. It can be difficult to diagnose with ultrasound and the appearance of a sarcoma may be identical to that of a leiomyoma, but the former tend to be more necrotic. If a fibroid grows quickly or has an unusual appearance, again, transvaginal-guided biopsies may be very useful in the differentiation between the two conditions. Parker et al.[8] reviewed 1302 women admitted between 1988 and 1992 for hysterectomy or myomectomy for uterine leiomyomas, and concluded that the incidence of sarcoma did not justify surgery where rapid growth had been observed. However, a simple procedure such as transvaginal biopsy may be justified in these circumstances, particularly where the patient is anxious about the possibility of cancer or when uterine artery embolization is being considered.

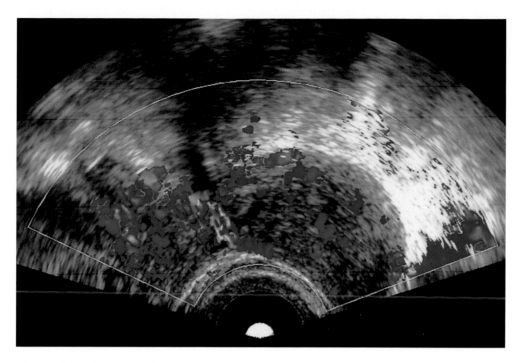

Figure 5.3 A pedunculated fibroid extending to the left. A typical hypervascular stalk indicates the nature of the lesion.

Colour duplex studies

Colour duplex studies are useful in the evaluation of leiomyomas, particularly in evaluating the relationship of the pseudocapsule to the endometrium, excluding arteriovenous malformation (AVM), and differentiating adnexal from uterine masses. Modern transvaginal scanners enable very accurate assessment of the vascularity of lesions and their blood flow characteristics. The resistivity index is particularly valuable, with pathological lesions tending to contain vessels of low resistance. With modern scanners a simultaneous real-time rendering of the target organ including the blood vessels and flow profile is possible. Unfortunately, in the author's experience, resistivity index and other parameters have been only marginally useful in the characterization of lesions because of a low specificity, particularly with regard to the differentiation of benign from malignant lesions; this has also been the experience of other authors, such as Tekay and Jouppila[9] and Carter et al.,[10] although some, such as Leeners et al.,[11] have found it useful.

Where the uterus is retroverted, transrectal scanning invariably gives better resolution than transvaginal scanning as the uterus is closer to the transducer and perpendicular along its axis to the sound beam, not axially orientated away from it. Sometimes fibroids, which are difficult to discern on a conventional scan because of a lack of echoic differentiation compared with normal uterine tissue, may be recognized by the typical peripheral hypervascularity shown when colour Doppler is utilized.

With regard to adnexal lesions, Doppler analysis may be helpful in the differentiation of, for example, intraligamentary fibroids from solid ovarian tumours.[12] Peripheral intramural spiral arteries have a very typical appearance, with high systolic velocity, a single prominent dichrotic notch and high resistance; the presence of such vessels adjacent to the extra-uterine wall is suggestive of a fibroid.

Exclusion of intracavity pathology

Unfortunately, dilatation and curettage has been shown to be unreliable in excluding intracavity pathology, particularly submucous myomas.[13–15] However, Fedele et al.[16] and Emanuel et al.[17] found transvaginal sonography to be accurate in the exclusion of intracavity pathology, and the accuracy is significantly increased when the examination is performed in the early proliferative phase. Hysterosonography, however, is probably the procedure of choice for the identification of endometrial polyps, submucous myomas and endometrial hyperplasia.

Technique of hysterosonography

For the delineation of these lesions the medium of choice is saline. Active inflammatory disease of the genital system is a contraindication to the procedure, which should only be carried out postmenstrually up to day 10 of the cycle. The cervix and vagina should be disinfected with iodine prior to introduction of a small balloon catheter into the cervical canal. Some investigators inflate the balloon within the cervical canal in the region of the internal os, whereas others (including the author) pass the catheter into the endometrial cavity, inflate the balloon and withdraw it to the internal os. A few millilitres of saline are used to inflate the balloon within the endometrial cavity, but in the cervical canal 1 ml usually suffices. Saline is then instilled into the endometrial cavity; the amount necessary is variable but generally should not exceed 20 ml. The cavity is then sufficiently distended to demonstrate the endometrial pathology. If the balloon has been inflated in the endometrial cavity it is then slowly withdrawn, reducing the amount of fluid within the balloon while saline is continuously infused to show the inferior cavity and supracervical area. It is in the latter position that these lesions are most likely to be missed. Submucous fibroids (Fig. 5.4) and polyps (Fig. 5.5) are readily shown, although occasionally it can be difficult to differentiate a pedunculated submucous fibroid from a polyp; usually, however, the texture of the fibroids is more heterogeneous than that of polyps. Hysterosonography not only facilitates the diagnosis of a polyp or a submucous myoma but also enables the depth of interstitial extension of the fibroid to be assessed (Fig. 5.4). This is useful in predicting the most appropriate surgical procedure, as hysteroscopy shows only the superficial element.

Cicincelli et al.,[18] in a series of 52 premenopausal women who underwent transabdominal sonohysterography, transvaginal sonography and hysteroscopy prior to hysterectomy, found that both *transabdominal* sonohysterography and hysteroscopy picked up *all* the submucous myomas, but that transabdominal sonohysterography included the added bonus of being better able to measure overall tumour size. Good results with transvaginal sonohysterography have also been obtained.[19,20]

Magnetic resonance imaging

As discussed above, MRI is based on the properties of the hydrogen proton. Tissues with low water content and/or low proton density, such as smooth muscle, fibrous or calcified tissue produce little MR signal. Thus, fibroids generally show as areas of low intensity on T2 sequences (Fig. 5.6) and are usually well circumscribed, with a well-demarcated pseudocapsule that appears as a rim of high signal in 36% of cases

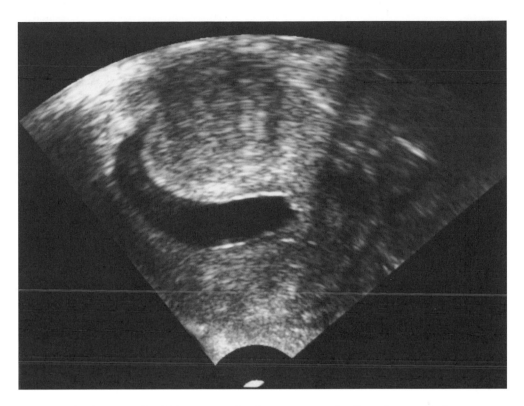

Figure 5.4 A submucous fibroid demonstrated on hysterosonography. Scan shows not only indentation of the cavity but also interstitial extent of the fibroid.

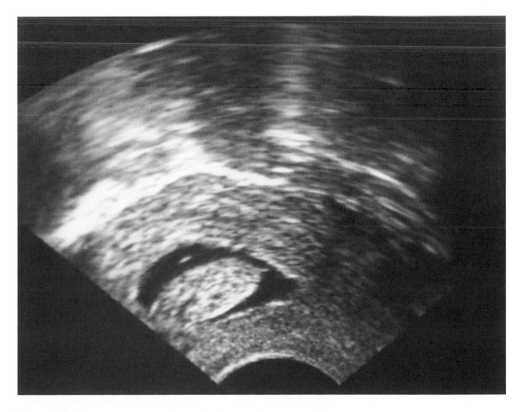

Figure 5.5 A hysterosonogram demonstrating a submucous polyp.

and is due to dilated lymphatics and veins adjacent to the tumour.[21] Degeneration within the fibroid is associated with an irregularly increased water content, producing a heterogeneous pattern of high and low signal on T2-weighted images (Fig. 5.7). Submucosal fibroids show particularly well when abutting or distorting the high-signal endometrium and interrupting the low-signal junctional zone (Fig. 5.8). Pedunculated fibroids and polyps also show well (Figs. 5.9, 5.10).

The other major advantage of MRI scanning is its ability to image the whole of the anterior and posterior pelvis and exclude concurrent ovarian pathology, lymphadenopathy and other pelvic lesions. The main criticism of MRI scanning is its expense and lack of availability. This is a peculiarly English criticism, illustrated by a quotation from a paper by Chapman and Chapman:[22] 'Magnetic resonance imaging is promising but it is an expensive method to employ to attempt to diagnose a non-malignant condition'. In reality, MRI scanning is widely available throughout most of the Western world and the improvement in the accuracy in pelvic imaging amply warrants its use in cases where transvaginal scanning does not clearly provide accurate or sufficient information.

A number of papers have indicated the superior accuracy of MRI compared with ultrasound in the diagnosis of uterine leiomyomas.[23,24] The problem is that these papers compare MRI with transabdominal scanning. In the author's opinion, the improved accuracy of transvaginal scanning over recent years renders such comparisons invidious. However, in a recent study by de Souza et al.[25] in a small number of cases even transvaginal scanning failed to detect submucous leiomyomas causing significant distortion of the uterine cavity and cornua that were clearly visualized on MRI scanning. A large series comparing MRI scanning with transvaginal scanning using 'state-of-the-art' equipment and experienced sonographers would give a more meaningful assessment of the relative accuracy of the two procedures.

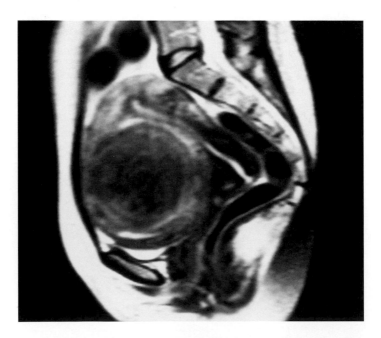

Figure 5.6 A T2 sagittal MRI sequence showing a large interstitial fibroid demonstrating typical low-signal intensity. Note the high-signal pseudocapsules containing the vessels extending to the junctional zone. This patient had menorrhagia.

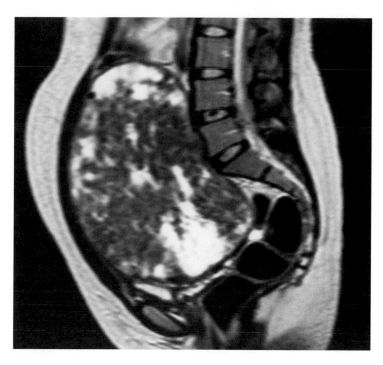

Figure 5.7 A T2 sagittal MRI scan showing a huge fibroid with extensive degeneration producing irregular areas of high signal.

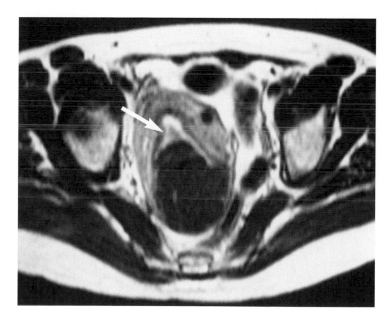

Figure 5.8 An axial T2 MRI scan showing a large full-thickness fibroid with an extensive submucous component. Note the normal junctional zone (arrowed).

In addition to the ability to map the position of fibroids more accurately and to show more clearly any distortion of the endometrium, MRI scanning better delineates fundal and cornual lesions which, in the case of large fibroid uteri, would be beyond the penetration capabilities of the transvaginal scanner; MRI is also better able to assess general pelvic pathology, including ovarian lesions, in such cases. In addition, MRI is more accurate in the assessment of endometriosis than is ultrasound.

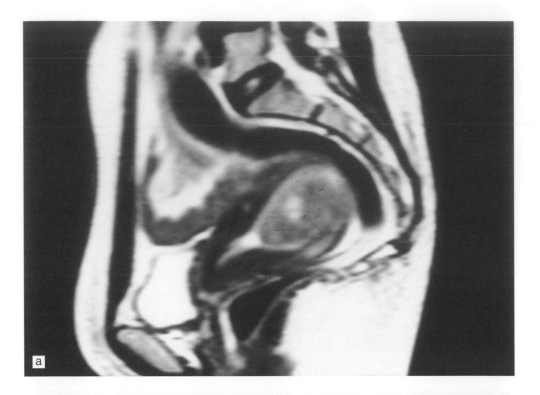

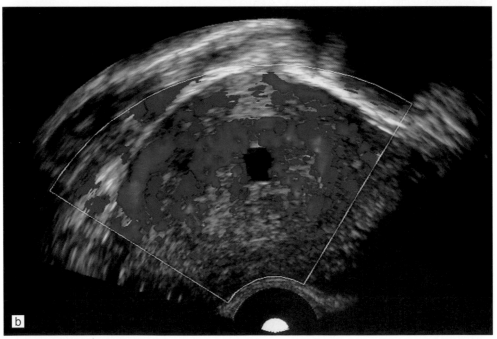

Figure 5.9 A patient who suffered severe menorrhagia unresponsive to drugs: (a) MRI scan showing a large intracavitary polyp; (b) colour Doppler ultrasound scan showing a hypervascular polyp in cavity.

Adenomyosis

Magnetic resonance imaging of adenomyosis

Unfortunately, the accuracy of the clinical diagnosis of adenomyosis is disappointingly low;[26] hysterography has been used in the past to attempt diagnosis but its sensitivity is low.[27] MRI, however, has been shown to possess a high degree

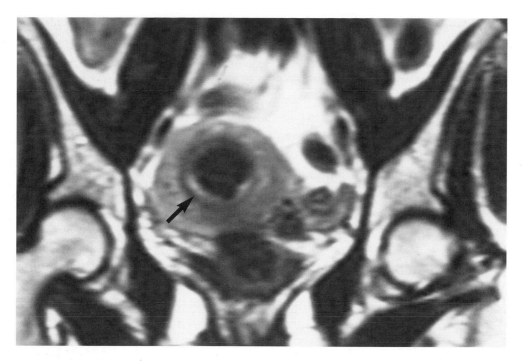

Figure 5.10 An axial T2 MRI scan showing a pedunculated intracavitary fibroid. Note the normal junctional zone (arrowed).

of accuracy in the diagnosis of adenomyosis. Togashi et al.[28] were able to differentiate adenomyosis from adenomyomas accurately in 92 of 93 patients: 15 cases of adenomyosis were correctly diagnosed, with one false negative. Hricak et al.[29] detected 15 of 19 cases of adenomyosis (79%). Mark and Hricak[30] found that, on examination of 23 women for whom there was a strong clinical suspicion of adenomyosis, MRI correctly diagnosed all eight cases of adenomyosis. It would appear that, with both transvaginal sonography and MRI, the diagnosis of adenomyosis is greatly improved when patients are selected on the basis of a strong clinical suspicion of this condition.

On MRI scans, adenomyosis is best diagnosed on the T2-weighted images. The normal uterus demonstrates three zones on MRI scanning: these are a high-signal endometrium, surrounded by a rim of low signal (called the junctional zone) that is the innermost layer of myometrium, and the mid and outer myometrium which is of intermediate signal. Brown et al.[31] have shown that the junctional zone (which appears to maintain the same thickness postmenopausally) consists of compact, smooth muscle fibres with little extracellular matrix compared with the rest of the myometrium. It is the extracellular matrix that contains the most fluid; therefore, the lack of extracellular matrix produces a low signal on MRI. The most consistent finding in adenomyosis of the uterus is the presence of an increased width of the junctional zone due to reactive hyperplasia of the muscle fibres. Reinhold et al.[32] have produced a value for the most consistent diagnosis of adenomyosis as a junctional-zone thickness of 12 mm or greater. Occasionally, small areas of high signal may be seen within the junctional zone, corresponding to hypoechoic areas seen on ultrasound scanning. These appear to be due to cystic dilatation of the ectopic endometrial glands, or haemorrhagic foci, or islands of ectopic endometrial tissue.[33]

Adenomyomas appear as areas of low signal on T2-weighted images but, in contrast to leiomyomas, their borders lack definition and are blurred.

Adenomyosis is a strange condition, the aetiology, histology, true incidence and correlation of symptoms of which are all controversial. Discussion of this is outside the brief of this chapter; however, there is little doubt that modern imaging techniques such as MRI are challenging previous assumptions about this condition. For example, de Souza et al.[25] carried out a limited study of the condition that challenged the concept that adenomyosis mainly affected multiparous women in the fourth and fifth decade: 71% of patients in their study were nulliparous and the average age of patients was only 34.4 years. If MRI criteria of diagnosis become accepted, then the true incidence of this condition will be easier to ascertain as, until now, selection bias has precluded determination of true incidence.

In addition, MRI has demonstrated that significant junctional-zone thickening and, therefore, reactive muscular hyperplasia, may be independent of endometrial penetration of the myometrium.[25,32] De Souza et al.[25] have postulated that the muscular hyperplasia of the myometrium causing the junctional-zone widening may precede the invasion of endometrium; an accurate correlation of junctional-zone width with symptomatology is therefore needed to further understanding of this condition. In patients with adenomyomas the junctional zone is of normal thickness.[25]

The modern treatment of menorrhagia and number of treatment options demands the accurate diagnosis of adenomyosis and, if present, an assessment of its extent. McCausland[34] has shown that the severity of menorrhagia in adenomyosis correlates with the depth of endometrial penetration. This can be assessed by MRI and is particularly important in cases where endometrial ablation is being considered,[35] as deep adenomyosis is associated with a poor result.

Ultrasound imaging of adenomyosis

It is generally accepted that transabdominal ultrasound imaging of the uterus provides insufficient resolution to detect the small and subtle architectural disturbances produced by adenomyosis and that the ultrasonic procedure of choice is transvaginal.

The more diffuse form of adenomyosis produces areas of mild echoic heterogenicity and/or the presence of anechoic areas less than 4 mm in diameter, termed myometrial cysts (Fig. 5.11).

In a recent article by Reinhold et al.,[32] it was felt that these anechoic areas appeared to be due to cystic dilatation of ectopic endometrial glands or haemorrhagic foci. However, Brosens et al.[36] have postulated that the heterogeneous areas are caused by irregular areas of hypertrophic/hyperplastic musculature rather than by glandular and stromal deposits.

In their series, Brosens et al.[36] also calculated an asymmetry ratio from the anterior and posterior wall thickness and found that increased posterior wall thickness compared with that of the anterior wall was helpful in the diagnosis of adenomyosis, but was not as accurate as the presence of myometrial heterogenicity.

The accuracy of ultrasound in the diagnosis of adenomyosis is difficult to assess. The modality is very operator dependent; in addition, the equipment is continually being updated, with significant improvements in imaging quality. A further

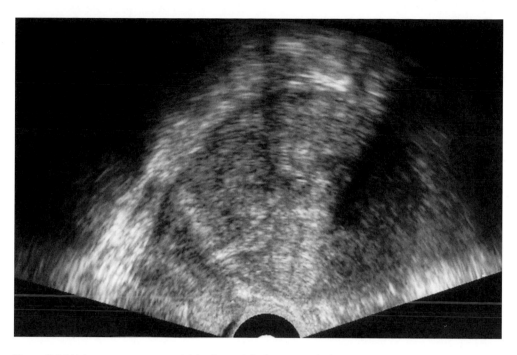

Figure 5.11 Heterogeneous myometrial echogenicity in a case of adenomyosis.

complication is that the sonographic features of adenomyosis are subtle and require experience for their diagnosis.

Some recent articles have reported good results in the detection of adenomyosis by transvaginal scanning in experienced hands. Reinhold et al.,[32] for example, comparing transvaginal ultrasound and MR imaging, showed a high degree of accuracy of ultrasound diagnosis. Reinhold et al.[32] studied 119 patients scheduled to undergo hysterectomy, with a variety of clinical symptoms (postmenstrual bleeding 35; metrorrhagia and/or menorrhagia 30; pelvic pain 16; abnormal cervical cytology 10; uterine prolapse 9; pelvic mass 8; urinary incontinence 7; miscellaneous 4). Investigators were blinded to other diagnostic tests. They found a sensitivity and specificity of 89% for MR imaging, which was the same as that for endovaginal ultrasound. The positive predictive value was 71% for ultrasound and 61% for MR imaging. The negative predictive value was 96% for ultrasound and 95% for MR imaging. False-positive diagnoses in both groups were the more common for reasons unknown, although some were due to muscular hypertrophy. It was concluded in that sense that endovaginal ultrasound was as accurate as MR imaging in the diagnosis of uterine adenomyosis. This series, however, consisted of highly selected patients who had been scheduled for hysterectomy. Nevertheless, Brosens et al.[36] found a specificity for ultrasound of only 50% for the diagnosis of adenomyosis. Ascher et al.[37] carried out a prospective study comparing MRI with transvaginal scanning (TVS) in the diagnosis of adenomyosis. The patients again had a prior clinical diagnosis of adenomyosis (including some with a previous TVS diagnosis of adenomyosis made by their gynaecologist); even so, eight of the 17 cases of adenomyosis were missed by TVS, despite the inherent bias to make the diagnosis. Of these eight false-positive cases, seven were due to adenomyosis being misinterpreted as leiomyomas. False-negative diagnoses are bad enough but false-positive diagnoses are more worrying, as anything but superficial adenomyosis would be treated by hysterectomy, whereas myomas may be treated by a less-invasive procedure. In a large series, Fedele et al.[16] compared TVS in the diagnosis of adenomyoma versus leiomyoma. The patients had a clinical diagnosis of 'symptomatic nodularities'. Worryingly, there were seven false-positive diagnoses of adenomyomas (the total number of pathologically confirmed adenomyomas in the series was 23) which, on pathological examination, were found to be leiomyomas with degeneration. Not only can degenerating leiomyomas simulate adenomyomas but also the diagnosis of adenomyosis can be extremely difficult where multiple fibroids are present.

Focal adenomyomas appear to arise from deep müllerian rests within the myometrium, whereas diffuse adenomyosis is a result of infiltration. The only real difference between a leiomyoma and an adenomyoma on ultrasound is marginal definition: leiomyomas are well defined by a vascular pseudocapsule around them whereas adenomyomas, which do not have a pseudocapsule but simply represent focal reactive muscular hyperplasia, blend around the margins with normal myometrium and have blurred edges. Unfortunately, some leiomyomas, particularly if degenerating, may also lack marginal distinction. In cases of doubt over the differentiation of leiomyoma and adenomyomas, the author has found targeted transvaginal or transabdominal gun biopsy extremely useful, whereas in the case of adenomyosis this technique is of limited value.

In conclusion, with regard to the accuracy of transvaginal scanning in the diagnosis of adenomyosis, the disparate results of recent series would indicate that the reliability of ultrasound is uncertain and that MRI is probably the procedure of choice.

Transvaginal guided biopsy of the uterus in the diagnosis of adenomyosis
In an article by Brosens et al.[36] it was noted that, if four 14 Fr needle biopsies were taken at random, one or more would be positive in 70% of uteri with deep underlying adenomyosis; however, if only superficial disease was present, the sensitivity of the technique fell to 5%. In a study by Popp et al.,[38] needle biopsies were taken immediately after hysterectomy, at the time of laparoscopy and transvaginally under ultrasound guidance. A single myometrial biopsy picked up only 8–19% of women with adenomyosis. From these results it can be concluded that transvaginal needle biopsy is useful in the case of deep adenomyosis but is of limited efficacy in the case of superficial disease. However, in the author's experience, the technique is particularly useful in focal lesions, where the differentiation between adenomyoma and leiomyoma is difficult.

Arteriovenous malformation of the uterus

AVM of the uterus is a rare condition. In a review of the literature, Fleming et al.[39] identified 15 congenital and 14 acquired cases; five of the latter were associated with trophoblastic disease, one with endometrial adenocarcinoma, five with previous surgery and three with maternal diethylstilboestrol (DES) administration. The lesions consisted of a tangle of arterial, venous or intermediate vessels with fistula formation. Menorrhagia is a common finding that may be punctuated by severe acute bleeds requiring transfusion. Bleeding has been attributed to the normal vessels eroding through the endometrium and becoming exposed when the endometrium is sloughed. Fleming et al.[38] have suggested that, if the malformation is deeply situated within the endometrium, the bleeding may be milder or non-existent. AVM may be restricted to the uterus or extend into the extra-uterine pelvis.

AVM is well demonstrated by angiography,[40] CT scanning,[41] and Doppler ultrasound.[42,43] MRI has also been reported as diagnostically useful.[43,44] In a recent article, Jain et al.[42] successfully diagnosed AVM in three cases using Doppler ultrasound. Huang et al.[43] reviewed 10 cases of acquired AVM and found that, in all cases, colour Doppler ultrasound was highly suggestive of the diagnosis. Grey-scale ultrasound alone commonly demonstrated small anechoic spaces within the myometrium, masses mimicking a fibroid, a polyp and a cervical fibroid or carcinoma. On colour duplex examination they found a combination of adjacent blue and red components, due to the intimate proximity of arterial and venous channels, and the presence of yellow and white components related to very high peak systolic velocities (96–201 cm/s) as opposed to the peak systolic velocity of normal intramural spiral arteries of 9–44 cm/s.[43]

Unfortunately, these findings, which are indicative of arteriovenous shunting, are not specific for AVM: they may be found in a number of conditions, including missed abortion, ectopic pregnancy, miscarriage[45] and, of course, in malignant trophoblastic disease.[46] However, where pregnancy complications are excluded and the serum beta human chorionic gonadotrophin (β-hCG) test is normal, then an AVM is very likely, particularly if there is a history of iatrogenic trauma. However, although colour Doppler ultrasound examination of the uterus may be highly suggestive of the presence of an AVM, it is not very accurate in determining the extent of extra-uterine spread of the malformation, and MRI is useful not only in demonstrating the AVM itself (which is indicated by the presence of signal voids within the lesion) but also in determining the extent of the lesion, particularly parametrial involvement, and in excluding other pelvic pathology. The assessment of the exact geography of the AVM is increasingly important as it may be treated conservatively by hysterectomy or by embolotherapy. With the introduction of uterine artery embolization for the treatment of fibroids, it is going to become increasingly important for radiologists to recognize AVM and, indeed, any cause of arteriovenous shunting as, in that situation, arterial embolization could be potentially dangerous.

References

1. Pourcelot L. Applications clinique de l'examen Doppler transcutane. In: Peronneau P (ed) Velocimetric ultrasonore Doppler. Paris: Inserm, 1974: 213–240

2. Tada S, Tsukioka M, Ishii C et al. Computed tomographic features of uterine myoma. J Comput Assist Tomogr 1981; 5: 866

3. Evans S, Kistner R W (eds) Gynecologic principles and practice, 4th edn. Chicago: Year Book Medical, 1986: 415

4. Emanuel M H, Verdel M J C, Stas H et al. An audit of true prevalence of intra-uterine pathology; the hysteroscopical findings controlled for patient selection in 1202 patients with abnormal uterine bleeding. Gynaecol Endosc 1995; 4: 237–241

5. Karasick S, Lev-Toaff A S, Toaff M. Imaging of uterine leiomyomas. AJR 1992; 158: 799–805

6. Goldstein S R. Incorporating endovaginal ultrasonography into the overall gynecologic examination. Am J Obstet Gynecol 1990; 162: 625–632

7. Lyons E A, Taylor P J, Zheng X H et al. Characterization of subendometrial myometrial contractions throughout the menstrual cycle in normal fertile women. Fertil Steril 1991; 55(4): 771–774

8. Parker W H, Fu Y S, Berek J S. Uterine sarcoma in patients operated on for presumed leiomyoma

and rapidly growing leiomyoma. Obstet Gynecol 1994; 83(3): 414–418

9. Tekay A, Jouppila P. Intraobserver variation in transvaginal Doppler blood flow measurements in benign ovarian tumors. Ultrasound Obstet Gynecol 1997; 9(2): 120–124

10. Carter J R, Lau M, Fowler J M et al. Blood flow characteristics of ovarian tumours: implications for ovarian cancer screening. Am J Obstet Gynecol 1995; 172(3): 901–907

11. Leeners B, Schild R L, Funk A et al. Colour Doppler sonography improves the pre-operative diagnosis of ovarian tumours made using conventional transvaginal sonography. Eur J Obstet Gynecol Reprod Biol 1996; 64(1): 79–85

12. Kurjak A, Kupesic S. Benign uterine conditions: what does color add? In: Osmers R, Jurjak A (eds) Ultrasound and the uterus. Carnforth: Parthenon, 1995: 99–103

13. Beazley J M. Dysfunctional uterine haemorrhage. Br J Hosp Med 1972; 7: 573–578

14. Brooks P G, Serden S P. Hysteroscopic findings after unsuccessful dilatation and curettage for abnormal uterine bleeding. Am J Obstet Gynecol 1988; 158: 1354–1357

15. Gimpelson R J, Rappold H O. A comparative study between panoramic hysteroscopy with directed biopsies and dilation and curettage. A review of 276 cases. Am J Obstet Gynecol 1988; 158: 489–492

16. Fedele L, Bianchi S, Dorta M et al. Transvaginal ultrasonography in the differential diagnosis of adenomyoma versus leiomyoma. Am J Obstet Gynecol 1992; 167: 603–606

17. Emanuel M H, Verdel M J C, Stas H et al. A prospective comparison of transvaginal ultrasonography and diagnostic hysteroscopy in the evaluation of patients with abnormal uterine bleeding: clinical implications. Am J Obstet Gynecol 1995; 172: 547–552

18. Cincinelli E, Romano F, Anastasio P S et al. Transabdominal sonohysterography, transvaginal sonography, and hysteroscopy in the evaluation of submucous myomas. Obstet Gynecol 1995; 85(1): 43–47

19. Lev-Toaff A S, Toaff M E, Liu J et al. Value of sonohysterography in the diagnosis and management of abnormal uterine bleeding. Genitourin Radiol 1996; 201(1): 179–184

20. Parsons A K, Lense J J. Sonohysterography for endometrial abnormalities: preliminary results. J Clin Ultrasound 1993; 21: 87–95

21. Mitil R L, Yeh I T, Kessell H Y. High signal-intensity rim surrounding uterine leiomyomas on MR images. Pathologic correlation. Radiology 1991; 180: 81–83

22. Chapman R, Chapman K. Review: An effective minimally invasive method of treating adenomyosis by interstitial laser photocoagulation with the KTP laser. Lasers Med Sci 1997; 2: 69–72

23. Dudiak C M, Turner D A, Patel S L et al. Uterine leiomyomas in the infertile patient: preoperative localization with MR imaging versus US and hysterosalpingography. Radiology 1988; 167: 627–630

24. Zawin M, McCarthy S, Scoutt L M, Comite F. High-field MRI and US evaluation of the pelvis in women with leiomyomas. Magn Reson Imaging 1990; 8: 371–376

25. De Souza N M, Brosens J J, Schwieson J E et al. The potential value of magnetic resonance imaging in infertility. Clin Radiol 1995; 50: 75–79

26. Gambone J C, Reiter R C, Lerich J B et al. The impact of a quality assurance process on the frequency and confirmation rate of hysterectomy. Am J Obstet Gynecol 1990; 163: 545–550

27. Marshak R H, Eliasoph J. The roentgen findings in adenomyosis. Radiology 1995; 64: 846–851

28. Togashi K, Ozasa H, Konishi I et al. Enlarged uterus: differentiation between adenoymosis and leiomyoma with MR imaging. Radiology 1991; 180: 81–83

29. Hricak H, Finck S, Honda G, Göranson H. MR imaging in the evaluation of benign uterine masses: value of gadopentetate dimeglumine-enhanced T1-weighted images. AJR 1992; 158: 1043–1050

30. Mark A S, Hricak H. Adenomyosis and leiomyoma: differential diagnosis with MR imaging. Radiology 1987; 163(2): 527–529

31. Brown H K, Stoll B S, Nicosia S V et al. Uterine junctional zone: correlation between histologic findings and MR imaging. Radiology 1991; 179(2): 409–413

32. Reinhold C, McCarthy S, Bret P M et al. Diffuse adenomyosis: comparison of endovaginal US and MR imaging with histopathologic correlation. Radiol 1996; 199: 151–158

33. Reinhold C, Atri M, Mehio A et al. Diffuse uterine adenomyosis: morphologic criteria and diagnostic accuracy of endovaginal sonography. Radiology 1995; 197: 609–614

34. McCausland A M. Hysteroscopic myometrial biopsy; its use in diagnosing adenomyosis and its clinical application. Am J Obstet Gynecol 1992; 174: 1619–1628

35. McCausland A M, McCausland V M. Depth of endometrial penetration in adenomyosis helps determine outcome of rollerball ablation. Am J Obstet Gynecol 1996; 174(6): 1786–1794

36. Brosens J J, de Souza N M, Barker F G et al. Endovaginal ultrasonography in the diagnosis of adenomyosis uteri: identifying the predictive characteristics. Br J Obstet Gynecol 1995; 102: 471–474

37. Ascher S M, Arnold L L, Pratt R H et al. Adenomyosis: prospective comparison of MR imaging and transvaginal sonography. Radiology 1994; 190: 803–806

38. Popp L W, Schwiedessen J P, Gaetje R. Myometrial biopsy in the diagnosis of adenomyosis uteri. Am J Obstet Gynecol 1993; 169: 546–549

39. Fleming H, Östör A G, Pickel H, Fortune D W. Arteriovenous malformations of the uterus. Obstet Gynecol 1989; 73(2): 209–213

40. Bottomley J P, Whitehouse G H. Congenital arteriovenous malformations of the uterus demonstrated by angiography. Liverpool; Department of Diagnostic Radiology, University of Liverpool, 1974: 43–48

41. Fakhri A, Fishman E K, Mitchell S E et al. The role of CT in the management of pelvic arteriovenous malformations. Cardiovasc Intervent Radiol 1987; 10: 96–99

42. Jain K A, Jeffrey R B, Sommer F G. Gynecologic vascular abnormalities: diagnosis with Doppler US. Radiology 1991; 178: 549–551

43. Huang M W, Muradali D, Thurston W A et al. Uterine arteriovenous malformations: gray-scale and droppler US features with MR imaging correlation. Radiology, 1998; 206: 115–123

44. Amparo E G, Higgins C B, Hricak H. Primary diagnosis of abdominal arteriovenous fistula by MR imaging. J Comput Assist Tomogr 1984; 8: 1140–1142

45. Borrell U, Fernstrom I. The ovarian artery. An angiographic study in human subjects. Acta Radiol 1954; 42: 253

46. Cockshott W P, Evans K T, Hendricks J P de V. Arteriography of trophoblastic tumours. Clin Radiol 1964; 15: 1

CHAPTER 6

Management of the pubertal patient

N. D. Motashaw

Introduction

In this chapter, menorrhagia at puberty and the adolescent period are not discussed separately.

At puberty, a series of changes occur that mark the evolution of childhood into adulthood. The child is transformed into a sexually active individual capable of reproduction. This period is stressful: there are physical and psychological changes, and the physician must appreciate this in the management of the pubertal patient.

It is interesting that scientific investigations have shown that the hypothalamus, anterior pituitary gland and gonads of the foetus, neonate and prepubertal child all secrete hormones. In utero at mid gestation the follicle-secreting hormone (FSH) and luteinizing hormone (LH) levels are as high as those in an adult but in the third trimester the placental steroids exert an inhibitory feedback.[1]

After birth, with the withdrawal of the maternal sex steroids, a prompt rise in FSH occurs, ovarian follicles mature and oestrogen is produced. A negative feedback depresses gonadotrophin in production and this remains low. The hypothalamopituitary system, termed the 'gonadostat', is highly sensitive to negative feedback of oestrogen, even at levels as low as 10 pg/ml. In addition to oestrogen, there exists a central non-steroidal suppresser of endogenous gonadotrophin-releasing hormone (GnRH).

As puberty approaches, the negative feedback from oestrogen and the central inhibition mechanism are relieved. Pulsatile GnRH is seen, followed by increased levels of gonadotrophins and steroids with the appearance of secondary sex characters. Initially, pulsatile LH patterns are seen during sleep, followed by the same throughout the day and night but of less amplitude. The gonad is stimulated, oestrogens appear later and the positive feedback between oestradiol and LH is established, leading to ovulatory cycles.[2]

Puberty is manifested by adrenarche, thelarche (breast development) and menarche. The growth of pubic and axillary hair is due to the production of adrenal androgens. Thelarche occurs in five stages, as defined by Marshall and Tanner.[3] The range for menarche is 8.5–15.7 years, the median being 12.8 years. The major determinant of the age of puberty is genetic, although other factors do operate: girls in tropical countries mature earlier than those in the temperate climates; girls in urban areas with good nutrition and better living conditions mature earlier than those in the rural areas. A good correlation exists between the times of menarche of mother, daughter and sisters. Of 500 adolescent girls analysed by Sheila et al.,[4]

54% attained menarche at 13.6 years; 3% of girls belonging to the higher income group attained menarche at 10.2–11 years; 90 girls who weighed less than 35 kg and were under 135 cm in height did not attain menarche by the age of 15. In this series, 5.6% had menorrhagia.

Frisch[5] believes that a critical body weight must be reached by a girl to achieve menarche. There is also a shift in body composition to a greater percentage of fat from 16 to 23.5%. Comerci,[6] in an article on symptoms associated with menstruation, has emphasized the profound emotional effects and psychological implications of abnormalities in the adolescent. Bourque et al.,[7] studying dysfunctional uterine bleeding (DUB) in the adolescent, stated that it is a frequent gynaecological problem in adolescent girls; in 75% of cases the dysfunction is due to inappropriate peripheral and central feedback mechanisms involved in the ovulatory process. As DUB is a diagnosis of exclusion, both systemic and local causes must be excluded.

Medical disorders associated with menorrhagia

Medical disorders associated with menorrhagia are a complex group. Bleeding disorders are relatively rare. Claessens and Cowell,[8] studying adolescents admitted with acute menorrhagia, found a coagulation disorder in 19% of patients; such a disorder can be idiopathic thrombocytopenic purpura ITP, von Willebrand's disease, Fanconi's anaemia, Glanzmann's disease and thrombocytopenia secondary to leukaemia. The incidence reported by Claessens and Cowell[8] is higher than usual as they analysed a selected group of patients. Von Willebrand's disease has been reported by several authors: Padte et al.[9] recently reported a case of menorrhagia due to von Willebrand's disease in a teenager. A rare cause of puberty menorrhagia is Schmidt's syndrome,[10] or polyglandular deficiency syndrome, which is the association of Addison's disease with hypothyroidism; other autoimmune disorders may coexist, such as vitiligo, diabetes mellitus and myasthenia gravis. Sharma et al.[10] have reported the occurrence of Schmidt's syndrome.

Hypothyroidism is associated with menorrhagia, whereas hyperthyroidism is usually associated with amenorrhoea. The menorrhagia responds promptly to thyroid replacement in doses insufficient to correct the other manifestations, suggesting that thyroxine in some way may have a direct effect on the spiral arterioles and on haemostasis at menstruation.[11] Other medical disorders associated with menorrhagia are infantile and adolescent cirrhosis of the liver, obesity and polycystic ovarian disease, and factors such as stress, crash diet and vigorous exercises.

Iatrogenic causes of abnormal bleeding in the pubertal patient are rare but need to be mentioned. Sex steroids, phenytoin, anticoagulants, hypothalamic depressants and the intra-uterine device (IUD) may play a role.

If adolescent menorrhagia persists with anovulatory bleeding, as it does in 5% of girls, it is responsible for chronic anaemia, ill health and, later, endometrial hyperplasia which may progress to frank carcinoma.

Pelvic pathology

Some 5% of patients have pelvic pathology. It is important to recognize early the ovarian tumour or cyst producing oestrogens and precocious puberty: 5% of granulosa cell tumours and 1% of theca cell tumours occur before puberty.

Teratomas, gonadoblastoma, lipid cell tumours, cystadenoma and ovarian cancers have been associated with menorrhagia and anovulatory cycles. An abdominal tumour mass may be palpable. The possibility of exposure to stilboestrol (diethylstilboestrol or DES), with its sequelae of vaginal and cervical adenosis and clear cell adenocarcinoma, is an important consideration in adolescents. The reported incidence of clear cell carcinoma is 0.14–1.4/1000 women exposed to DES;[12] it is rare but lethal.

Endometriosis has been described in girls as young as 10 years of age. Motashaw[13] has reported on the occurrence of adolescent endometriosis. The predominant symptom is pelvic pain, but irregular or profuse bleeding may coexist.

In a series of girls under 20 years with abnormal uterine bleeding, Sutherland[14] found eight cases of unsuspected tuberculous endometritis.

An ultrasound examination, a CT scan, magnetic resonance imaging (MRI), tumour markers and hormone assays are useful. An office hysteroscope (2.9 mm; Karl Storz, Tuttlingen) can be used as a vaginoscope. Cervical polyps, sarcoma botryoides, endodermal carcinomas and other rare lesions can be visualized and biopsied; foreign bodies can be identified and removed.

Adolescent DUB[8] can be of varying degrees, classified as follows:

Group I (minor)
This group is characterized by normal haemoglobin and no heavy bleeding, but there is the inconvenience of erratic menses. Nature usually corrects this condition within one or two years. Watchful waiting is recommended, with a proper diet and iron.

Group II (major)
This group is characterized by profuse, prolonged periods and low haemoglobin content (but not less than 10 g/dl). It should be determined if the patient is sexually active; if necessary, she should be given oral contraceptives. Progestogens will also control excess of blood loss; supplementary oral iron should also be given.

Group III (severe)
The characteristics of this group are severe bleeding episodes and haemoglobin level less than 10 g/dl. Coagulopathies should be excluded in such cases. Hospitalization and active management to achieve haemostasis are required; if necessary, blood transfusion is given.

It is important to realize that these patients can have life-threatening complications, even with their first menstrual period. Kuvin's report on the subject[15] was aptly entitled 'Near-fatal menarche'.

Treatment of pubertal menorrhagia due to DUB

Once systemic causes and local pathology have been excluded, medical therapy is almost always successful. Between 1970 and 1984, 89 patients under 18 years of age were treated by Pepe et al.[16]: 12 cases were of DUB at menarche, while 68 cases of menorrhagia or menometrorrhagia occurred 2 months to 6 years after menarche.

Oral contraceptives for three or more cycles and progestational agents constitute the first line of treatment. Progestational agents such as norethisterone acetate 5 mg daily administered from day 5 to day 25 of the cycle, or medroxyprogesterone 10 mg daily from day 15 for 10 days, together with oral iron and correction of malnutrition, are effective methods of reducing the blood loss. When endometrial hyperplasia is present, medroxyprogesterone should be administered for nine or more cycles.

Prostaglandin synthetase inhibitors[17] reduce menstrual blood loss, particularly in ovulatory menorrhagia where there is increased prostaglandin $(PG)I_2$ production. Their advantage is that they are to be administered for only 1–2 days of the month. In a paper comparing ethamsylate and mefenamic acid, Chamberlain et al.[18] reported significant decrease in blood loss with both these drugs.

Danazol was first advocated by Chimbira:[19] 200 mg given daily for 12 weeks reduces the blood loss more effectively than oral contraceptives and antifibrinolytic agents.

When coagulation disorders are present, the expertise of a haematologist is needed. Ahuja et al.[20] and others have treated patients with menorrhagia and von Willebrand's disease successfully with hormone therapy.

Desmopressin[21] is a synthetic analogue of arginine vasopressin. It is used to treat abnormal uterine bleeding in patients with coagulation disorders, and rapidly increases coagulation factor VIII, the effect lasting for 6 hours. The route of administration is intravenous or intranasal, the former (0.3 µg/kg diluted in 50 ml saline and administered over 15–30 min) being more effective than the intranasal route.

Endometrial ablation is an option for the management of menstrual problems in the young girl who is intellectually disabled: Wingfield et al.[22] have used endometrial ablation in eight such patients.

GnRH agonists provide short-term relief from a bleeding problem in patients with renal failure or blood dyscrasia, and after organ transplantation. The toxicity of immunosuppressive drugs makes the use of sex steroids less desirable.

The intra-uterine device that releases levonorgestrel may be used in sexually active adolescents with ovulatory menorrhagia who are averse to oral contraceptives. An unwanted teenage pregnancy is avoided and blood loss is considerably reduced. In a trial comparing a prostaglandin synthetase inhibitor, an antifibrinolytic agent and the levonorgestrel-releasing IUD, the latter outperformed the medical treatment dramatically;[23] it is also useful in adolescents with chronic illness such as renal failure.

The prognosis[24] for adolescent DUB is nevertheless good, in that 40–50% of cases resolve at 2 years and 70–80% in up to 10 years. In about 5% of the patients DUB will persist, owing to chronic anovulation.

References

1. Kaplan S C, Geusnbach M M, Audebert M L. The ontogenesis of pituitary hormones and hypothalamic factors in the human foetus: maturation of the central nervous system regulation of anterior pituitary function. Recent Prog Horm Res 1976; 32: 161–243

2. Speroff L, Glass R H, Kase N G. Abnormal puberty and growth problems. In: Speroff L, Glass R H, Kase N G (eds) Clinical gynecologic endocrinology and infertility, 5th edn. Baltimore: Williams and Wilkins, 1994: 361–388

3. Marshall W A, Tanner J M. Variations in the pattern of pubertal changes in girls. Arch Dis Child 1969; 44: 291–301

4. Sheila W, Malathy K, Premila S. Menstrual and gynaecological disorders in 500 school girls in Madras city. J Obstet Gynecol India 1993; 43: 950–955

5. Frisch R E. Body fat, menarche and reproductive ability. Semin Reprod Endocrinol 1985; 3: 45

6. Comerci C D. Symptoms associated with menstruation. Pediatr Clin North Am 1982; 29: 177–200

7. Bourque J, Gaspard U, Bourguignon J P, Lambotte R. Dysfunctional uterine bleeding in the adolescent. J Gynecol Obstet Biol Reprod (Paris) 1986; 15: 173–184

8. Claessens E A, Cowell C A. Dysfunctional uterine bleeding in the adolescent. Med Clin North Am 1981; 28: 369–378

9. Padte K M, Padte J, Couto F et al. Perimenarchal menorrhagia: von Willebrand disease. J Obstet Gynaecol India 1995; 45: 789–790

10. Sharma J B, Tiwari S, Gulati N, Sharma S J. Schmidt's syndrome: a rare cause of puberty menorrhagia. Int J Gynaecol Obstet 1990; 33: 373–375

11. Davey D A. Dysfunctional uterine bleeding. In: Whitfield C R (ed) Dewhurst's Textbook of obstetrics and gynecology, 5th edn. London: Blackwell Science, 1995: 590–608

12. Herbst A L, Robboy S J, Scully R E, Poskanzer D C. Clear cell adenocarcinoma of the vagina and cervix in girls. An analysis of 170 registered cases. Am J Obstet Gynecol 1974; 119: 713–724

13. Motashaw N D. Endometriosis in young girls. In: Bruhat M A, Canis M (eds) Contributions to gynecology and obstetrics. Basel: Karger, 1987; 16: 22–27

14. Sutherland A M. Functional uterine haemorrhage in puberty and adolescence: Scott Med J 1953; 34: 496–509

15. Kuvin S F. Near fatal menarche. Clin Pediatr 1964; 3: 177–178

16. Pepe F, Iachello R, Panella M et al. Dysfunctional uterine bleeding in adolescents. Clin Exp Obstet Gynecol 1987; 14: 182–184

17. Anderson A B M, Haynes P J, Guillebaud J et al. Reduction of menstrual blood loss by prostaglandin synthetase inhibitors. Lancet 1976; 1: 774–776

18. Chamberlain G, Freeman R, Price F et al. A comparative study of ethamsylate and mefenamic acid in dysfunctional uterine bleeding. Br J Obstet Gynaecol 1991; 98: 707–711

19. Chimbira T H, Cope E, Anderson A B M et al. The effect of Danazol on menorrhagia, coagulation mechanisms, haematological indices and body weight. Br J Obstet Gynaecol 1979; 86: 46–50

20. Ahuja R, Kripalani A, Choudhary V P, Takkar D. Von Willebrand disease a rare cause of puberty menorrhagia. Aust N Z J Obstet Gynaecol 1995; 35: 337–338

21. Kubrinsky N L, Tulloch H. Treatment of refractory thrombocytopenic bleeding with 1-desamino-8-D-arginine vasopressin (desmopressin). J Pediatr 1988; 112: 993–996

22. Wingfield M, McClure N, Mamers P M et al. Endometrial ablation: an option for the management of menstrual problems in the intellectually disabled. Med J Aust 1994; 160: 533–536

23. Milson I, Anderson K, Andersch B, Rybo G. A comparison of flurbiprofen, tranexamic acid and a levonorgestrel releasing intrauterine contraceptive device in the treatment of idiopathic menorrhagia. Am J Obstet Gynecol 1991; 164: 879–883

24. Southam A L, Richart R M. Prognosis for adolescents with menstrual abnormalities. Am J Obstet Gynecol 1966; 94: 637–645

CHAPTER 7

Management of menorrhagia in women of childbearing age

R. W. Shaw and K. Duckitt

Introduction

Menorrhagia (excessive menstrual blood loss) has an enormous impact on many women's lives and may affect up to 20–30% of women at some point during their childbearing years.[1–3] In the United Kingdom, one in 20 women aged 30–49 consult their GP each year with menorrhagia.[4,5] The consultation rate is rising, suggesting either an increased incidence, or more likely, a decreased tolerance of this problem.[6] There are wide variations in general practice management of menorrhagia,[5,7] in referral patterns for this condition[8] and in population-based rates of hysterectomy.[9,10] Once the patient has been referred to a gynaecologist, surgical intervention is highly likely.[8] One in five women in the United Kingdom will have a hysterectomy before the age of 60,[6] and at least one-half of these will be for menorrhagia.[4,11] About one-half of all women that have a hysterectomy for menorrhagia have a normal uterus removed.[12,13] The treatment objectives in menorrhagia are to alleviate the burden of heavy menstrual flow and consequently to improve quality of life and prevent iron-deficiency anaemia.

Definition

Menorrhagia is defined as heavy cyclical menstrual bleeding taking place over several consecutive cycles. Menorrhagia can be caused by (1) pelvic pathology,[14] such as fibroids, adenomyosis, endometriosis or endometrial polyps, (2) systemic disorders such as inherited clotting deficiencies,[14,15] thrombocytopenia, chronic liver failure or hypothyroidism, (3) iatrogenic causes such as the intra-uterine contraceptive device (IUCD),[16] or warfarin therapy. Management of menorrhagia secondary to any of these pathological disorders should be directed at treatment of the primary cause. However, 80% of women complaining of menorrhagia will have idiopathic menorrhagia or dysfunctional uterine bleeding (DUB), which is the diagnosis after these specific causes have been excluded. Most women with idiopathic menorrhagia have regular ovulatory cycles,[17,18] and the excessive bleeding is attributed to a disorder of the local control of menstruation. Although menorrhagia can be due to anovulatory cycles, this tends to occur at the extremes of reproductive life[19,20] and does not usually affect women of childbearing age unless they have an underlying disorder such as polycystic ovaries. One study[21] has shown that adolescents with menorrhagia, whether ovulatory or not, have an increased risk of an underlying coagulopathy.

Menorrhagia can be defined subjectively or objectively. Objective menorrhagia is taken to be a total menstrual blood loss (MBL) of 80 ml or more per cycle; this was the 95th centile in Hallberg and colleagues' classic population study of 476 women in Gothenberg.[1] Two-thirds of women with an MBL in excess of 80 ml will have evidence of iron-deficiency anaemia.[1,22] Subjectively, menorrhagia is defined by the woman's complaint of excessive MBL.

History

Many women who seek treatment for heavy bleeding do not have objectively heavy menstrual loss. Indicators in the patient's history, such as length of period or amount of sanitary protection used, do not correlate with objective measurements of MBL. Hallberg et al.[1] found that 14% of women who had a measured MBL of less than 20 ml thought that their periods were heavy. Chimbira et al.[23] also found that women's subjective assessment of their periods did not agree with the objective loss: of the women who had an MBL of 80 ml, or more, 34% thought their periods were light and 47% of women who complained of heavy periods had a loss of less than 80 ml. Haynes et al.[24] found no relationship between the length of the menstrual period and the total blood lost, as 72% of the total blood loss was passed by the end of the second day and 90% by the end of the third day. Chimbira came to the same conclusion,[23] and also found that MBL was not correlated with the total number of sanitary towels and tampons used; this seemed to vary more with age, social class and the woman's individual perception of hygiene. Fraser et al.[25] found that, of 69 women complaining of menorrhagia, only 47% had an objective MBL of 80 ml or more; again, there was no correlation between length of period or number of sanitary towels and tampons used when compared with measured MBL.

The purpose of history taking in a woman presenting with subjective menorrhagia is to exclude pathology that would need management differing from that of idiopathic menorrhagia. Therefore, it is important to verify that the bleeding is *regular*, with no intermenstrual bleeding, post-coital bleeding or *sudden* increase in loss. In addition, the presence of pelvic pain — either constant, pre-menstrually or with intercourse — may suggest adenomyosis or endometriosis. The presence of risk factors for endometrial cancer, such as obesity, polycystic ovaries, tamoxifen or unopposed oestrogen administration, should be noted, as endometrial sampling may be indicated before medical treatment is started. In addition, thyroid disease or clotting disorders should be excluded as possible causes of the menorrhagia. It is important to discuss the woman's contraceptive needs or intention of having children in the future, as this will greatly influence treatment.

Examination

An abdominal and pelvic examination is required to ensure that there is no obvious pelvic pathology present before treatment is initiated. A breast examination is indicated if hormonal therapy is contemplated. The presence of a pelvic mass, an enlarged uterus (≥10 weeks size), or significant pelvic tenderness should alert the practitioner to the presence of other pathology. If a cervical smear is due, it would be good practice to take one at the same time. A speculum examination may also show a forgotten IUCD, gross cervical lesions, or a prolapsing endometrial fibroid or polyp.

Investigations

Objective measurement of menstrual blood loss

The alkaline haematin method for measuring MBL, described originally by Hallberg and Nilsson in 1964,[26] has since been modified[27] and validated in several studies,[28,29] and has become the 'gold standard' for the objective measurement of MBL. It involves mixing the collected sanitary items with a known volume of sodium hydroxide, which forms alkaline haematin from the haemoglobin in the menstrual loss. The concentration of alkaline haematin is then calculated from its optical density as measured by spectrophotometry. The MBL in millilitres is calculated from a known standard of venous blood. This method is sensitive down to 0.1 ml blood, is accurate (as it recovers at least 98% of the MBL),[29] and is a very reproducible method. Sanitary items with coloured contents must not be used as this alters the optical density of the solution.

Vasilenko et al.[30] modified the alkaline haematin method to avoid large volumes of caustic solutions and unpleasant odours. The haemoglobin was eluted from the pads and tampons with a detergent and then a known volume of sodium carbonate was added to the supernatant. The optical density was again measured spectrophotometrically and the MBL in millilitres calculated. This method of objective measurement also seemed to perform well and has recently been used by Gannon et al.[31] in a study of 372 women offered endometrial resection. The criticism of both these methods is that they need to be hospital based and require specialized equipment and staff to perform the procedures. However, the technology is by no means complicated and should not be beyond the capabilities of most hospitals.

In order to obtain a semi-quantitative measurement of the MBL, better suited to general practice or non-research gynaecological outpatient settings, a pictorial blood loss assessment chart (PBAC) was developed.[32] The chart took into account the degree to which each item of sanitary protection was soiled with blood, as well as the number used. Set scores were assigned to different degrees of soiling of pads and tampons. Clots were also scored and the score for the period totalled. This was found to correlate well with objective MBL as determined by the alkaline haematin method, regardless of whether the patient completed the chart or the score was determined by the gynaecologist after studying the collected sanitary wear. A score of 100 or more was found to correlate with an MBL of 80 ml or more. Deeny and Davis[33] found that the PBAC was better than the woman's subjective assessment as a test for menorrhagia, but the plotting of a receiver-operating characteristic (ROC) curve indicates that the PBAC has only intermediate discriminatory power in detecting excessive menstrual loss. This means that the PBAC may still be useful in the clinical situation but does not replace the alkaline haematin method as the gold standard for objective measurement of MBL.

Other methods to measure menstrual blood loss include weight measurements,[34,35] when the weight of sanitary wear is determined before and after use. Since it is known that the percentage contribution of blood to the total menstrual discharge varies greatly between individuals,[36] this method is not the method of choice. Radioisotopic methods have also been used: ^{59}Fe- or ^{51}Cr-labelled red blood cells in used sanitary wear are detected and compared with venous blood.[37,38] These methods are laborious and invasive, and their accuracy has not been described.

Full blood count

Although Hallberg[1] showed that 66% of women with a menstrual blood loss of 80 ml or more had haematological indices indicative of iron-deficiency anaemia, not all women, even if proven to have objective menorrhagia, will have anaemia as defined by WHO (<12 g/dl). This is not, therefore, a perfect screening test for objective menorrhagia. Janssen et al.[34] found that a low haemoglobin predicted objective menorrhagia better than the woman's subjective assessment, but not as well as a PBAC. Likelihood ratios calculated from Janssen's study[34] and the reported values in Hallberg's study[1] show that a low haemoglobin makes the diagnosis of objective menorrhagia more likely, but a normal haemoglobin does not absolutely exclude objective menorrhagia. However, a full blood count will also give extra information about the haematological indices and may reveal an iron-deficiency state before anaemia is reached. It will also give information about the platelet count. As symptoms and signs of anaemia do not correlate well with the haemoglobin level until the patient is moderately to severely anaemic, a full blood count should be performed in all women complaining of menorrhagia to aid recognition of objective menorrhagia and to allow early recognition and treatment of iron-deficiency anaemia.

Thyroid function tests

There is no evidence linking menorrhagia with thyrotoxicosis,[39] but there have been several small series of hypothyroid patients reporting an excess of menstrual irregularities, particularly menorrhagia;[40] however, these involved known hypothyroid patients and only subjective menorrhagia was reported. A case report in 1992 demonstrated how objectively measured menorrhagia in a hypothyroid patient improved with thyroxine replacement.[41] It has also been suggested that some women with menorrhagia have subclinical hypothyroidism and that thyroxine replacement may decrease their menstrual blood loss.[42,43] These studies did not objectively measure menstrual blood loss in the subjects and both relied on the response to a thyrotrophin-releasing hormone (TRH) test in women with normal free thyroxine and thyrotrophin (TSH) levels; this area requires further study.

Routine screening for thyroid disease with thyroid function tests is not recommended for asymptomatic adults,[44] and there is no evidence to suggest that the situation differs in women complaining of menorrhagia; nevertheless, as always with thyroid disorders, a high level of clinical suspicion should exist and thyroid function should be measured in any woman with symptoms of hypothyroidism.

Other endocrine tests

Other endocrine investigations, such as progesterone, luteinizing hormone (LH) and follicle-stimulating hormone (FSH) levels, are of no value in women with heavy, regular menstrual cycles, as 80% of women with three or more consecutive regular menstrual cycles were found to be ovulatory[17] and there were no significant differences in the plasma concentrations of LH, FSH or 17β-oestradiol (E2) or in the salivary concentrations of progesterone between women with objectively heavy loss and those with normal loss.[45]

Endometrial sampling

The Pipelle sampler is a type of endometrial sampler that is in common use in the United Kingdom. It has been shown to be an accurate and acceptable means of obtaining endometrial histological samples in order to exclude endometrial hyperplasia and carcinoma in symptomatic women,[46–48] and is as good as (or better than) other endometrial sampling devices.[49–54] The use of blind endometrial sampling to screen for endometrial cancer in asymptomatic women has not been recommended;[55,56] endometrial cancer is rare in premenopausal women, and diagnostic endometrial sampling procedures are not cost effective in women under the age of 40 without specific risk factors.[57] Although the incidence of endometrial cancer does rise after the age of 40, it still tends to present with some form of irregular bleeding rather than regular heavy menstrual loss. Rather than arbitrarily choosing an age at which endometrial sampling should be done to evaluate abnormal bleeding, each woman should be judged according to her individual risk factors for developing endometrial adenocarcinoma and its precursors. Some women are at high risk of endometrial cancer and would need endometrial sampling (i.e. those with polycystic ovary syndrome or obesity, or those receiving tamoxifen or unopposed oestrogen treatment) but there is not enough evidence to justify performing an endometrial biopsy in everyone over 40 complaining of menorrhagia alone. Endometrial biopsy cannot determine the presence, or otherwise, of intra-uterine pathology such as submucous fibroids or polyps. Therefore, if a woman complaining of menorrhagia has not improved with effective drug therapy, a further assessment of her uterine cavity with either transvaginal ultrasound or diagnostic hysteroscopy is warranted. A directed endometrial biopsy can then be performed.

Is treatment indicated or required?

Some women may merely want an explanation of their heavy periods and may be reassured after being examined and investigated. After their first consultation for menorrhagia, 4% of 518 patients studied in general practice[58] wanted advice or minimal treatment only. The effectiveness of reassurance and counselling is not known; it is currently being studied in a randomized controlled trial in Oxford. However, if the patient is anaemic, iron therapy and treatment to reduce menstrual blood loss are indicated. In practice, menstrual blood loss is very rarely measured outside research studies and, therefore, treatment is based on the woman's subjective complaint. This may be reasonable, as the woman's quality of life may be affected even though her MBL does not exceed 80 ml. However, if medical management fails, it may be because the loss was not truly heavy in the first place. The woman may then be subjected to further investigation and, ultimately, definitive surgery, with its attendant risk of mortality, in the absence of objectively diagnosed disease.

Initial treatment

Drug treatment is the preferred initial option for women in their childbearing years as it is reversible and preserves fertility. However, it is important that only drugs known to be effective in reducing menstrual blood loss are used. Several surveys[5,7] have shown that general practitioners prescribe ineffective drug treatments for menorrhagia. This results in patient dissatisfaction with drug therapy in general, and may contribute to unnecessary surgical intervention. The treatment options, which need to be individualized for each woman, have been divided into three areas dependent on patient preferences and contraceptive requirements. Before initiating any drug therapy, any possible contraindications should be excluded. At least three menstrual cycles should be evaluated before a treatment is deemed to be ineffective.

The woman who does not require hormonal contraception or who prefers non-hormonal treatment

The two most effective drugs for women who fall into this category are tranexamic acid and mefenamic acid. The reduction in MBL is greater with tranexamic acid, but mefenamic acid should be used preferentially if dysmenorrhoea is a significant problem. These drugs have the advantages of being non-hormonal, with administration being necessary only during menstruation; they can also be used, therefore, if the woman is trying to conceive. It is possible that the reduction in MBL may be even greater if these two drugs are used together. However, no studies could be found that addressed this question.

Tranexamic acid

Tranexamic acid competitively inhibits the activation of plasminogen to plasmin and counteracts the high fibrinolytic activity in the endometrium that may be one of the causes of menorrhagia.[59] Coulter et al.,[5] in a meta-analysis of tranexamic acid treatment for menorrhagia, found that, when compared with pretreatment MBL, tranexamic acid reduced mean MBL by 46.7% [reported 95% confidence interval (CI) 45–46.7]. Some of the studies included in the meta-analysis involved women with subjective menorrhagia. In other randomized controlled trials, not included in this meta-analysis, MBL reduction varied from 33% and 41% with a prodrug of tranexamic acid given four times daily or twice daily, respectively[60] (the prodrug is rapidly converted to the active drug, tranexamic acid, but has the advantage of better gastrointestinal absorption and therefore increased bioavailability of the active drug) to 53%[61] and 54%[62] with tranexamic acid.

Tranexamic acid fared better when compared with placebo or with other treatments: the reduction was significantly greater than that found during treatment with diclofenac sodium,[63] mefenamic acid,[62] flurbiprofen,[59,61] norethisterone[64] or ethamsylate.[62] The dosage tested in the majority of the studies was 1 g three times a day from day 1 for the days of heaviest flow; however, the maximum dosage that can be used is 1.5 g four times a day. Side effects are nausea, vomiting and diarrhoea, which seem to be dose related.

Tranexamic acid is contraindicated in women with a history of thrombo-embolic disorders; however, it does not seem to cause thromboses, as large-scale studies in Scandinavia have shown that the incidence of thrombosis in women treated by tranexamic acid does not differ from the spontaneous incidence of thrombosis in untreated women.[65]

Mefenamic acid

Mefenamic acid is a prostaglandin synthetase inhibitor. Coulter et al.,[5] in a meta-analysis of 11 studies of mefenamic acid treatment for menorrhagia, found that, compared with pretreatment MBL, mefenamic acid reduced mean MBL by 29% (95% CI 27.9–30.2). The range of reduction in MBL varied between 20%[66] and

47.7%,[67] with an indication that a proportionally greater reduction is seen in those with the highest initial MBL.[68] In a more recent randomized controlled trial, not included in the meta-analysis mentioned above, the reduction in MBL with mefenamic acid was 20%.[62] Compared with other treatments, mefenamic acid fared significantly better than ethamsylate,[62] but significantly worse than danazol.[66] The effect observed with mefenamic acid can be sustained as long as treatment is continued.[69]

If successful in reducing MBL, these drugs can be continued indefinitely as long as the pattern of bleeding does not change and the woman does not report any different symptoms that suggest the presence of pathology.

The woman who requires contraception

Combined oral contraceptives   Combined oral contraceptives (COCs) can be useful in reducing menstrual bleeding. Although their mode of action is unclear, they probably induce endometrial atrophy.[70] The height of the endometrium is less than in an ovulatory cycle and there is less proliferation in the glandular epithelium, so the amount of blood loss is reduced at the time of menstrual shedding.[71]

The paper most commonly cited in support of the use of COCs for the treatment of menorrhagia dates back to 1971 and is based on a study of a series of 164 women with objective menorrhagia who were administered COCs for a period of 284 cycles.[72] The COCs used were all high-dose preparations containing either 0.15 mg mestranol or 50 μg ethinyloestradiol given in the usual 21- out of 28-day schedule. There was an overall 52.6% reduction in MBL: in 68% of the patients MBL was normalized after COC treatment; this represented 88.5% of those with MBL less than 100 ml prior to treatment, 69% of those with MBL between 100 and 200 ml before treatment and 44.5% of those with initial MBL of more than 200 ml.

The only trial to address low-dose COCs in menorrhagia was that by Fraser and McCarron,[73] who performed a randomized cross-over study of two hormonal and two prostaglandin-inhibiting agents in women with subjective menorrhagia. In the group randomized to mefenamic acid and then COC, a highly significant reduction of 43% in blood loss was obtained for the COC; this did not differ significantly from the 38% MBL reduction obtained with mefenamic acid. The COCs used in this study were ethinyloestradiol 30 μg and levonorgestrel 150 μg daily for 21 days of 28.

Despite the wide variety of COCs in use, no other controlled trials could be found in which COCs were evaluated in patients with objective or subjective menorrhagia. Other non-randomized, non-controlled studies,[16,74,75] and large prospective series of COC users,[76,77] add supporting evidence that COCs do reduce MBL both in women with subjectively normal periods and in women complaining of menorrhagia.

It seems clear that COC preparations can reduce MBL and consequently increase haemoglobin concentrations and reduce iron-deficiency anaemia. What is less clear is whether the COCs that are in common use today (i.e. low-dose preparations containing 30 μg ethinyloestradiol) are as effective in reducing MBL as the higher-dosage preparations used in many of these studies, and whether the particular progestogen used makes any difference. Although there is some indication that the frequency of menstrual disturbances, such as spotting and breakthrough bleeding, is less when the COC contains a relatively high dose of progestogen,[78] no evidence could be found to suggest that changing the progestogen influenced total MBL. Further research in these areas is needed.

Progestogen-releasing intra-uterine devices   There is only one progestogen-releasing intra-uterine device (IUD) available in the United Kingdom at present: this is the levonorgestrel intra-uterine system (LNG–IUS) known as Mirena. However, it is likely that other progestogen-releasing IUDs will be developed in the future. The LNG–IUS consists of a plastic T-shaped device with a steroid reservoir around the vertical stem which regulates the intra-uterine release of levonorgestrel to 20 μg per 24 hours. In the United Kingdom, the LNG–IUS is licensed for contraception for 3 years, but this is likely to be extended to 5 years shortly and an application for a licence for use in menorrhagia is in progress. Currently, it can be used in a woman complaining of menorrhagia as long as she also requires contraception. European countries that have the LNG–IUS have issued licences for both contraception and menorrhagia. The contraceptive and therapeutic effect of the LNG–IUS is based on the local effects of the released levonorgestrel on the uterine cavity, which leads to a high local tissue concentration in the endometrium. Endometrial proliferation is prevented[79] and the cervical mucus becomes thicker.[80] During the first year of LNG–IUS use, a few women stop ovulating but thereafter most cycles are ovulatory.[81,82] Luukkainen[83] reports that published studies covering more than 10,000 woman-years show an annual pregnancy rate, in all age groups, of less than 0.2 per 100 women.

The strong suppression of endometrial growth results in the reduction of the amount of MBL and of the duration of menstrual bleeding; this effect can be used for treatment of menorrhagia. During the first few months of use, the total number of bleeding days (menstrual bleeding plus intermenstrual bleeding plus spotting) increases in most women;[84] however, by 12 months most women bleed lightly for only 1 day a month, while about 15% of women are amenorrhoeic.[83] After removal of the LNG–IUS, the morphological changes in the endometrium revert to normal[79] and menstruation returns within 30 days.[85] The return of fertility is also rapid.[86]

Most of the studies concerning all types of progestogen-releasing IUCDs have looked primarily at their contraceptive efficacy rather than objectively measuring their effect on MBL. The studies that have measured MBL in association with these IUCDs have all been small and non-randomized;[59,83,85,87,88] however, they all show a consistent effect in significantly reducing MBL. Andersson and Rybo[87] found an 86% decrease in MBL after 3 months' use, which increased to 97% after 12 months' use. Tang and Lo[88] found that the MBL had decreased by 95% after 6 months.

As with all long-acting progestogen-only contraceptive methods, abnormal bleeding patterns are the most common side effect. Oligomenorrhoea and amenorrhoea are the commonest of these abnormal patterns in users of progestogen-releasing IUCDs and contribute to the therapeutic effect in women with menorrhagia. It is possible that the acceptance of these abnormal bleeding patterns will vary between women using it solely for contraception and those with menorrhagia, and may also depend on the quality of the pre-insertion counselling.

Comparing the LNG–IUS with other drug treatments, Milsom et al.[59] found that it achieved a significantly greater reduction in MBL than either tranexamic acid or flurbiprofen, although this was not a randomized controlled trial. Comparisons between progestogen-releasing IUCDs and non-drug treatments of menorrhagia are scarce. However, Crosignani et al.[89] found that the LNG–IUS and endometrial resection were equally effective in a randomized trial of 70 women with dysfunctional uterine bleeding. In two other studies[90,91] the LNG–IUS was inserted into women awaiting hysterectomy or transcervical resection of the endometrium after a failed trial of medical therapy for menorrhagia. In the first of these studies, 67% of women randomized to LNG–IUS cancelled their planned hysterectomy, as opposed to 15% of the controls,[90] while 82% were removed from the waiting list in the other study.[91]

Progestogen-releasing IUCDs can offer an alternative to both medical and surgical treatments of menorrhagia. They preserve fertility and are inexpensive compared with surgical options. The cost of one LNG–IUS, used for 3 years, is £33/year, although the costs of counselling, insertion, follow-up visits and removal are additional.[84]

Long-acting progestogens   Medroxyprogesterone acetate is available as a depot injection for contraception at a dose level of 150 mg administered every 3 months. It is likely to cause unpredictable, irregular spotting and bleeding in the first few months of use,[92,93] and has been estimated to cause heavy bleeding in 1–2% of women.[94] However, with repeated administration, amenorrhoea becomes common and haemoglobin levels increase with prolonged usage.[93] After 1 year of use, 45–50% of women are likely to be amenorrhoeic.[92,93] Subdermal implants that release levonorgestrel over several years are another way of administering long-acting progestogens for contraceptive purposes. Like depot medroxyprogesterone acetate, bleeding disturbances such as irregular bleeding and periods of prolonged bleeding are common with levonorgestrel, although, again, the frequency of such disturbances decreases considerably after the first year of use.[95] The acceptability and effectiveness of long-acting progestogens as treatments for menorrhagia, in view of their highly variable bleeding patterns, has not yet been addressed. However, these methods may be suitable for women with menorrhagia who also require effective long-term contraception.

The woman who has a copper intra-uterine device

Inert IUDs have been shown to at least double the MBL, while copper devices increase MBL by an average of 40–50% over 6–12 months compared with pre-insertion values.[96] Inert devices are seldom used in the United Kingdom. Removal of the IUD is often necessitated by this excessive or irregular bleeding and/or pain.[96] Two types of problems arise with bleeding due to IUD use: these are (1) inconvenience due to heavy menstrual loss and (2) iron depletion produced by loss of excessive volumes of blood.[97]

Several of the drugs that have been effective in treating idiopathic menorrhagia have been investigated to see whether they can also reduce MBL in women with IUDs. Randomized controlled trials consistently show that tranexamic acid reduces MBL in users of both inert and copper IUDs.[63,98] Neither of the studies showed a reduction in MBL that persisted after treatment. Non-steroidal anti-inflammatory drugs (NSAIDs) also seem to be effective: mefenamic acid,[99] ibuprofen,[100] naproxen[101] and diclofenac[63] have all been shown to reduce MBL in IUD users by between 23 and 37%.

Less-effective drug treatments

Oral low-dose luteal-phase progestogens Norethisterone (NET), a progestogen derived from 19-nortestosterone, has been used to treat menstrual disorders since Bishop and de Almeida[102] described a subjective improvement in 34 of 52 treated cycles in 13 patients suffering from menorrhagia. Their hypothesis was that menorrhagia was caused by an inadequate progesterone influence on the endometrium; therefore, a progestogen such as NET might be expected to induce full secretory changes in the endometrium and give rise to normal shedding and normal menstrual loss.

A meta-analysis[5] of four randomized trials, all using NET 5 mg two or three times a day in the luteal phase of the cycle, found that NET had a combined percentage reduction in menstrual blood loss of −3.6, suggesting that it actually increases menstrual blood loss. In three of the randomized trials women with objective menorrhagia of more than 80 ml entered the studies, the exception being that by Cameron et al.,[103] which had an entry criterion of more than 50 ml. Two of these studies found that NET increased MBL by 12% and 20%, respectively;[64,103] and the other two showed reductions in MBL of only 20% and 4%.[104,105] NET did not perform better than any of the drugs with which it was compared. Fraser,[106] in a non-randomized trial, found a significant reduction in the mean MBL in ovulatory cycles of 32–36% when NET was used, but this could have been due to the higher dosage (up to 10 mg three times a day) and longer administration period (days 5–25). Therefore, in the dosages and timings currently recommended in the British National Formulary and in the data sheets, norethisterone is not an effective treatment for menorrhagia.

Dydrogesterone, a progestogen licensed for treatment of menorrhagia in the United Kingdom, has not been subject to evaluation of its effectiveness in menorrhagia.

Ethamsylate Ethamsylate is a non-hormonal agent that is thought to act by increasing capillary vascular wall resistance and platelet adhesiveness in the presence of a vascular lesion. It is used for the duration of the heavy period and has minimal side effects.

Four studies[62,107–109] have looked at ethamsylate in the treatment of menorrhagia and have objectively measured MBL. Two of these studies[108,109] included IUD users as well as women with unexplained menorrhagia, but did not demand that the women had MBL of over 80 ml before entry, whereas the other two studies looked only at women with a pretreatment MBL exceeding 80 ml.[62,107] The results were conflicting: Kasonde[109] and Chamberlain et al.[107] found that ethamsylate 500 mg four times daily during menstruation decreased MBL by 7% and 20%, respectively. Bonnar and Sheppard[62] found that the same dosage had no effect on MBL at all. In contrast, Harrison and Campbell[108] found that ethamsylate reduced MBL by 50% in women with 'primary menorrhagia' and by 19% in IUD users. Interestingly, this was the only study to determine MBL by a method other than the normally accepted alkaline haematin method of Hallberg and Nilsson,[26] and the women started the ethamsylate treatment 5 days prior to the expected start of their period, instead of on day 1 as in the other reports. However, when these trials were combined,[5] an overall reduction of 13.1% (95% CI 10.9–15.3) was calculated. In the studies that compared ethamsylate with other drugs used to treat menorrhagia, it was less effective than aminocaproic acid[109] or than mefenamic acid and tranexamic acid.[62] Chamberlain et al.[107] found that ethamsylate and mefenamic acid reduced MBL by a similar amount (20% vs 24%).

In summary, it seems that ethamsylate in this dosage, when taken only during menstruation, is not particularly effective in reducing MBL. On the basis of the results outlined above, it should not be used as first-line treatment in menorrhagia.

What if initial treatment fails?

Several studies that have looked at the effectiveness of drug therapy have found that, if drug therapy fails to reduce MBL to an acceptable level, intra-uterine pathology, such as the presence of submucous fibroids, is more likely to be present.[68,72,110] Fraser[111] also demonstrated that women with the highest measured MBL were more likely to have pathology; therefore, further investigation is essential if initial drug therapy with an effective agent fails. Hysteroscopy with directed endometrial biopsy would be the procedure of choice.[112]

Second-line drug treatments

The following drugs have been shown to be effective in reducing MBL but are limited in their usage by side effects or by cost, or both. They should, therefore, be used only after first-line drug therapy has failed and when intra-uterine pathology has been excluded. With these drugs, as with all those used to treat menorrhagia, the MBL will eventually return to pretreatment levels after therapy has stopped. Danazol and gonadotrophin-releasing hormone (GnRH) analogues can also be used for thinning the endometrium before ablation or resection.

Danazol Danazol is an isoxazol derivative of 17α-ethinyl testosterone. It inhibits ovulation and causes low circulating oestrogen levels and endometrial atrophy.[113] It has mild androgenic properties.

Several trials have assessed the effects of danazol in the treatment of menorrhagia. The criterion for entry into the studies has varied between 50, 60 and 80 ml of MBL and the dosage of danazol used has also varied between studies. However, the beneficial effect of danazol in reducing MBL is consistent across all studies.

All the randomized trials[66,73,103,104,114,115] examining the effects of danazol in cases of menorrhagia show a significant reduction in MBL (range 22–99%) when danazol is administered daily. The reduction depends on the dosage of danazol administered (as the dose in the studies ranges from 50 to 400 mg daily) and on the length of treatment, as the MBL is reduced more in the second and third treatment cycles than in the first. The preferred dose for the treatment of menorrhagia seems to be 200 mg daily,[104,114,115] as light, regular cycles are produced; the higher dose of 400 mg daily tends to produce amenorrhoea and is associated with a greater incidence of side effects;[116] lower doses result in lower MBL reductions and can cause irregular bleeding.[114,115] A meta-analysis[5] of five of the studies discussed previously[66,73,103,104,114] found an overall reduction in MBL of 49.7% (95% CI 47.9–51.6) for danazol treatment. However, all the studies that measured post-treatment cycles[104,114–116] found that the MBL gradually returned towards pretreatment levels during the first 3 months after treatment had ended, regardless of which dose was used initially.

The main disadvantages of danazol therapy are its side effects. Although withdrawals due to side effects were not higher with danazol in those studies that detailed side effects, the proportion of subjects reporting the presence of side effects was higher. Dockeray et al.[66] found that side effects occurred in 75% of the group given danazol compared with 30% of the group on mefenamic acid; 40% of these side effects were unacceptable. An average weight gain of 2–4 kg is common with 3 months treatment.[66,114,116] Other side effects include androgenic effects such as acne, seborrhoea, hirsutism and hoarseness, and general complaints including irritability, musculoskeletal pains and tiredness. Hot flushes and breast atrophy can sometimes result. Most side effects are reversible on stopping treatment. Women must be advised to use barrier methods of contraception because of potential virilization of a foetus if pregnancy occurs while on treatment. It is suggested in the data sheet that treatment is restricted to 6 months maximum because of adverse androgenic effects on lipid levels.

Gestrinone Gestrinone is a synthetic 19-nortestosterone derivative that is an antiprogesterone and anti-oestrogen with some androgenic activity. It interacts with the hypothalamic and pituitary steroid receptors to decrease the secretion of FSH and LH.[110] It induces amenorrhoea as a result of ovulation inhibition, thereby producing endometrial atrophy.[117] Although Turnbull and Rees[110] conducted a randomized, single-blind placebo-controlled trial and found that gestrinone, 2.5 mg twice weekly, was effective in treating objective menorrhagia (MBL >80 ml) in 15 of the 19 women studied, it is not at present licensed for use in menorrhagia, only in endometriosis. It is also nearly five times the price of danazol.

GnRH analogues Synthetic GnRH analogues bind to the same receptor as naturally occurring GnRH, but with a greater affinity, so prolonged use leads to desensitization of the gonadotrophin-releasing cells in the anterior pituitary which leads to hypo-oestrogenism and results in endometrial atrophy;[118] this is the basis of their effect on MBL.

Only a few studies, involving small numbers of women, have investigated GnRH analogues in menorrhagia alone; most involve their action on fibroids or on thinning the endometrium prior to ablation or resection. Shaw and Fraser[119] administered buserelin intranasally to four women (with MBL of more than 80 ml and no pelvic pathology) for 3 months. The pretreatment range of MBL was 95–198 ml; by the second and third months of treatment, this had decreased to 4–30 ml, with an associated rise in haemoglobin level. Menses returned within 16–27 days of stopping treatment and the measured blood loss returned towards pretreatment levels. Gardner and Shaw[118] also investigated the effect of a different GnRH analogue, goserelin, on MBL in six women with proven menorrhagia. A subcutaneous depot injection of goserelin (3.6 mg) was administered monthly for 3 months. The MBL decreased in the first cycle and, by the second cycle, five of the six women had become amenorrhoeic while the sixth woman had an MBL of 2 ml. There was no loss in the third treatment cycle or in the first post-treatment cycle. It took longer for menses to return than with buserelin, but by 7–10 weeks menses had returned and had started to approach pretreatment values.

Although hot flushes can be an unpleasant side effect, treatment with GnRH analogues also results in bone loss. Up to 5% of bone loss has been demonstrated with 6 months goserelin treatment, although this has not been associated with an increased risk of fracture and may be equivalent to 6 months of breast-feeding.[120] Consequently, treatment for longer than 6 months is not recommended for benign disorders. To try to reduce these side effects, Thomas et al.[121] added Cyclo-Progynova 1 mg to monthly goserelin treatment for 20 women with a subjective complaint of menorrhagia and a normal pelvis on clinical examination. In those women with pretreatment MBL of more than 80 ml, MBL was significantly reduced from a median pretreatment loss of 171 ml to 73.5 ml by the third month of treatment. In the other women, the MBL was significantly reduced from a median of 53 ml before treatment to 8.5 ml by month 3. Subjective complaints of clots, flooding, dysmenorrhoea and symptoms of premenstrual tension all improved but 17 of the 20 women still experienced hot flushes despite the hormone replacement treatment (HRT), with two women rating them as severe.

GnRH analogue treatment is effective in reducing MBL but can be considered only as a temporary treatment, perhaps while awaiting surgery or the natural menopause. Further studies are needed to see if regimens consisting of GnRH analogues with 'add back' HRT are effective in reducing MBL while minimizing side effects and bone loss.

Summary

Drug treatment is the first choice of treatment for women of childbearing age with menorrhagia. However, therapy must be with drugs of proven effectiveness and the choice individualized to each woman, depending on her fertility concerns or contraceptive needs. If drug treatment fails despite at least 3 months of treatment, further evaluation of the uterine cavity must take place. However, it must be remembered that one reason for treatment failure may be an objectively normal menstrual loss and it then becomes necessary to explore further the woman's concerns and expectations regarding menstruation and the expected outcomes with treatment.

References

1. Hallberg L, Hogdahl A, Nilsson L, Rybo G. Menstrual blood loss — a population study: variation at different ages and attempts to define normality. Acta Obstet Gynecol Scand 1966; 45: 320–351

2. Gath D, Osborn M, Bungay G et al. Psychiatric disorder and gynaecological symptoms in middle aged women: a community survey. Br Med J 1987; 294: 213–218

3. Jacobs A, Butler E B. Menstrual blood loss in iron deficiency anaemia. Lancet 1965; ii: 407–409

4. Vessey M P, Villard-Mackintosh L, McPherson K et al. The epidemiology of hysterectomy: findings in a large cohort study. Br J Obstet Gynaecol 1992; 99: 402–407

5. Coulter A, Kelland J, Peto V, Rees M C. Treating menorrhagia in primary care. An overview of drug trials and a survey of prescribing practice. Int J Technol Assess Health Care 1995; 11: 456–471

6. Coulter A, McPherson K, Vessey M. Do British women undergo too many or too few hysterectomies? Soc Sci Med 1988; 27: 987–994

7. Taskforce to Improve the Management of Menorrhagia. GP Survey on Menorrhagia. 35 Findon Road, London W12 9PP: Secretariat to the Taskforce to Improve the Management of Menorrhagia, 1997

8. Coulter A, Bradlow J, Agass M et al. Outcomes of referrals to gynaecology out-patients clinics for menstrual problems: an audit of general practice records. Br J Obstet Gynaecol 1991; 98: 789–796

9. Doherty L, Harper A, Russell M. Menorrhagia management options. Ulster Med J 1995; 64: 64–71

10. McPherson K, Strong P, Epstein A, Jones L. Regional variation in the use of common surgical procedures within and between England and Wales, Canada and the United States of America. Soc Sci Med 1981; 15a: 273–288

11. Coulter A, Klassen A, McPherson K. How many hysterectomies should purchasers buy? Eur J Public Health 1995; 5: 123–129

12. Clarke A, Black N, Rowe P et al. Indications for and outcome of total abdominal hysterectomy for benign disease: a prospective cohort study. Br J Obstet Gynaecol 1995; 102: 611–620

13. Grant J M, Hussein I Y. An audit of abdominal hysterectomy over a decade in a district hospital. Br J Obstet Gynaecol 1984; 91: 73–77

14. Fraser I S, McCarron G, Markham R et al. Measured menstrual blood loss in women with menorrhagia associated with pelvic disease or coagulation disorder. Obstetr Gynecol 1986; 68: 630–633

15. Greer I A, Lowe G D O, Walker J J, Forbes C D. Haemorrhagic problems in obstetrics and gynaecology in patients with congenital coagulopathies. Br J Obstet Gynaecol 1991; 98: 909–918

16. Hefnawi F, Askalani H, Zaki K. Menstrual blood loss with copper intrauterine devices. Contraception 1974; 9: 133–139

17. Haynes P J, Anderson A B, Turnbull A C. Patterns of menstrual blood loss in menorrhagia. Res Clin Forums 1979; 1: 73–78

18. Cameron I T. Dysfunctional uterine bleeding. Baillieres Clin Obstet Gynaecol 1989; 3: 315–327

19. Fraser I S, Michie E A, Wide L, Baird D T. Pituitary gonadotrophins and ovarian function in adolescent dysfunctional uterine bleeding. J Clin Endocrinol Metab 1973; 37: 407–414

20. Van Look P F A, Lothian H, Hunter W M et al. Hypothalamic–pituitary–ovarian function in perimenopausal women. Clin Endocrinol 1977; 7: 13–31

21. Claessens E A, Cowell C A. Acute adolescent menorrhagia. Am J Obstet Gynecol 1981; 139: 277–280

22. Cole S K, Billewicz W Z, Thomson A M. Sources of variation in menstrual blood loss. J Obstet Gynaecol Br Commonw 1971; 78: 933–939

23. Chimbira T H, Anderson A B, Turnbull A C. Relation between measured menstrual blood loss and patient's subjective assessment of loss, duration of bleeding, number of sanitary towels used, uterine weight and endometrial surface area. Br J Obstet Gynaecol 1980; 87: 603–609

24. Haynes P J, Hodgson H, Anderson A B, Turnbull A C. Measurement of menstrual blood loss in patients complaining of menorrhagia. Br J Obstet Gynaecol 1977; 84: 763–768

25. Fraser I S, McCarron G, Markham R. A preliminary study of factors influencing perception of menstrual blood loss volume. Am J Obstet Gynecol 1984; 149: 788–793

26. Hallberg L, Nilsson L. Determination of menstrual blood loss. Scand J Clin Lab Invest 1964; 16: 244–248

27. Newton J, Barnard G, Collins W. A rapid method for measuring menstrual blood loss using automatic extraction. Contraception 1977; 16: 269–285

28. Shaw S T, Aaronson D E, Moyer D L. Quantitation of menstrual blood loss. Further evaluation of the alkaline hematin method. Contraception 1972; 5: 497–513

29. van Eijkeren M A, Scholten P C, Christiaens G C et al. The alkaline hematin method for measuring menstrual blood loss — a modification and its clinical use in menorrhagia. Eur J Obstet Gynecol Reprod Biol 1986; 22: 345–351

30. Vasilenko P, Kraicer P F, Kaplan R et al. A new and simple method of measuring menstrual blood loss. J Reprod Med 1988; 33: 293–297

31. Gannon M J, Day P, Hammadieh N, Johnson N. A new method for measuring menstrual blood loss and its use in screening women before endometrial ablation. Br J Obstet Gynaecol 1996; 103: 1029–1033

32. Higham J M, O'Brien P M S, Shaw R W. Assessment of menstrual blood loss using a pictorial chart. Br J Obstet Gynaecol 1990; 97: 734–739

33. Deeny M, Davis J A. Assessment of menstrual blood loss in women referred for endometrial ablation. Eur J Obstet Gynecol Reprod Biol 1994; 57: 179–180

34. Janssen C A, Scholten P C, Heintz A P. A simple visual assessment technique to discriminate between menorrhagia and normal menstrual blood loss. Obstet Gynecol 1995; 85: 977–982

35. Pendergrass P B, Scott J N, Ream L J. A rapid non-invasive method for evaluation of total menstrual loss. Gynecol Obstet Invest 1984; 17: 174–178

36. Fraser I S, McCarron G, Markham R. Blood and total fluid content of menstrual discharge. Obstet Gynecol 1985; 65: 194–198

37. Baldwin R M, Whalley P J, Pritchard J A. Measurement of menstrual blood loss. Am J Obstet Gynecol 1961; 81: 739–742

38. Tauxe W N. Quantitation of menstrual blood loss: a radioactive method using a counting dome. J Nucl Med 1962; 3: 282–287

39. Krassas G E, Pontikides N, Kaltsas T et al. Menstrual disturbances in thyrotoxicosis. Clin Endocrinol 1994; 40: 641–644

40. Scott J C, Mussey E. Menstrual patterns of myxedema. Am J Obstet Gynecol 1964; 90: 161–165

41. Higham J M, Shaw R W. The effect of thyroxine replacement on menstrual blood loss in a hypothyroid patient. Br J Obstet Gynaecol 1992; 99: 695–696

42. Blum M, Blum G. The possible relationship between menorrhagia and occult hypothyroidism in IUD-wearing women. Adv Contracept 1992; 8: 313–317

43. Wilansky D L, Greisman B. Early hypothyroidism in patients with menorrhagia. Am J Obstet Gynecol 1989; 160: 673–677

44. U.S. Preventive Services Task Force. Report of the U.S. Preventive Service Task Force: Guide to clinical preventive services, 2nd edn. Baltimore: Williams and Wilkins, 1996: 209

45. Eldred J M, Thomas E J. Pituitary and ovarian hormone levels in unexplained menorrhagia. Obstet Gynecol 1994; 84: 775–778

46. Ben-Baruch G, Seidman E S, Shiff E et al. Outpatient endometrial sampling with the pipelle curette. Gynecol Obstet Invest 1994; 37: 260–262

47. Goldchmit R, Katz Z, Blickstein I et al. The accuracy of endometrial Pipelle sampling with and without sonographic measurement of endometrial thickness. Obstet Gynecol 1993; 82: 727–730

48. Stovall T G, Photopulos G J, Poston W N. Pipelle endometrial sampling in patients with known endometrial carcinoma. Obstet Gynecol 1991; 77: 954–956

49. Eddowes H. Pipelle: a more acceptable technique for outpatient endometrial biopsy. Br J Obstet Gynaecol 1990; 97: 961–962

50. Kaunitz A M, Masciello A, Ostrowski M, Rovira E Z. Comparison of endometrial biopsy with the endometrial Pipelle and Vabra aspirator. J Reprod Med 1988; 33: 427–431

51. Koonings P P, Moyer D L, Grimes D A. A randomized clinical trial comparing Pipelle and Tis-u-trap for endometrial biopsy. Obstet Gynecol 1990; 75: 293–295

52. Lipscomb G H, Lopatine S M, Stovall T G, Ling F W. A randomized comparison of the Pipelle, Accurette, and Explora endometrial sampling devices. Am J Obstet Gynecol 1994; 170: 591–594

53. Silver M M, Miles P, Rosa C. Comparison of Novak and Pipelle endometrial biopsy instruments. Obstet Gynecol 1991; 78: 828–830

54. Stovall T G, Ling F W, Morgan P L. A prospective, randomized comparison of the Pipelle endometrial sampling device with the Novak curette. Am J Obstet Gynecol 1991; 165: 1287–1290

55. Ferry J, Farnsworth A, Webster M, Wren B. The efficacy of the Pipelle endometrial biopsy in detecting endometrial carcinoma. Aust N Z J Obst Gynaecol 1993; 33: 76–78

56. Mettlin C, Jones G, Averette H et al. Defining and updating the American Cancer Society guidelines for the cancer-related checkup: prostate and endometrial cancers. CA 1993; 43: 42–46

57. Coulter A, Kelland J, Long A. The management of menorrhagia. Volume 9. Effect Health Care, 1995

58. Coulter A, Peto V, Doll H. Patients' preferences and general practitioners' decisions in the treatment of menstrual disorders. Fam Pract 1994; 11: 67–74

59. Milsom I, Andersson K, Andersch B, Rybo G. A comparison of flurbiprofen, tranexamic acid, and a levonorgestrel-releasing intrauterine contraceptive device in the treatment of idiopathic menorrhagia. Am J Obstet Gynecol 1991; 164: 879–883

60. Edlund M, Andersson K, Rybo G et al. Reduction of menstrual blood loss in women suffering from idiopathic menorrhagia with a novel antifibrinolytic drug (Kabi 2161). Br J Obstet Gynaecol 1995; 102: 913–917

61. Andersch B, Milsom I, Rybo G. An objective evaluation of flurbiprofen and tranexamic acid in the treatment of idiopathic menorrhagia. Acta Obstet Gynecol Scand 1988; 67: 645–648

62. Bonnar J, Sheppard B L. Treatment of menorrhagia during menstruation: randomised controlled trial of ethamsylate, mefenamic acid, and tranexamic acid. Br Med J 1996; 313: 579–582

63. Ylikorkala O, Viinikka L. Comparison between antifibrinolytic and antiprostaglandin treatment in the reduction of increased menstrual blood loss in women with intrauterine contraceptive devices. Br J Obstet Gynaecol 1983; 90: 78–83

64. Preston J T, Cameron I T, Adams E J, Smith S K. Comparative study of tranexamic acid and norethisterone in the treatment of ovulatory menorrhagia. Br J Obstet Gynaecol 1995; 102: 401–406

65. Rybo G. Tranexamic acid therapy is effective treatment in heavy menstrual bleeding: clinical update on safety. Ther Adv 1991; 4: 1–8

66. Dockeray C J, Sheppard B L, Bonnar J. Comparison between mefenamic acid and danazol in the treatment of established menorrhagia. Br J Obstet Gynaecol 1989; 96: 840–844

67. Hall P, Maclachlan N, Thorn N et al. Control of menorrhagia by the cyclo-oxygenase inhibitors naproxen sodium and mefenamic acid. Br J Obstet Gynaecol 1987; 94: 554–558

68. Fraser I S, Pearse C, Shearman R P et al. Efficacy of mefenamic acid in patients with a complaint of menorrhagia. Obstet Gynecol 1981; 58: 543–551

69. Fraser I S, McCarron G, Markham R et al. Long-term treatment of menorrhagia with mefenamic acid. Obstet Gynecol 1983; 61: 109–112

70. Shaw R W. Assessment of medical treatments for menorrhagia. Br J Obstet Gynecol 1994; 101 (suppl 11): 15–18

71. Mishell D R Jr. Noncontraceptive health benefits of oral steroidal contraceptives. Am J Obstet Gynecol 1982; 142: 809–816

72. Nilsson L, Rybo G. Treatment of menorrhagia. Am J Obstet Gynecol 1971; 110: 713–720

73. Fraser I S, McCarron G. Randomized trial of 2 hormonal and 2 prostaglandin-inhibiting agents in women with a complaint of menorrhagia. Aust N Z J Obstet Gynaecol 1991; 31: 66–70

74. Nilsson L, Solvell L. Clinical studies on oral contraceptives — a randomised, doubleblind crossover study of 4 different preparations. Acta Obstet Gynecol Scand 1967; 46(suppl 8): 1–31

75. Callard G V, Litofsky F S, DeMerre L J. Menstruation in women with normal or artificially controlled cycles. Fertil Steril 1966; 17: 684–688

76. Royal College of General Practitioners. Oral contraceptives and health. London: Pitman Medical, 1974

77. Ramcharan S, Pellegrin F A, Ray M R, Hsu J. The Walnut Creek Contraceptive Drug Study — A prospective study of the side effects of oral contraceptives. Volume III. An interim report: A comparison of disease occurrence leading to hospitalization or death in users and nonusers of oral contraceptives. J Reprod Med 1980; 25(suppl 6): 345–372

78. Gray R H. Patterns of bleeding associated with the use of steroidal contraceptives. In: Endometrial bleeding and steroidal contraception. Diczfalusy E, Fraser I S, Webb F T G (eds) Bath: Pitman Press, 1980: 14–49

79. Silverberg S G, Haukkamaa M, Arko H et al. Endometrial morphology during long-term use of levonorgestrel releasing intrauterine devices. Int J Gynecol Pathol 1986; 5: 235–241

80. Barbosa I, Bakos O, Olsson S E et al. Ovarian function during use of a levonorgestrel-releasing IUD. Contraception 1990; 42: 51–66

81. Luukkainen T, Toivonen J. Levonorgestrel-releasing IUD as a method of contraception with therapeutic properties. Contraception 1995; 52: 269–276

82. Nilsson C G, Lahteenmaki P, Luukkainen T. Ovarian function in amenorrheic and menstruating users of a levonorgestrel-releasing intrauterine device. Fertil Steril 1984; 41: 52–55

83. Luukkainen T. The levonorgestrel-releasing IUD. Br J Fam Plann 1993; 19: 221–224

84. Anon. Long-acting progestogen-only contraception. Drug Ther Bull 1996; 34: 93–96

85. Nilsson C G. Comparative quantitation of menstrual blood loss with a d-norgestrel-releasing IUD and a Nova-T-copper device. Contraception 1977; 15: 379–387

86. Andersson K, Batar I, Rybo G. Return to fertility after removal of a levonorgestrel-releasing intrauterine device and Nova-T. Contraception 1992; 46: 575–584

87. Andersson J K, Rybo G. Levonorgestrel-releasing intrauterine device in the treatment of menorrhagia. Br J Obstet Gynaecol 1990; 97: 690–694

88. Tang G W, Lo S S. Levonorgestrel intrauterine device in the treatment of menorrhagia in Chinese women: efficacy versus acceptability. Contraception 1995; 51: 231–235

89. Crosignani P G, Vercellini P, De Giorgi O et al. A levonorgestrel-releasing intrauterine device versus hysteroscopic endometrial resection in the treatment of dysfunctional uterine bleeding (abstr). Hum Reprod 1996; 11 (abstract bk 1). 9–10

90. Puolakka J, Nilsson C G, Haukkamaa M et al. Conservative treatment of excessive uterine bleeding and dysmenorrhoea with levonorgestrel intrauterine system as an alternative to hysterectomy. Acta Obstet Gynecol Scand 1996; 75 (suppl): 82

91. Barrington J W, Bowen-Simpkins P. The levonorgestrel intrauterine system in the management of menorrhagia. Br J Obstet Gynaecol 1997; 104: 614–616

92. Belsey E M. Vaginal bleeding patterns among women using one natural and eight hormonal methods of contraception. Contraception 1988; 38: 181–206

93. Schwallie P C, Assenzo J R. Contraceptive use–efficacy study utilizing Depo-Provera administered as an injection every 90 days. Fertil Steril 1973; 24: 331–342

94. Fraser I S. A survey of different approaches to management of menstrual disturbances in women using injectable contraceptives. Contraception 1983; 28: 385–397

95. Olsson S E. Contraception with subdermal implants releasing levonorgestrel. A clinical and pharmacological study. Acta Obstet Gynecol Scand 1987; supplement 142: 1–45

96. Andrade A T E, Pizarro Orchard. Quantitative studies on menstrual blood loss in IUD users. Contraception 1987; 36: 129–144

97. Shaw S T, Andrade A T, Souza J P et al. Quantitative menstrual and intermenstrual blood loss in women using Lippes loop and copper T intrauterine devices. Contraception 1980; 21: 343–352

98. Westrom L, Bengtsson L P. Effect of tranexamic acid (AMCA) in menorrhagia with intrauterine contraceptive devices. J Reprod Med 1970; 5: 154–161

99. Guillebaud J, Anderson A B, Turnbull A C. Reduction by mefenamic acid of increased menstrual blood loss associated with intrauterine contraception. Br J Obstet Gynaecol 1978; 85: 53–62

100. Roy S, Shaw S T. Role of prostaglandins in IUD-associated uterine bleeding — effect of a prostaglandin synthetase inhibitor (Ibuprofen). Obstet Gynecol 1981; 58: 101–106

101. Davies A J, Anderson A B, Turnbull A C. Reduction by naproxen of excessive menstrual bleeding in women using intrauterine devices. Obstet Gynecol 1981; 57: 74–78

102. Bishop P M F, Cabral de Almeida J C. Treatment of functional menstrual disorders with norethisterone. Br Med J 1960; 1: 1103–1105

103. Cameron I T, Leask R, Kelly R W, Baird D T. The effects of danazol, mefenamic acid, norethisterone and a progesterone-impregnated coil on endometrial prostaglandin concentrations in women with menorrhagia. Prostaglandins 1987; 34: 99–110

104. Higham J M, Shaw R W. A comparative study of danazol, a regimen of decreasing doses of danazol, and norethindrone in the treatment of objectively proven unexplained menorrhagia. Am J Obstet Gynecol 1993; 169: 1134–1139

105. Cameron I T, Haining R, Lumsden M A et al. The effects of mefenamic acid and norethisterone on measured menstrual blood loss. Obstet Gynecol 1990; 76: 85–88

106. Fraser I S. Treatment of ovulatory and anovulatory dysfunctional uterine bleeding with oral progestogens. Aus N Z J Obstet Gynaecol 1990; 30: 353–356

107. Chamberlain G, Freeman R, Price F et al. A comparative study of ethamsylate and mefenamic acid in dysfunctional uterine bleeding. Br J Obstet Gynaecol 1991; 98: 707–711

108. Harrison R F, Campbell S. A double-blind trial of ethamsylate in the treatment of primary and intrauterine-device menorrhagia. Lancet 1976; 2: 283–285

109. Kasonde J M. Effect of ethamsylate and aminocaproic acid on menstrual blood loss in women using intrauterine devices. Br Med J 1975; iv: 21–22

110. Turnbull A C, Rees M C. Gestrinone in the treatment of menorrhagia. Br J Obstet Gynaecol 1990; 97: 713–715

111. Fraser I S. Hysteroscopy and laparoscopy in women with menorrhagia. Am J Obstet Gynecol 1990; 162: 1264–1269

112. Gimpelson R J, Rappold H O. A comparative study between panoramic hysteroscopy with directed biopsies and dilatation and curettage. Am J Obstet Gynecol 1988; 158: 489–492

113. Jeppsson S, Mellquist P, Ranneisk G. Short term effects of danazol on endometrial histology. Acta Obstet Gynecol Scand 1984; 123: 41–44

114. Chimbira T H, Anderson A B, Naish C et al. Reduction of menstrual blood loss by danazol in unexplained menorrhagia: lack of effect of placebo. Br J Obstet Gynaecol 1980; 87: 1152–1158

115. Need J A, Forbes K L, Milazzo L, McKenzie E. Danazol in the treatment of menorrhagia: the effect of a 1 month induction dose (200 mg) and 2 month's maintenance therapy (200 mg, 100 mg, 50 mg or placebo). Aust N Z J Obstet Gynaecol 1992; 32: 346–352

116. Chimbira T H, Cope E, Anderson A B, Bolton F G. The effect of danazol on menorrhagia, coagulation mechanisms, haematological indices and body weight. Br J Obstet Gynaecol 1979; 86: 46–50

117. Stovall T G. Gonadotrophin-releasing hormone agonists: utilization before hysterectomy. Baillieres Clin Obstet Gynaecol 1993; 36: 642–649

118. Gardner R L, Shaw R W. LHRH analogues in the treatment of menorrhagia. In: Shaw R W (ed) Dysfunctional uterine bleeding. Carnforth: Parthenon Press, 1990: 149–159

119. Shaw R W, Fraser H M. Use of a superactive luteinizing hormone-releasing hormone (LHRH) agonist in the treatment of menorrhagia. Br J Obstet Gynaecol 1984; 91: 913–916

120. Miller R M, Frank R A. Zoladex (goserelin) in the treatment of benign gynaecological disorders: an overview of safety and efficacy. Br J Obstet Gynaecol 1992; 99(suppl 7): 37–41

121. Thomas E J, Okuda K J, Thomas N M. The combination of a depot gonadotrophin releasing hormone agonist and cyclical hormone replacement therapy for dysfunctional uterine bleeding. Br J Obstet Gynaecol 1991; 98: 1155–1159

CHAPTER 8

Management of women of perimenopausal age

S. S. Sheth and K. R. Damania

Introduction

Perimenopausal (Greek *peri*: around; *meniaia*: menstruation; *pause*: cessation) means 'around menopause' or 'around the cessation of menstruation'. It is well known that menopause occurs between 46 and 50 years of age; the perimenopausal age is thus often designated to be around 46–50 years.[1] Age of menopause depends on racial, nutritional and socio-economic factors. Bharadwaj et al.[2] found the age of menopause among Indian women to be 45.03 ± 5.17 years. Thus the perimenopausal age in these women would frequently be earlier than that of Western women.

Epidemiologically, Brambilla et al.[3] have defined perimenopause based on self-reported data of 1550 women aged between 45 and 55 years. The authors defined its inception as that period in a woman's menstrual history characterized by 3–11 months of amenorrhoea and increased menstrual irregularity for those without amenorrhoea. They described its cessation with the onset of menopause.

Endocrinologically, the perimenopausal woman is one whose hormonal features are characterized by lower levels of oestradiol (E_2), higher levels of follicle-stimulating hormone (FSH), with still-normal luteinizing hormone (LH) levels emphasizing the complexity of the hypothalamopituitary–ovarian regulating system.[4]

The boundaries of the perimenopausal period appears to last for about 4 years.[5] It is that transient phase in a woman's life when affective disorders may occur coincidentally or perimenopause itself may present as a non-specific stressor, precipitating an affective disorder.[6] Considering menorrhagia, both the aforementioned relationships could be true: coincidental leiomyomas or, rarely, even an abnormality of pregnancy, can occur to cause menorrhagia, or perimenopause itself with its peculiar altered menstrual physiology could precipitate menorrhagia (Table 8.1). Consultations among perimenopausal patients for menstrual irregularities could be as high as 69%.[7]

Evaluation today is often assisted by the technological advances of imaging sciences (endovaginal ultrasound and sonohysterography) with that of advanced hysteroscopic surgery. Better understanding of the pathophysiology has brought a shift from the traditional management of dilatation and curettage, often followed by hysterectomy, to a treatment protocol directed towards treating the appropriate cause of menorrhagia. Furthermore, many associated medical problems, such as hypertension or diabetes, could compound treatment in these patients. Management in the perimenopausal woman is thus often custom-made.

Table 8.1 Causes of menorrhagia in perimenopausal women

Type	Cause
Endocrine	DUB
	Thyroid dysfunction
	Adrenal disorders
	Metabolic disorders, including obesity
Pathological	Malignant and premalignant lesion of the uterus
	Adenomyosis
	Leiomyomas
	Endometrial polyps
	Ovarian tumours
	Rarely: • tuberculous endometritis
	• forgotten IUD
	• blood dyscrasias
	• abnormalities of pregnancy

DUB, dysfunctional uterine bleeding; IUD, intra-uterine device.

Pathophysiology of DUB in the perimenopause

Perimenopause starts with a phase of physiological transition characterized by a drop in oestrogen and progressive rise in FSH. The initial short luteal phase from a low follicular response to gonadotrophins among women still ovulating leads to low oestradiol levels and luteal defects.[4,8] The endometrium in this phase undergoes irregular shedding or ripening, leading to abnormal menstrual bleeds. Subsequently, a short luteal phase ensues with eventual aluteal cycles[9] from unopposed anovulation. This unopposed oestrogen stimulation leads to endometrial hyperplasia, leading to eventual loss of stromal support and bleeding.

Ovulatory menorrhagia from dysfunctional uterine bleeding (DUB) occurs in 15% of women whereas, in the remaining 85%, it is the result of anovulation.[9] After menopause, too, for a few years the ovary may produce small quantities of oestrogen. Extragonadal sources of oestrogen arise from conversion of androstenedione to oestrone.[10,11] This allows the endometrium to reach a threshold level but is not enough to produce the usual proliferative pattern; atrophic endometrium therefore results. This, too, could lead to annoying uterine haemorrhage.

Organic pathological causes

Organic pathologies occur to a greater extent in perimenopausal women and it is mandatory to exclude premalignant and malignant lesions, which are the foremost pathologies in this group of patients. Seltzer et al.[12] found that 19% of perimenopausal women with abnormal bleeding had premalignant or malignant lesions of the endometrium; 20% of women undergoing a hysterectomy for endometrial hyperplasia were found to have coexisting endometrial carcinoma.[13]

Adenomyosis, too, is a frequent cause of menorrhagia among perimenopausal women. However, it is difficult to diagnose accurately: in fact, only 48% of preoperative diagnoses were confirmed by histopathological study. In 360 cases diagnosed preoperatively as DUB, histopathological examination revealed adenomyosis in 236 (65.6%), in contrast to 48 (21.4%) proved to be DUB out of 224 diagnosed preoperatively as having adenomyosis (see Chapter 3). Adenomyosis is commonly found in women undergoing hysterectomy for DUB unresponsive to treatment.[14] Furthermore, 40% of women undergoing endometrial resection with a diagnosis of DUB have superficial adenomyosis.[15]

Leiomyomas are found to occur in about 20% of women above 35 years of age and 30% of these have abnormal uterine bleeding. Endometrial polyps are most frequently encountered in women of perimenopausal years and benign polyps can coexist with endometrial cancer in menopausal women.[16]

Rarely, even in perimenopausal women, tuberculous endometritis, a forgotten intra-uterine device (IUD), blood dyscrasias and abnormalities of early pregnancy can lead to abnormal uterine haemorrhage.

Obesity, which is frequently encountered among perimenopausal women, can be considered as an organic or endocrine-related cause of menorrhagia. Obesity induces hyperinsulinaemia; the insulin activates immunoglobulin (IG)F_1 and IGF_2 receptors, leading to increased production of androgens from ovarian stroma. The rise in androgens affects the local ovarian micro-environment and leads to anovulation, in addition to systemic effects of hyperandrogenism. The extent of aromatization increases with obesity, leading to oestrogen excess and subsequent endometrial hyperplasia.[17]

Evaluation

Assessment of blood loss is often subjective. What is often reported by the patient may not be a correct measure of menstrual loss: in fact, only 38% of women with subjective complaints of hypermenorrhoea were found actually to have excessive blood loss.[18,19] Often, passage of blood clots suggests heavy bleeding, as the fibrinolytic mechanisms are overwhelmed by the volume of bleeding. Pictorial charts, if reliably completed, have been found to be helpful in making a diagnosis objectively and monitoring treatment.[20]

The patient's history should be evaluated, bearing in mind medical disorders such as diabetes, thyroid disorders, liver or adrenal dysfunction, past treatments with drugs (including hormones) and previous contraceptive use. Other symptoms suggesting a decline in ovarian function, such as vasomotor symptoms, declining bone mass, urinogenital changes and psychosexual dysfunction should be inquired about. A physical examination should include examination of the breast (especially for discharge), thyroid enlargement or abdominal masses. A thorough pelvic inspection and evaluation must try to rule out organic causes of menorrhagia. Adenomyosis is best suspected in a perimenopausal woman with a history of severe dysmenorrhoea associated with a generalized enlarged uterus that is often tender during menses.

Diagnosis

If associated medical disorders or coagulopathy are suspected, then these must be first ruled out by an estimation of thyroid-stimulating hormone (TSH), serum prolactin, prothrombin time, partial thromboplastin time and platelets. Subsequent evaluation aims at ruling out a malignant or premalignant uterine lesion. The

Papanicolaou smear associated with colposcopy should be carried out in every perimenopausal patient to screen for cervical cancers.

Traditionally, dilatation and curettage (D&C) has been the 'gold standard' diagnostic aid in evaluating perimenopausal women with menorrhagia. However, the D&C often misses small focal pathologies, giving a false-negative rate of 10–15%.[21] The D&C, too, gives rise to problems of uterine perforation and infection, with a complication rate of around 2%.[21] Today, office endometrial sampling, which utilizes a disposable flexible Pipelle or simpler procedure, has been shown to be as accurate as the D&C in detecting intra-uterine pathologies; these techniques are well tolerated and are more cost effective.[22–24]

The advent of office hysteroscopy, with newer, smaller-diameter hysteroscopes requiring no dilatation or anaesthesia, has made direct inspection of the uterine cavity superior to blind endometrial curettage.[25,26]

Endovaginal ultrasonography, too, has been used to investigate patients with perimenopausal bleeding. Nasri et al.[27] reported that, if the endometrial thickness was less than 5 mm, histopathological examination would reveal either inactive or no endometrial tissue; if the endometrial thickness was greater than 8 mm, or if the interface between the endometrium and myometrium appeared truncated or not well delineated, a fractional curettage would be warranted.

Transvaginal sonography is particularly helpful in looking at endometrial thickness in postmenopausal women. In menopausal patients, an endometrial thickness of more than 4 mm in the absence of oestrogen or tamoxifen therapy requires investigation.[28] Any postmenopausal woman on oestrogen or tamoxifen with an endometrial thickness of 8–10 mm or more needs histopathological study; a thickness less than 4 mm means absence of cancer or hyperplasia.

Goldstein et al.[29] evaluated perimenopausal patients with abnormal uterine bleeding by an ultrasonographic-based triage. If a distinct endometrial echo of 5 mm or less (double layer) was imaged by endovaginal sonography on days 4–6 of the bleeding cycle, DUB was diagnosed; if the thickened endometrial echo was more than 5 mm or if no endometrial echo was reliably visualized, saline-infused sonohysterographic examination was performed: 13% of patients had focal polypoidal masses that were subsequently hysteroscopically removed and confirmed pathologically. These authors concluded that a non-directed office biopsy would have missed the diagnosis of focal lesions such as polyps, submucous myomas or focal hyperplasia in 18% of patients. Botsis et al.[30] found measurement of endometrial thickness with endovaginal ultrasonography better than Doppler velocimetry in discriminating between benign and malignant endometrium of the uterine arteries. Better results were obtained with the uterine artery resistance index than with pulsatility index in detecting malignant endometrial changes.

Reinhold et al.[31] evaluated the role of endovaginal sonography in the diagnosis of adenomyosis. Adenomyosis was correctly identified in 25 of 29 pathologically proved cases of adenomyosis, with a positive predictive value of 71%; it also correctly ruled out adenomyosis in 61 of 71 patients, with a negative predictive value of 86%. Adenomyosis was diagnosed when the myometrium demonstrated heterogeneous and hypoechoic areas with or without the presence of cysts (84%), hypoechoic areas with cysts (12%) and heterogeneous areas within the myometrium (4%). Brosens et al.[32] also evaluated the diagnosis of adenomyosis by endovaginal ultrasound and found that uterine measurements alone were not

Table 8.2 Perimenopausal women at high risk of malignancy

Site of malignancy	Risk factor
Uterine corpus	• Long-term history suggestive of oligo-ovulation or anovulation • Unopposed oestrogen stimulation • Persistent intermenstrual or postcoital bleeding • Obese, diabetic or hypertensive patient • Family history of endometrial carcinoma
Ovary	• Early menarche or late menopause • Increased ovulatory age (number of years spent menstruating less than those years pregnant or having ovulation suppressed) • Genetic predisposition • Diet of high quantity of fibre or Vitamin A • Perineal use of talc with asbestos particles

significant in making a diagnosis: ill-defined myometrial echogenicity was the best predictor of adenomyosis.

Thus, in most perimenopausal patients with menorrhagia, an accurate diagnosis can be made by office endometrial sampling supplemented by either hysteroscopy or endovaginal ultrasonography. The combined use of hysteroscopy and endometrial sampling leads to a near-100% accuracy in the diagnosis of endometrial neoplasia and its precursors.[33] This is the protocol recommended most often to rule out malignancy and arrive at a diagnosis as to the cause of menorrhagia. In centres where the level of competence in endovaginal sonography is high, a combination of Pipelle aspiration with ultrasonographic endometrial thickness of 5 mm or less[34] could well be used. If these show conflicting results or are inconclusive, or if adequate samples cannot be obtained, or if the patient has a high risk factor for malignancy of the uterine corpus (Table 8.2), it is best that she should undergo hysteroscopy and conventional fractional curettage. Patients at risk of ovarian malignancy (Table 8.2) should undergo screening for the same, with tumour markers such as CA125 and sonographic evaluation of the ovaries.

Treatment

General principles of management should include the following:

1. Search and treat organic reproductive or systemic disease;
2. If the cause thus identified is dysfunctional, document the functional defect;
3. Individualize treatment modality according to severity and nature of underlying endometrial defect.

Current treatments opt for a more conservative approach to surgery, even in the perimenopausal patient. Decisions as to medical or surgical modality, minimally invasive treatment or hysterectomy, depend on the pathology, failure of previous treatment, side effects and acceptability to the patient. Explanations and counselling regarding advantages, disadvantages and expectations of cure can make patient decisions easier. In certain cases, as in leiomyomas, premalignant or malignant lesions, the treatment options are in the form of clear-cut recommendations. However, where organic pathology does not exist (especially in DUB), offering a particular regimen by the physician should take into account factors such as the patient's education and compliance, and treatment acceptability. Consideration that physiological menopause is just around the corner should also be borne in mind; in such cases, a trial of medical management for 4–6 months should be carried out before resorting to surgical options. Lynestrenol or norethisterone with haematinics for 3–4 weeks will prepare an anaemic patient to undergo major surgery.

Medical options

For patients opting to await spontaneous menopause, reassurance and treatment with medical drugs can tide over this transitional period.

Progestin therapy has been considered the mainstay treatment for menstrual disorders. Such drugs bring about pseudodecidualization of the oestrogen-primed endometrium. However, anovulatory bleeds accompanied by their low levels of oestrogen in the perimenopause may not be helped by progestins alone. These patients can be treated by cyclic use of conjugated oestrogen (CE) (0.625 or 1.25 mg) given for 25 days, with medroxyprogesterone acetate added to CE from day 15 to day 25. The conjugated oestrogen will also relieve the patient of other perimenopausal symptoms related to low oestrogen.[35] Prolonged progestogen therapy can be used to treat the more refractory ovulatory bleeds. A 19-nortestosterone derivative such as lynestrenol (5 mg/day) from day 5 to day 25 of the cycle is helpful: the androgenic effect of 19-nortestosterone derivatives has a more atrophic effect on the endometrium.

The use of the oral contraceptive pill (OCP) in the perimenopause has been restricted to temporary management. With the availability of low-dose OCPs, the risk of developing myocardial infarcts has abated especially in low-risk women. The OCP is an effective option for decreasing the frequency of DUB. The menstrual blood flow is reduced by 60%.[36] The OCP also provides effective contraception right through to menopause and, at a time in perimenopausal years when ovulation is unpredictable, it avoids the risk of an unplanned pregnancy. The OCP has other advantages — a reduced risk of ovarian/endometrial cancers and protection against endometriosis and benign breast disease; also noted is higher bone density, which may be protective against future osteoporosis.[37]

Slow-release progesterone-medicated intra-uterine devices such as the levonorgestrel-releasing intra-uterine device (LNG–IUD) have been shown to reduce blood loss in 97% of patients at one year of use.[38] The device was effective and acceptable amongst Chinese perimenopausal women, who preferred the device to a hysterectomy:[39] the device could help them through to menopause without having to undergo surgery. If, subsequently, these menopausal women decide to take hormone replacement therapy in the form of oestrogen replacement, the device can offer local endometrial protection. However, discontinuation due to menstrual irregularities among Indian IUD users was highest with the LNG–IUD than with other types of IUD, indicating that acceptability may not be universal.[40]

In a patient at high risk from surgery or hormonal management, medical treatments in the form of non-steroidal anti-inflammatory agents (NSAIDs) such as mefenamic acid, or antifibrinolytics such as epsilon-aminocaproic acid (EACA) can be tried. Short-term relief can be obtained from gonadotrophin-releasing hormone (GnRH) agonist and danazol. Their side-effect profiles and cost are the main reasons why these agents are utilized only for short-term relief; they are poor choices for chronic treatment, owing to postmenopausal side effects of bone demineralization and altered lipid profile that raise coronary artery disease risk. Danazol therapy is a good treatment, especially in low doses of 100–200 mg daily, for 3-month periods; the effect usually carries over for an additional 3–6 months. This is particularly useful for patients over the age of 47 who are perimenopausal.[41]

Surgical options

The D&C and/or hysterectomy have been the standard surgical options for treatment of menorrhagia. Today, the focus is towards minimal invasive options: their advantages of reduced morbidity, shorter hospital stay and the ensuing satisfaction from rapid recovery and return to normal activities, makes these procedures popular amongst women keen to preserve their uterus. These factors, coupled with a 90% chance of improvement in symptoms, have made these procedures an acceptable alternative to hysterectomy.[42] The type of surgical option depends on the doctor's training, his confidence and ease at performing the procedure and his personal conviction about its merits.

The D&C is still the most rapid way to stop a torrential haemorrhage and provide relief from profuse bleeding, especially if the patient is becoming hypovolaemic. It does not usually prevent the recurrence of excessive uterine bleeding unless it is followed by additional hormonal management.[43] The therapeutic efficacy of the D&C is in subsequent regeneration of new endometrium under hormonal influence and its ability to remove foci of endometrial polyps.

The hysterectomy has the advantage of a one-time cure and often ensures patient satisfaction.[44] Hysterectomy is the first choice in the presence of leiomyoma or premalignant lesions (complex or atypical hyperplasia). It is often undertaken in cases of DUB after medical treatments have failed or adenomyosis is strongly suspected. Coexisting symptomatology such as pelvic pain, dysmenorrhoea, premenstrual syndrome (PMS) or prolapse may alter the patient's preference towards hysterectomy.[45] The presence of associated high-grade cervical intra-epithelial neoplasia (high CIN) in a perimenopausal woman with menorrhagia is also an indication for hysterectomy.[45] Preservation of the uterus needs consideration, even in the absence of adnexa, in these days of oöcyte donation programmes; this can help a woman who has plans of future marriage.

Today, there is little doubt that a vaginal hysterectomy (VH) is the easiest, quickest and safest method of removing the uterus.[46] An experienced vaginal surgeon does not usually contradict VH when the uterus size is up to 12–14 weeks. Oöphorectomy is often performed in perimenopausal patients, especially in those at risk of ovarian cancers (Table 8.1). This avoids the risk of development of a subsequent ovarian malignancy. Oöphorectomy performed vaginally would not pose a problem for the experienced surgeon;[46] however, if technical problems occur, there should be no hesitation in undertaking laparoscopic assistance. If, however, the uterus is enlarged beyond a size when the concerned surgeon would find a VH technically difficult, or there are associated pathologies such as large leiomyomas or tubovarian masses or malignancies, laparoscopically assisted vaginal hysterectomy (LAVH) or an exploratory laparotomy with appropriate surgical procedure would be correct.

Laparoscopy has demonstrated unequivocally the superiority of the vaginal route over the abdominal route by reducing the latter and promoting the former. LAVH is designed to replace or reduce the number of abdominal hysterectomies. A study of VH, total abdominal hysterectomy (TAH) and LAVH procedures[47] resulted in higher scores on tests in favour of VH, which conferred a better postoperative quality of life, and postoperative outcomes, and earlier recovery.

Subtotal hysterectomy has a place only when (a) the surgical situation indicates it (e.g. the patient's condition at surgery or inseparable adhesions), or (b) when a woman insists on retaining her cervix.

Minimally invasive options such as transcervical resection of the endometrium (TCRE), performed by using an electrocautery loop/roller ball/laser,[48,49] radiofrequency ablation[50] or thermal balloon endometrial ablation,[51] have all come into vogue with their earlier-mentioned advantages. Success rates of 85–90% in alleviating symptoms makes them alternatives to hysterectomy — especially in women at anaesthetic risk, as these procedures can be performed even under local anaesthesia. Procedures such as thermal ablation, with their sophisticated yet costly ancillaries, require less expertise than TCRE and would be preferred by physicians not well versed in the same. Thermal balloon endometrial ablation appears to be safe as well as effective in properly selected women with menorrhagia, and is potentially an outpatient procedure, thus reducing the cost and increasing the convenience.[52]

Conclusions

In the perimenopausal years, disruption of normal menstrual patterns is associated with a high incidence of pelvic pathologies, especially malignancies. It is, therefore, imperative that the gynaecologist should use the latest tools available to identify the cause and arrive at an accurate diagnosis; only then will treatment be successful and rewarding. Technological advances have given a far wider range of therapeutic options than those that were available in the past. To choose wisely and appropriately will be the physician's responsibility; to offer a wide variety of treatments, while explaining their relative merits, constitutes the physician's duty to each individual patient. In every case, treatment should be on the basis of clinical findings and on the patient's compliance to the treatment offered, and it should provide the best quality of life thereafter.

References

1. Agnew L R C, Avialdo D M, Brody J I et al. (eds) Dorland's illustrated medical dictionary, 24th edn. Philadelphia: Saunders, 1965: 898
2. Bharadwaj J A, Kendurkar S M, Vaidya P R. Age and symptomatology of menopause in Indian women. J Postgrad Med 1983; 29: 218–222
3. Brambilla D J, McKinlay S M, Johannes C B. Defining the perimenopause for application in epidemiologic investigations. Am J Epidemiol 1994; 140: 1091–1095
4. Sherman B M, West J H, Korenman S G. The menopausal transition: analysis of LH, FSH, estradiol and progesterone concentrations during menstrual cycles of older women. J Clin Endocrinol Metab 1976; 42: 629–636

5. McKinlay S M, Brambilla D J, Posner J G. The normal menopause transition. Am J Hum Biol 1992; 4: 37–46

6. Schmidt P, Rubinow D R. Mood and the perimenopause. Contemp Ob Gyn — The Healthy Woman 1993, 34: 68–75

7. Mencaglia L, Perino A, Hamou J. Hysteroscopy in perimenopausal and postmenopausal women with abnormal uterine bleeding. J Reprod Med 1987; 32: 577–582

8. Lenton E A, Landgren B M, Sexton L et al. Normal variation in the length of the follicular phase of the menstrual cycle: effect of chronologic age. Br J Obstet Gynaecol 1984; 91: 681–684

9. Awwad J T, Toth T I, Schiff I. Abnormal uterine bleeding in the perimenopause. Int J Fertil 1993; 38: 261–269

10. Richards-Kustan C J, Kase N G. Diagnosis and management of perimenopausal and postmenopausal bleeding. J Obstet Gynecol Clin North Am 1987; 14: 169–189

11. Vermeulen A. The hormonal activity of the postmenopausal ovary. J Clin Endocrinol Metab 1976; 42: 247–253

12. Seltzer V L, Benjamin F, Deutsch S. Perimenopausal bleeding patterns and pathologic findings. J Am Med Womens Assoc 1990; 45: 132–134

13. Gusberg S B, Kaplan A L. Precursors of corpus cancer. Am J Obstet Gynecol 1963; 87: 662–676

14. Lee N C, Dicker R C, Rubin G L et al. Confirmation of the preoperative diagnosis for hysterectomy. Am J Obstet Gynecol 1984; 150: 283–287

15. Fraser I S. Menorrhagia — a pragmatic approach to the understanding of the causes and the need for investigations. Br J Obstet Gynaecol 1994; 101(suppl 11): 3–7

16. Jutras M C, Cowan B D. Abnormal bleeding in the climacteric. J Obstet Gynecol Clin North Am 1990; 17: 409–425

17. MacDonald P C, Edman C D, Hemsell D L et al. Effect of obesity on conversion of plasma androstenedione to estrone in postmenopausal women with and without endometrial cancer. Am J Obstet Gynecol 1978; 130: 448–455

18. Chimbira T M, Anderson A B M, Turnbull A C. Relation between measured blood loss and patient's subjective assessment of loss, duration of bleeding, number of sanitary towels used, uterine weight and endometrial surface area. Br J Obstet Gynaecol 1980; 87: 603–609

19. Fraser I S, McCarron G, Markham R. A preliminary study of factors influencing perception of menstrual blood loss volume. Am J Obstet Gynecol 1984; 149: 788–793

20. Higham J M, O'Brien P M S, Shaw R W. Assessment of menstrual blood loss using a pictorial chart. Br J Obstet Gynaecol 1990; 97: 734–739

21. Preston J T, Smith S K. Investigation of menorrhagia. Curr Obstet Gynecol 1992; 2: 129–135

22. Stovall T G, Photopulos G J, Poston W M et al. Pipelle endometrial sampling in patients with known endometrial carcinoma. Obstet Gynecol 1991; 77: 954–956

23. Ben-Baruch G, Seidman D S, Schiff E et al. Outpatient endometrial sampling with the Pipelle curette. Gynecol Obstet Invest 1994; 37: 260–262

24. Ong S, Duff T, Lenehan P et al. Endometrial pipelle biopsy compared to conventional dilatation and curettage. Ir J Med Sci 1997; 166: 47–49

25. Burnett J E. Hysteroscopy controlled curettage for endometrial polyps. Obstet Gynecol 1964; 24: 621–625

26. Gimpleson R J, Rappold H O. A comparative study between panoramic hysteroscopy of 276 cases with directed biopsies and dilatation and curettage. Am J Obstet Gynecol 1988; 158: 489–492

27. Nasri M N, Shepherd J H, Setchell M E. The role of vaginal scan in measurement of endometrial thickness in postmenopausal women. Br J Obstet Gynaecol 1991; 98: 470–475

28. Goldstein S R, Nachtigall M, Synder J R et al. Endometrial assessment by vaginal ultrasonography before endometrial sampling in patients with postmenopausal bleeding. Am J Obstet Gynecol 1990; 163: 119–123

29. Goldstein S R, Zeltser I, Hovan C K. Ultrasonography based triage for perimenopausal patients with abnormal uterine bleeding. Am J Obstet Gynecol 1977; 177: 102–108

30. Botsis D, Kassanos D, Antonion G et al. Endometrial thickness and Doppler velocimetry in women with peri- and postmenopausal bleeding, before endometrial sampling. Eur Menopause J 1996; 3: 42–46

31. Reinhold C, Atri M, Mehio A et al. Diffuse uterine adenomyosis: morphologic criteria and diagnostic accuracy of endovaginal sonography. Radiology 1995; 197: 609–614

32. Brosens J J, de Souza N M, Barker F G et al. Endovaginal ultrasonography in the diagnosis of adenomyosis uteri: identifying the predictive characteristics. Br J Obstet Gynaecol 1995; 102: 471–474

33. Mencaglia L. Hysteroscopy and adenocarcinoma. Obstet Gynecol Clin North Am 1995; 22: 573–579

34. Goldchmit R, Katz Z, Blickstein I et al. The accuracy of endometrial Pipelle sampling with and without sonographic measurement of endometrial thickness. Obstet Gynecol 1993; 82: 727–730

35. Mishell D R. Abnormal uterine bleeding. In: Herbst A L, Mishell D R, Stenchever M A, Droegemueller W (eds) Comprehensive gynecology, 2nd edn. St Louis: Mosby Year Book, 1992: 1079–1100

36. Nilsson L, Rybo G. Treatment of menorrhagia. Am J Obstet Gynecol 1971; 110: 713–720

37. Enzelsberger H, Metka M, Heytmanck G. Influence of oral contraceptive use on bone density in climacteric women. Maturitas 1988; 9: 375–378

38. Andersson J K, Rybo G. Levonorgestrel releasing intrauterine device in the treatment of menorrhagia. Br J Obstet Gynaecol 1990; 97: 690–694

39. Tang G W, Lo S S. Levonorgestrel intrauterine device in the treatment of menorrhagia in Chinese women: efficacy versus acceptability. Contraception 1995; 51: 231–235

40. Baveja R, Bichille L K, Coyaji K J et al. Randomized clinical trial with intrauterine devices (levonorgestrel intrauterine device (Lng), CuT 380Ag, CuT 220C and CuT 200B) — a 36 month study. Contraception 1989; 39: 37–52

41. Shah A A, Grainger D A. Contemporary concepts in managing menorrhagia. Medscape Women's Health 1996; 1: 12

42. Magos A L. Evaluation of endometrial ablation as an alternative to hysterectomy. In: Expert perspectives in menorrhagia. Worthing, W. Sussex: Cambridge Medical, 1992: 15–21

43. Chuong C J Management of abnormal uterine bleeding. Am J Obstet Gynecol 1996; 175: 787–792

44. Carlson K J, Miller B A, Fowler F J. The Maine Women's Health Study: II Outcomes of nonsurgical management of leiomyomas, abnormal bleeding and chronic pelvic pain. Obstet Gynecol 1994; 83: 566–572

45. Phipps J H. The place of hysterectomy in the management of menorrhagia. Curr Obstet Gynecol 1992; 2: 146–148

46. Sheth S S. Vaginal hysterectomy. In: Studd J (ed) Progress in obstetrics and gynecology, 10th edn. London: Churchill Livingstone, 1993: 317–340

47. Van Den Eeden S K, Glasser M, Mathias S D et al. Quality of life, health care utilization and costs among women undergoing hysterectomy in a managed care setting. Am J Obstet Gynecol 1998; 178: 91–110

48. Magos A L, Baumann R, Turnbull A C et al. Transcervical resection of endometrium in women with menorrhagia. Br Med J 1989; 298: 1209–1212

49. Goldrath M H, Fuller T A, Segal S. Laser photovaporization of endometrium for the treatment of menorrhagia. Am J Obstet Gynecol 1981; 140: 14–19

50. Phipp J H, Lewis B V, Roberts T. Treatment of functional menorrhagia by radiofrequency induced thermal endometrial ablation. Lancet 1990; 335: 374–376

51. Vilos G A, Fortin C A, Sanders B et al. Clinical trial of the uterine balloon for treatment of menorrhagia. J Am Assoc Gynecol Laparosc 1997; 4: 559–565

52. Amso N N, Seth S A, McFraul P et al. Uterine thermal balloon therapy for the treatment of menorrhagia: the first 300 patients from a multicentric study. Br J Obstet Gynaecol 1998; 105: 517–523

CHAPTER 9

Place of intra-uterine delivery of progestogen and progesterone

N. Panay and J. Studd

Introduction

The recent government-funded Effective Health Care Bulletin entitled *The Management of Menorrhagia* states that data from Scandinavia point to the effectiveness of the hormone-releasing intra-uterine device as a first-line treatment for menorrhagia.[1] This chapter describes how the progestogen and progesterone intra-uterine systems have at last provided the physician with a medical treatment for menorrhagia that is a truly effective long-term alternative to hysterectomy. The systems can also be used in hormone replacement therapy (HRT) regimens to minimize bleeding and adverse progestogenic effects, thus maximizing compliance. In addition, there is evidence that dysmenorrhoea may be improved, pelvic inflammatory disease (PID) and ectopic rates reduced and fibroid growth inhibited. Of course, there is no such thing as the universal panacea and the systems are not without their problems, such as initial cost, occasional difficulty in insertion and continued bleeding problems in some users. However, the authors wish to show that the benefit–risk ratio is such that almost every patient should be offered the option of an intra-uterine system before hysterectomy is undertaken.

Structure and mechanism of action of intra-uterine systems

Structure

Two intra-uterine systems are currently in use. The system currently licensed in the United Kingdom for contraception is the levonorgestrel intra-uterine system, Mirena (LNG–IUS), which consists of a plastic T-shaped frame with a steroid reservoir around the vertical stem of polydimethylsiloxane (Fig. 9.1). The stem contains 52 mg levonorgestrel, the laevo-isomer of norgestrel, derived from the 19 nortestosterone progestogens (Fig. 9.2), released at a rate of 20 µg/day. The Progestasert intra-uterine progesterone system (PIPS) (Fig. 9.1) is not yet licensed in the United Kingdom but is being used in phase III trials. It consists of a polymeric T-shaped platform with a reservoir containing 38 mg progesterone released at a rate of 65 µg/day. The total quantity of progesterone contained in one Progestasert system is less than the amount produced in one day by the corpus luteum during the latter part of the menstrual cycle. The drug is distributed in silicone (polydimethylsiloxane) fluid in both systems with a rate-limiting membrane allowing slow diffusion of the drug into the endometrium (Fig. 9.3).[2] Both frames are rendered radio-opaque by impregnated barium sulphate. The LNG–IUS is currently licensed for contraception for 3 years but there are data for

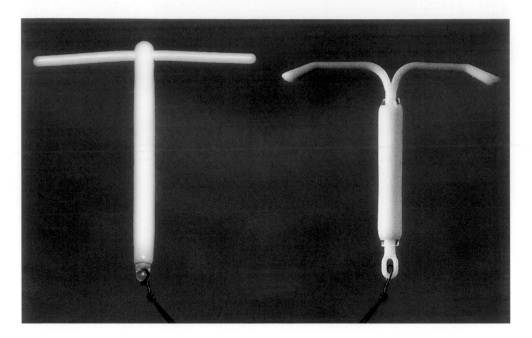

Figure 9.1 Progesterone-releasing (left) and levonorgestrel-releasing (right) intra-uterine systems.

7-year bioavailability; the PIPS is licensed in the United States for 1 year's usage with up to 2-year bioavailability.

Endometrial effects

The effect of all progestogens on the endometrium is mediated via a decrease in oestrogen receptors and an increase in the 17α-oxoreductase activity that converts oestradiol to oestrone. Progestogens inhibit mitotic activity, as evidenced by the decrease in number of mitoses in both the glandular epithelium and stroma; they also induce the secretory transformation. In women using oestrogen therapy, the incidence of hyperplasia is reduced to 4% with 7 days of oral progestogen and 0% with 12 days of oral progestogen if it is prescribed at an adequate daily dosage.[3,4] Although the effect of progestogen is protective to the endometrium in a dose- and duration-dependent manner, the exact relationship remains largely unknown because of considerable interindividual variability,[5] complex oestrogen/progestogen interactions[6] and the absence of an appropriate animal model. This would explain why some patients experience problems with heavy, prolonged periods and endometrial hyperplasia where the same duration, dose and type of progestogen would produce atrophy in another patient.

The LNG–IUS has been shown to be effective at controlling endometrial hypertrophy by suppressing endometrial growth. After a few weeks the endometrial glands atrophy, the stroma becomes swollen and decidual, the mucosa thins and the epithelium becomes inactive. There is also suppression of spiral arterioles, capillary thrombosis and a local inflammatory response.[7] As a result of the suppression caused by the local release of hormone, also mediated by the regulatory action of high local levels of progestogen on endometrial oestrogen receptors,[8] the endometrium becomes unresponsive to oestrogen with no menstrual shedding. It has also been shown that there is no effect on endometrial endothelial factor VIII activity, which is reduced by ordinary coils, leading to a bleeding tendency.[9] The

Figure 9.2 Chemical classification of progestogens.

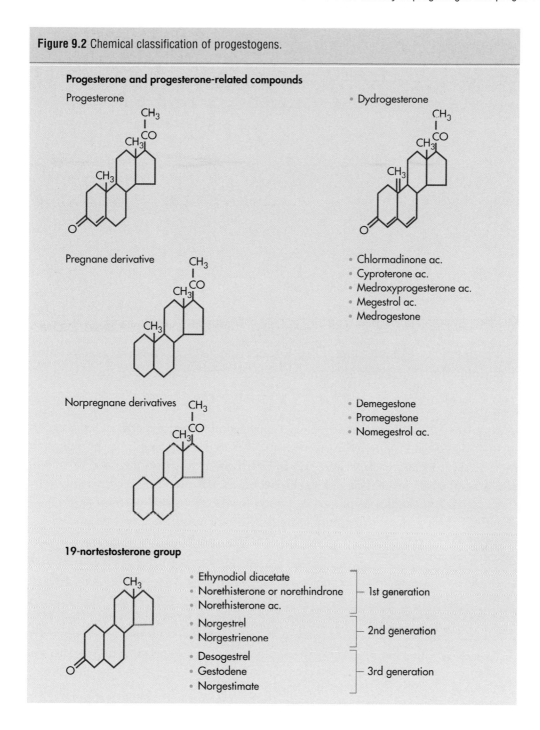

Progesterone and progesterone-related compounds

Progesterone

• Dydrogesterone

Pregnane derivative

• Chlormadinone ac.
• Cyproterone ac.
• Medroxyprogesterone ac.
• Megestrol ac.
• Medrogestone

Norpregnane derivatives

• Demegestone
• Promegestone
• Nomegestrol ac.

19-nortestosterone group

• Ethynodiol diacetate
• Norethisterone or norethindrone   — 1st generation
• Norethisterone ac.

• Norgestrel
• Norgestrienone   — 2nd generation

• Desogestrel
• Gestodene   — 3rd generation
• Norgestimate

endometrial changes are uniform within three cycles after insertion of the system,[8] with no further histological development over the long term.[10] After removal of the system, the morphological changes in the endometrium return to normal and menstruation returns within 30 days.[11]

Endometrial suppression with decidual transformation is also the main mechanism of action with the PIPS, with equally rapid return to normal of the morphological changes.[12] The PIPS has been shown to be effective at controlling endometrial hypertrophy by suppressing endometrial growth,[13–15] and can be even used to treat endometrial hyperplasia.[16] Endometrial biopsy studies indicate that continuous application of progesterone to the uterus results in changes indicative

Figure 9.3 Delivery of levonorgestrel from an intra-uterine system to the uterine wall. (Adapted from ref. 2.)

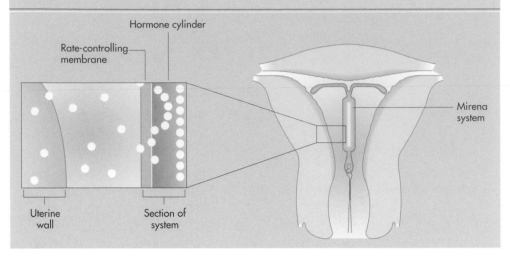

of an inactive endometrium. The changes appear to reverse rapidly after discontinuation. No cellular abnormalities were attributed to use of the system.[17]

Ovulation

During the first year of LNG–IUS use some women may experience changes in ovarian function, but after this women usually have completely normal ovulatory cycles.[18] Menstrual bleeding does not reflect ovarian function, average oestradiol and progesterone levels being the same in amenorrhoeic and menstruating users (Table 9.1).[19,20] Studies of plasma hormone levels, menstrual patterns and blood chemistry in various patient groups using the PIPS demonstrated no systemic effects of the system, even on the progesterone-sensitive hypothalamic–pituitary–ovarian axis.[21,22]

Pharmacokinetics

Plasma concentrations achieved by the LNG–IUS are lower than those seen with the LNG implant, combined oral contraceptive or minipill[23–26] (Fig. 9.4).

Table 9.1 Mean plasma 17β-oestradiol (E2) and levonorgestrel (LNG) concentrations in menstruating and amenorrhoeic women using the LNG–IUS*

Patient status	Plasma concentration (pg/ml)	
	E2	LNG
Menstruating	103.9 (n = 66)	175.2 (n = 62)
Amenorrhoeic	132.7 (n = 20)	179.9 (n = 20)

*LNG–IUS, levonorgestrel intra-uterine system. (Adapted from ref. 19.)

Although there is marked interindividual variation in serum levonorgestrel levels (1–200 pg/ml), the serum and endometrial levels remain stable for 6–7 years. Also, the levels with the LNG–IUS, unlike the oral contraceptives, do not display peaks and troughs. Endometrial concentrations after 6 years are still in excess of the capacity of the local progesterone receptors.

Results of studies with baboons show that intra-uterine systems delivering 65 μg/day of labelled progesterone do not produce detectable changes in concentrations of circulating progesterone. Progesterone released by the system is quickly metabolized to steroid intermediates. Unlike the metabolites of synthetic analogues, progesterone catabolites have little or no endocrine function and do not accumulate in the tissues.

Premenopausal bleeding problems and hysterectomy

Until recent years, only a small range of medical treatments were available for menorrhagia, of limited or no benefit, usually failing and leaving no option between putting up with the symptoms and hysterectomy. Most hysterectomies are performed for benign reasons, usually for intractable menorrhagia and pain where medical therapy has failed. For a while there was optimism that the hysterectomy rate could be dramatically reduced by resection or ablation of the endometrium, but enthusiasm waned when it was realized that the procedures were not without their own complications: bleeding disorders returned in over one-third of cases, often necessitating hysterectomy to solve the problem, and women wishing to use oestrogen therapy still required progestogenic opposition.

There is now enthusiasm that the hysterectomy rate can be reduced with hormone-releasing intra-uterine systems, which originally were developed for use as contraceptives. It was subsequently realized that these systems could dramatically reduce the amount of blood loss and lead to amenorrhoea in a substantial number

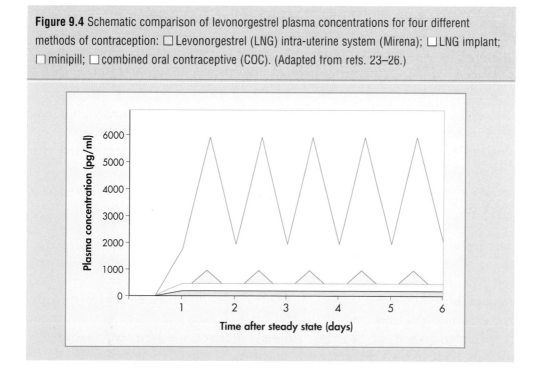

Figure 9.4 Schematic comparison of levonorgestrel plasma concentrations for four different methods of contraception: ☐ Levonorgestrel (LNG) intra-uterine system (Mirena); ☐ LNG implant; ☐ minipill; ☐ combined oral contraceptive (COC). (Adapted from refs. 23–26.)

of cases. The intra-uterine systems have been shown to be highly effective in reducing menstrual loss in premenopausal women. In a study by Andersson and Rybo,[27] menstrual loss was significantly reduced in women with dysfunctional menorrhagia (> 80 ml loss per period). After 3 months' usage of the LNG–IUS there was an 85% reduction in menstrual loss, and a 97% reduction after 12 months, as measured by extraction of blood. There was a significant increase in serum ferritin in the first year of use. At the end of the first year, 35% of women were amenorrhoeic. In a more recently reported study by Andersson et al.,[28] it was shown that haemoglobin concentrations increased as a result of the reduction in menstrual loss produced by the LNG–IUS, thus demonstrating another positive health benefit for the system. The progesterone-releasing system has also been shown to reduce menstrual blood loss,[29] but not to the same extent as the LNG–IUS (65% reduction, 12 months after insertion).

A reduction in menstrual loss brought about by the LNG–IUS was also demonstrated by Barrington and Bowen-Simpkins[30] in a group of 50 women in whom medical therapy had failed and who were awaiting hysterectomy or transcervical resection of the endometrium. The treatment was so effective that it was possible to take 41 of these women off the waiting list — i.e. 82% were able to avoid major surgery. In another prospective study of 54 women on the waiting list for hysterectomy for menorrhagia, 67% came off the waiting list because they were satisfied with their treatment, compared with only 15% of those on medical therapy.[31]

The reduction in menstrual blood loss with the hormone-releasing intra-uterine systems is far superior to anything achieved with medical treatments such as the prostaglandin inhibitors and the anti-fibrinolytics, which at very best reduce blood loss by 50%.[1] Although amenorrhoea can be achieved with the gonadotrophin-releasing analogues and danazol, their side effects and risks associated with a long-term hypo-oestrogenic state make them unacceptable for long-term usage.

Although the hormone-releasing systems are not, strictly speaking, licensed for treatment of menorrhagia, there is no reason why a premenopausal non-sterilized woman could not be given the LNG–IUS for contraception, which, coincidentally, might have a beneficial effect on her heavy periods. Also, a large and ever-growing number of gynaecologists and general practitioners are using the LNG–IUS on a 'named patient basis' for non-contraceptive indications such as menorrhagia and as progestogenic opposition to oestrogen therapy. It is important to note that it is legal for a practitioner to prescribe an unlicensed product to a fully informed and consenting patient if he/she is adopting a practice that would be endorsed by a responsible body of professional opinion.[32] However, the authors look forward to the day when the hormone systems can be officially registered for indications for which they are already known to be of benefit.

Dysmenorrhoea

There is evidence that other gynaecological conditions that could necessitate hysterectomy are resolved by the intra-uterine systems. Both Sivin and Stern[33] and Barrington and Bowen-Simpkins[30] reported that, in their groups of patients, dysmenorrhoea was alleviated by the LNG–IUS: 80% of patients had improvement in the latter study group. The mechanism of action could be a combination of a relaxant effect on the uterine smooth muscle and a reduction in menstrual loss.

Endometrial hyperplasia

Workers first used the PIPS to reverse endometrial hyperplasia and associated bleeding problems.[16] In a subsequent study, the PIPS was found to be successful in 81% of cases but there was quite a high recurrence rate after removal.[34] There are also good data for regression of endometrial hyperplasia[35,36] with the LNG–IUS, which can be achieved more rapidly than with the PIPS, probably owing to the greater efficacy of androgenic progestogens over progesterone in achieving secretory transformation. The LNG–IUS would therefore be the IUS of choice for this indication unless the woman is severely progestogen intolerant, in which case the PIPS would be a better choice.

The hormone-releasing intra-uterine systems may also have a preventative and therapeutic role in women using tamoxifen for breast cancer. It is a well-recognized complication of tamoxifen therapy that the partial oestrogenic agonistic effect of the drug often induces endometrial hyperplasia, which can lead to erratic/heavy bleeding and uterine cancer.[37] Studies are currently being conducted to determine the effectiveness of the LNG–IUS in both preventing and treating hyperplasia in this situation.

Prevention and treatment of uterine fibroids

Uterine fibroids, particularly submucous ones, are a well-known cause of menorrhagia and intermenstrual bleeding. Prevention of fibroid growth with long-term intra-uterine system usage was suggested by the Population Council Study, which detected a significantly lower incidence of fibroids in LNG–IUS users than in users of copper IUCDs.[33] A prospective pilot study of five women, reported in the same year,[38] suggested not only a preventative but also a therapeutic effect for the LNG–IUS in that fibroids were actually reduced in size after 6–18 months' usage. It has been postulated that these findings may be due to the effect of levonorgestrel on insulin-like endometrial growth factors and their binding proteins.[39,40] The obvious restriction to usage of the system in women with fibroids would be if a cervical fibroid prevented IUS insertion or if a submucous fibroid was so large that there was insufficient space within the uterine cavity for the IUS.

Menopausal bleeding problems on HRT

The intolerance of progestogenic bleeding problems is one of the main reasons for poor compliance with HRT,[41,42] leading to high discontinuation rates.[43] Not infrequently, women request hysterectomy so that unopposed oestrogens may be used and bleeding can be completely avoided.[44] In the last few years, workers have shown that the LNG–IUS can provide progestogenic opposition with minimal bleeding in users of oral,[45] transdermal[46] and implanted oestrogens.[47] Transvaginal ultrasound and endometrial biopsy were used in the studies to confirm atrophy; there were no cases of endometrial hyperplasia in any of the LNG–IUS users. The proportion of amenorrhoeic IUS users after 1 year was high, Raudaskoski's patients achieving an 80% rate[46] and Suhonen's a 75% rate[47] of amenorrhoea.

In principle, the lowest effective dose of progestogen should be used for opposition to oestrogen therapy in order to avoid progestogenic premenstrual syndrome (PMS)-like side effects.[48,49] Use of the hormone-releasing intra-uterine systems, rather than an oral progestogen, as progestogenic opposition, should also be an ideal way of avoiding progestogenic side effects as well as of minimizing bleeding. Despite the favourable bleeding and progestogenic side effect data in HRT usage, the LNG–IUS is currently licensed only as a contraceptive in the United Kingdom, whereas Finland allows its use for up to 5 years as progestogenic opposition for oestrogen therapy. There appears to be no lipid metabolic advantage of the LNG–IUS compared with cyclical oral administration of progestogen in HRT, although data are scarce.[50,51]

Results of two recent studies[52,53] indicate that the PIPS also suppresses endometrial proliferation in postmenopausal women taking 0.625 mg oral conjugated oestrogen daily. Shoupe et al.[52] reported a progestational effect of the system on the endometrium (late secretory changes, decidualized stroma, atrophic glands) after 12 months; prior to the study, biopsy had shown a proliferative endometrium. Archer et al.[53] reported similar progestational effects after 18 months' use of the system with oestrogen therapy. In these studies there was no systemic absorption of progesterone; both Shoupe et al.[52] and Archer et al.[53] reported unchanged levels of serum progesterone compared with baseline during use of the system with oestrogen therapy. This differs from the LNG–IUS, where some systemic absorption of levonorgestrel does occur, producing levels of around 200 pg/ml.[48] Shoupe et al.[52] reported a beneficial effect on lipids with a 22% increase in high-density lipoprotein (HDL) levels and a 21% decrease in low-density lipoprotein (LDL) levels from baseline with the combined regimen.

Work recently completed in the authors' unit showed that both adverse progestogenic effects and severity of bleeding were reduced to a minimum when patients using mainly oestradiol implants and who were progestogen intolerant were switched from oral progestogens to the LNG–IUS (Fig. 9.5a). Endometrial suppression was uniform, with no cases of endometrial proliferation or hyperplasia at one year (Fig. 9.5b) and a greater than 50% rate of amenorrhoea. At time of data analysis, all but one of the 20 women who said they wanted hysterectomy (because of either bleeding problems or progestogenic side effects) were able to avoid this by LNG–IUS usage.[54]

Premenstrual syndrome
Recent work suggests that the LNG–IUS on its own may benefit premenstrual symptoms.[30] This effect may possibly be due to improvement in menorrhagia and dysmenorrhoea, which reduces the depression associated with the premenstrual expectancy of these symptoms.

Problems of the hormone-releasing intra-uterine systems
Fitting of systems
The initial drawback of both systems is their slightly wider diameter vertical stem, which is a consequence of the steroid reservoir. This necessitates a wider insertion tube in the case of the LNG–IUS. The insertion diameter is even greater in the case of the PIPS because the arms are initially folded down against the stem. These features can lead to difficulty in fitting the systems, particularly in nulliparous women, and may require some cervical dilatation prior to insertion. The requirement for dilatation can usually be determined at time of uterine sounding by judgement of the ease with which the sound passes. Should it be deemed necessary to dilate the cervix, it is vital that adequate analgesia is administered first if the patient's confidence is to be retained and insertion is not to fail. This can usually

Figure 9.5 (a) Visual analogue scales (VAS) of global progestogenic side effects (□) and bleeding (□) severity in women using oestrogens with the levonorgestrel intra-uterine system (Mirena) for progestogenic opposition; (b) effect of LNG–IUS on endometrium after 1 year: □ no specimen; □ atrophic; □ secretory/decidual; □ proliferative. (Reproduced from ref. 54.)

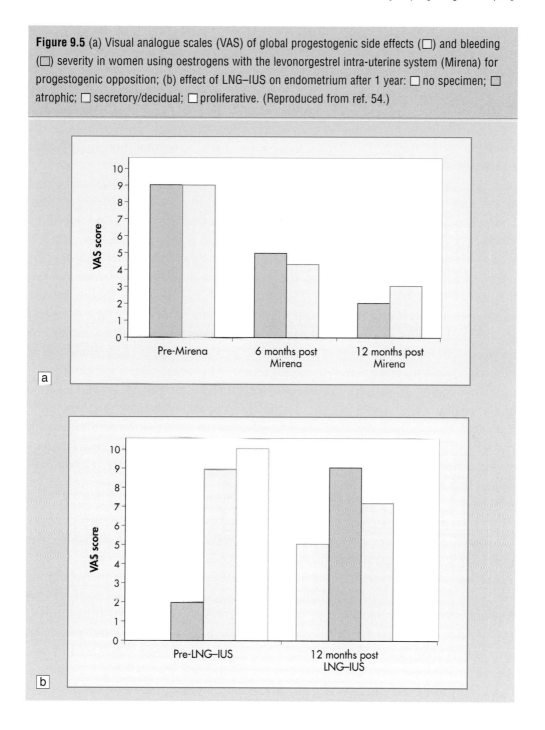

be achieved either by the administration of a non-steroidal analgesic (e.g. mefenamic acid 500 mg) 1 hour before insertion, or by use of a paracervical block via a dental syringe of either 1% lignocaine or xylocaine without adrenaline, 5 minutes before insertion. The same care should be taken when inserting the intra-uterine systems as with other IUDs, and complications such as perforation, embedment, expulsion and fragmentation are all possible. Interestingly, the expulsion and perforation rates of the LNG–IUS do not differ significantly from those of the Nova-T IUCD.

Bleeding problems

Before insertion of the system in a woman with bleeding problems, at the very least a transvaginal ultrasound examination should be performed to detect significant endometrial or uterine pathology. If the woman is over 40 years of age and/or if the scan is suspicious, endometrial sampling should also be performed either with a Pipelle or, ideally, following hysteroscopy. A problem with both the currently available intra-uterine systems is that, even with a normal non-hyperplastic endometrium, it takes approximately 3 months for the endometrium to atrophy under the influence of the released hormone. During this time, bleeding can be very erratic and heavy at times, but almost always settles after 3–6 months' usage.[55] Pre- and perimenopausal women experience more episodes of spotting and bleeding. Good counselling is vital if treatment discontinuation is to be avoided. In the PIPS studies by Wan et al.,[22] Shoupe et al.[52] and Archer et al.,[53] bleeding and spotting were common in patients during the first 3 months following insertion but diminished substantially thereafter. No patients withdrew from the studies because of adverse events. It may be of benefit to use tranexamic acid for the first 3 months to reduce bleeding until atrophy of the endometrium has occurred under the influence of the IUS hormone. It would be prudent to perform a transvaginal ultrasound scan for endometrial thickness followed by hysteroscopy and curettage if problems continue and/or if the scan is suspicious, for example, of a thickened endometrium or a polyp. These diagnostic procedures would be particularly indicated if they had not been performed prior to insertion of the system. If pathology has been excluded and bleeding continues for more than a year, it can be assumed that the system is not going to be effective and an alternative treatment should be sought.

Adverse progestogenic effects: physical and metabolic

Despite the very low constant serum levels of progestogen produced by the LNG–IUS, some women still seem to experience adverse progestogenic effects. These can be both physical — such as oedema, headache, breast tenderness, acne and hirsutism[19,28] — and metabolic — such as decreased LDL levels.[51] This is probably because the progestogen within the LNG–IUS is derived from the 19-nortestosterone group of progestogens, which have more physical and metabolic side effects than the C21 progesterone group of progestogens (Fig. 9.2). There appears to be no significant effect on carbohydrate metabolism, coagulation parameters or liver enzymes.[56] The physical effects have been shown to subside after the first few months of usage. It is important that patients are sympathetically counselled and reassured that most side effects are transient, and are reminded that the serum hormone levels are much lower than those produced by other hormonal contraceptives such as the progestogen-only pill. Side effects related to fluid retention, such as oedema and bloating, may respond to a mild diuretic such as 25 mg of either spironolactone or hydrochlorothiazide.[57] Addition of an androgen (e.g. a 100 mg testosterone implant every 6 months) may occasionally ameliorate breast tenderness. Headaches are unlikely to occur if oestrogens are used continuously but, if they do occur, they may be improved by the addition of a mild diuretic or of androgen.

From studies of plasma hormone levels, menstrual patterns and blood chemistry in various patient groups,[21,22] it was found that the PIPS produced no significant systemic effects. Shoupe et al.[52] reported that serum HDL increased by 22% and LDL decreased by 21% from baseline with the combined oestrogen/PIPS regimen. Archer et al.[53] and Spellacy et al.[58] reported no change in total cholesterol, although triglycerides did increase between 6 and 12 months in Archer's study. Spellacy et al.[58] surprisingly detected an increase in insulin secretion, suggesting a systemic effect from the progesterone released by PIPS. However, there do not appear to be adverse physical or psychological progestogenic side effects with the PIPS and, as such, it is ideal for women who are exquisitely progestogen sensitive.

Ectopic pregnancy

The absolute ectopic rate is extremely low with the LNG–IUS, being the lowest of any intra-uterine method of contraception. In one study by Andersson et al.,[28] the rate of 0.02 per 100 woman-years compared very favourably with that for Nova-T users (0.25 per 100 woman-years) and sexually active women not using contraception (1.2–1.6 per 100 woman-years). However, because the LNG–IUS is so effective at preventing intra-uterine pregnancy, if a pregnancy does occur with the IUS in situ then there is a high risk of this being ectopic (one of five pregnancies in the study by Andersson et al.[28] of 1821 coil insertions). The risk of an ectopic pregnancy with the PIPS appears to be higher than that with other non-hormone-releasing IUDs and is about the same as that for women not using contraceptive methods. However, if the PIPS is used as progestogenic opposition for oestrogen therapy in perimenopausal women, particularly with patches and implants that can inhibit ovulation, the ectopic rate should be negligible.

Pelvic inflammatory disease

The system appears to be protective because of the thickening effect on cervical mucus, preventing ascending infection, endometrial suppression and reduced bleeding. The incidence of pelvic inflammatory disease (PID) with the LNG–IUS is very low: at 5 years the rate is less than 1 per 100 woman-years. The difference in PID incidence between the LNG–IUS and copper IUCD was greatest in women less than 25 years of age, the age group most associated with an increased risk of PID.[28,59] However, not all studies have confirmed these findings; nevertheless at worst they have found the incidence of PID to be comparable to that with traditional IUCDs.[8,33] The PIPS does not appear to have this protective effect, the relative risk of PID being the same as that with other IUDs at about 1.6 per 100 woman-years. In view of the favourable PID data for the LNG–IUS, this system might be slightly favoured in cases where there is a past history of PID.

Functional ovarian cysts

Functional ovarian cysts have been shown to be commoner in LNG–IUS users than in copper IUCD users (1.2 vs 0.4 per 100 woman-years).[33] This finding is not surprising, considering the higher incidence of cysts in progestogen-only pill users. What must be remembered is that these cysts can almost always be managed conservatively.

Amenorrhoea

If inadequately counselled prior to insertion of the system, a woman may regard the reduction in bleeding or cessation of periods as being pathological; this has led to unnecessary system removal in some cases.[28,33] It is vital that patients and practitioners are aware that the amenorrhoea is due purely to a local effect of hormone on the endometrium, producing atrophy. Patients should be made aware of the health benefits of reduced bleeding. If a woman feels strongly about maintaining regular bleeds, then the hormone-releasing intra-uterine systems are an inappropriate therapeutic option. As discussed earlier, ovulation is affected only rarely and oestrogen levels are identical in menstruating and non-menstruating users.[19,20]

Cost effectiveness

The cost of the LNG–IUS to the National Health Service in the UK is £99.25, an initially high price. However, to make its use cost effective as treatment for menorrhagia, which might otherwise lead to hysterectomy (costing the National Health Service approximately £4000), only one in 40 hysterectomies would have to be saved. Furthermore, the longer the duration of use of HRT, the greater the cost effectiveness.[60] Since bleeding problems and progestogenic side effects are the major reasons for women dropping out from therapy, the hormone-releasing coils easily justify their initial expense by increasing continuation rates, preventing hysterectomy to allow the use of unopposed oestrogens and ultimately maximizing the cost effectiveness of HRT. It is unfortunate therefore that many health care trusts, gynaecologists and general practitioners still object to the initial cost of the systems when they have the potential to be cost effective by reducing patient morbidity, and specifically, the need for hysterectomy.

Conclusions

Until recently, approximately 100,000 hysterectomies per annum were being performed in the UK for benign causes, mainly for menorrhagia. This figure is already being reduced by the beneficial effects of the levonorgestrel intra-uterine system and the progesterone-releasing intra-uterine systems on menorrhagia,

Table 9.2 Summary of possible non-contraceptive uses of the hormone-releasing intra-uterine systems

Potential application	Most appropriate IUS
Menorrhagia	LNG–IUS
Dysmenorrhoea	LNG–IUS/PIPS
Endometrial hyperplasia	LNG–IUS/PIPS
Prevention/treatment of fibroids	LNG–IUS
HRT bleeding problems	LNG–IUS
HRT progestogenic side effects	PIPS/LNG–IUS
Progestogenic opposition for E2 in PMS	PIPS/LNG–IUS
Prevention of ectopic pregnancy	LNG–IUS
Prevention of PID	LNG–IUS

E2, 17β-oestradiol; HRT, hormone replacement therapy; IUS, intra-uterine system; LNG–IUS, levonorgestrel intra-uterine system; PID, pelvic inflammatory disease; PIPS, Progestasert intra-uterine progesterone system; PMS, premenstrual syndrome.

dysmenorrhoea and fibroids. When, to this, is added the reduction of PID and ectopic pregnancy and avoidance of progestogenic side effects in HRT users, the result is one of the most significant developments in gynaecological management of the 20th century (Table 9.2). In many cases the systems will not be appropriate — for instance, in a patient who wishes to be absolutely certain that she will not have any further bleeding. For some patients the systems may not be effective enough, or may produce unacceptable side effects (Table 9.3). For these reasons there will always be a place for endometrial ablation or resection and hysterectomy. However, the hormone-releasing systems provide the first true medical alternative to hysterectomy for intractable menstrual and HRT-associated bleeding problems which, at the very least, can be tried while the patient is on the waiting list for hysterectomy. Future work should focus on confirming the efficacy, safety and cost effectiveness of these systems, thus building confidence amongst gynaecologists, general practitioners and patients regarding their first-line use for menorrhagia.

Table 9.3 Summary of potential problems with hormone-releasing intra-uterine systems and possible solutions

Potential problem	Relevant IUS	Possible solution(s)
Difficulty fitting	PIPS/LNG–IUS	(1) Premedicate with non-steroidals (2) Paracervical block (3) Cervical dilatation (4) Consider GA
Bleeding problems	PIPS/LNG–IUS	(1) Pre- and post-insertion counselling (2) Tranexamic acid
Progestogenic side effects	LNG–IUS	(1) Pre- and post-insertion counselling (2) Reassure that usually transient (3) Symptomatic relief, e.g.: (a) Evening primrose oil/low-dose androgen for breast tenderness (b) Mild diuretics for fluid retention
Functional cysts	LNG–IUS	Manage conservatively if possible; ultrasound follow-up
Amenorrhoea	LNG–IUS/PIPS	Pre- and post-insertion counselling
Perforation/embedment/expulsion	LNG–IUS/PIPS	Manage as with other IUCDs
Pregnancy with IUS in situ	PIPS/LNG–IUS	Manage as with other IUCDs (no evidence of foetal abnormality)

GA, general anaesthesia; IUS, intra-uterine system; IUCD, intra-uterine contraceptive device; LNG–IUS, levonorgestrel intra-uterine system; PIPS, Progestasert intra-uterine progesterone system.

References

1. Coulter A, Kelland J, Long A et al. The management of menorrhagia. Effective Health Care: Bulletin No.9. Leeds: University of Leeds, 1995

2. Davie J. New hormone delivery systems. Diplomate 1996; 3(3): 184–190

3. Sturdee D W, Wade-Evans T, Paterson M E L et al. Relations between bleeding pattern, endometrial histology and oestrogen treatment in menopausal women. Br Med J 1978; I: 1575–1577

4. Paterson M E L, Wade-Evans T, Sturdee D W et al. Endometrial disease after treatment with oestrogens and progestogens in the climacteric. Br Med J 1980; I: 822–824

5. Lane G, Siddle N C, Ryder T A et al. Dose dependent effects of oral progesterone on the oestrogenised postmenopausal endometrium. Acta Obstet Gynecol Scand 1983; 106: 17–22

6. Henderson B E, Ross R K, Lobo R A et al. Re-evaluating the role of progestogen therapy after the menopause. Fertil Steril 1988; 49: 9S–15S

7. Zhu P, Hongzhi L, Ruhua X et al. The effect of intrauterine devices, the stainless steel ring, the copper T220 and releasing levonorgestrel, on the bleeding profile and the morphological structure of the human endometrium — a comparative study of three IUDs. Contraception 1989; 40: 425–438

8. Luukkainen T, Allonen H, Haukkamaa M et al. Five year's experience with levonorgestrel releasing IUD's. Contraception 1986; 33: 139–148

9. Zhu P, Hongzhi L, Wenliang S et al. Observation of the activity of factor VIII in the endometrium of women pre- and post-insertion of three types of IUD's. Contraception 1991; 44: 367–387

10. Silverberg S G, Haukkamaa M, Arko H et al. Endometrial morphology during long-term use of levonorgestrel-releasing intrauterine devices. Int J Gynecol Pathol 1986; 5: 235–241

11. Nilsson C G, Lahteenmaki P. Recovery of ovarian function after the use of a d-norgestrel releasing IUD. Contraception 1977; 15: 389–400

12. Hagenfeldt K, Landgren B M, Edstrom K, Johanisson E. Biochemical and morphological changes in the human endometrium induced by the Progestasert device. Contraception 1977; 16: 183–197

13. Martinez-Manautou J, Aznar R, Maqueo M, Pharriss B B. Uterine therapeutic system for long term contraception: II. Clinical correlates. Fertil Steril 1974; 25(11): 922–926

14. Martinez-Manautou J, Maqueo M, Aznar R et al. Endometrial morphology in women exposed to uterine systems releasing progesterone. Am J Obstet Gynecol 1975; 121: 175–179

15. Sievers S, Dallenbach-Hellweg. Clinical and morphological studies in patients following insertion of progesterone containing IUD (Progestasert system). Geburtshilfe Frauenheilkd 1976; 36: 334–340

16. Volpe A, Botticelli A, Abrate M et al. An intrauterine progesterone contraceptive system (52mg) used in pre- and peri-menopausal patients with endometrial hyperplasia. Maturitas 1982; 4: 73–79

17. Erickson R E, Mitchell C, Pharriss B B, Place V A. The intrauterine progesterone contraceptive system. In: Advances in planned parenthood. Princeton; Excerpta Medica, 1976: 167–174

18. Luukkainen T. Levonorgestrel-releasing intrauterine device. Ann N Y Acad Sci 1991; 626: 43–49

19. Luukkainen T, Lahteenmaki P, Toivonen J. Levonorgestrel-releasing intrauterine device. Ann Med 1990; 22: 85–90

20. Nilsson C G, Lahteenmaki P L A, Luukkainen T. Ovarian function in amenorrhoeic and menstruating users of a levonorgestrel-releasing intrauterine device. Fertil Steril 1984; 41: 52–55

21. Tillson S A, Marian M, Hudson R et al. The effect of intrauterine progesterone on the hypothalamic–hypophyseal–ovarian axis in humans. Contraception 1975; 11(2): 179–192

22. Wan L S, Ying-Chih H, Manik G, Bigelow B. Effects of the Progestasert® on the menstrual pattern, ovarian steroids and endometrium. Contraception 1977; 16(4): 417–434

23. Diaz S, Pavez M, Miranda P et al. Long term follow-up of women treated with Norplant® implants. Contraception 1987; 35: 551–567

24. Kuhnz W, Al-Yacoub G, Fuhrmister A. Pharmacokinetics of levonorgestrel and ethinylestradiol in 9 women who received a low-dose oral contraceptive over a treatment period of 3 months, and, after a washout phase, a single oral administration of the same contraceptive formulation. Contraception 1992; 46: 455–469

25. Weiner E, Victor A, Johansson E D B. Plasma levels of d-norgestrel after oral administration. Contraception 1976; 14: 563–570

26. Nilsson C G, Lahteenmaki P L A, Luukkainen T et al. Sustained intrauterine release of levonorgestrel over five years. Fertil Steril 1986; 45: 805–807

27. Andersson J K, Rybo G. Levonorgestrel-releasing intrauterine device in the treatment of menorrhagia. Br J Obstet Gynaecol 1990; 97: 690–694

28. Andersson K, Odlind V, Rybo G et al. Levonorgestrel-releasing and copper-releasing IUD's during 5 years of use: a randomised comparative trial. Contraception 1994; 49: 56–72

29. Bergkvist A, Rybo G. Treatment of menorrhagia with intrauterine release of progesterone. Br J Obstet Gynaecol 1983; 90: 255–258

30. Barrington J W, Bowen-Simpkins P. The levonorgestrel intrauterine system in the management of menorrhagia. Br J Obstet Gynaecol 1997; 104: 614–616

31. Puolakka J, Nilsson C, Haukkamaa M et al. Conservative treatment of excessive uterine bleeding and dysmenorrhoea with levonorgestrel intrauterine system as an alternative to hysterectomy. Acta Obstet Gynecol Scand 1996; 75(s): 82

32. Mann R. Unlicensed medicines and the use of drugs in unlicensed indications. In: Goldberg A, Dodd-Smith I (eds) Pharmaceutical medicine and law, Vol 8. London: Royal College of Physicians, 1991: 103–110

33. Sivin I, Stern J. Health during prolonged use of levonorgestrel 20 µg/d and the Copper T Cu 380 Ag intrauterine contraceptive devices: a multicentre study. Fertil Steril 1994; 61, 70–77

34. Gasparri F, Scarselli G, Colafranceschi M et al. Management of precancerous lesions of the endometrium. In: Ludwig H, Thomsen K (eds) Gynaecology and obstetrics. Berlin: Springer-Verlag, 1986

35. Perino A, Quartararo P, Catinella E et al. Treatment of endometrial hyperplasia with levonorgestrel releasing intrauterine devices. Acta Eur Fertil 1987; 18: 137–140

36. Scarselli G, Tantini C, Colafranceschi M et al. Levonorgestrel-Nova T and precancerous lesions of the endometrium. Eur J Gynaecol Oncol 1988; IX: 284–286

37. Neven P, De Muylder X, Van Belle Y et al. Tamoxifen and the uterus. Br Med J 1994; 309; 1313–1314

38. Singer A, Ikomi A. Successful treatment of fibroids using an intrauterine progesterone device (abstract). 14th World Congress of Gynaecology and Obstetrics (FIGO); Montreal, Canada; 24–30 Sept 1994

39. Pekonen F, Nyman T, Lahteenmaki P et al. Intrauterine progestin induces continuous insulin-like growth factor binding protein-1 production in the human endometrium. J Clin Endocrinol Metab 1992; 75; 660–664

40. Sturridge F, Guillebaud J. Gynaecological aspects of the levonorgestrel-releasing intrauterine system. Br J Obstet Gynaecol 1997; 104: 285–289

41. Ferguson K J, Hoegh C, Johnson S. Estrogen replacement therapy: a survey of women's knowledge and attitudes. Arch Intern Med 1989; 149: 133

42. Studd J W W. Complications of hormone replacement therapy in post-menopausal women. J R Soc Med 1992; 85: 376–378

43. Barlow D H, Grosset K A, Hart H, Hart D M. A study of the experience of Glasgow women in the climacteric years. Br J Obstet Gynaecol 1989; 96: 1192–1197

44. Studd J W W. Shifting indications for hysterectomy. Lancet 1995; 345: 388

45. Andersson K, Mattsson L A, Rybo G et al. Intrauterine release of levonorgestrel — a new way of adding progestogen in hormone replacement therapy. Obstet Gynecol 1992; 79: 963–967

46. Raudaskoski T H, Lahti E I, Kauppila A J et al. Transdermal estrogen with a levonorgestrel-releasing intrauterine device for climacteric complaints: clinical and endometrial responses. Am J Obstet Gynecol 1995; 172: 114–119

47. Suhonen S P, Holmstrom T, Allonen H O et al. Intrauterine and sub-dermal progestin administration in postmenopausal hormone replacement therapy. Fertil Steril 1995; 63: 336–342

48. Rozenbaum H. How to choose the correct progestogen. In: Birkhauser M H, Rozenbaum H (eds) Menopause. European Consensus Development Conference, Montreux, Switzerland. Paris: Editions ESKA, 1996: 243–256

49. Panay N, Studd J W W. Progestogen intolerance and compliance with HRT in menopausal women. Hum Reprod Update 1997; 3(2): 159–171

50. Andersson K, Stadberg E, Mattsson L A et al. Intrauterine or oral administration of levonorgestrel in combination with estradiol to perimenopausal women — effects on lipid metabolism during 12 months of treatment. Int J Fertil 1996; 41: 476–483

51. Raudaskoski T H, Tomas E I, Paakkari I A et al. Serum lipids and lipoproteins in postmenopausal women receiving transdermal oestrogen in combination with a levonorgestrel intrauterine device. Maturitas 1995; 22(1): 47–53

52. Shoupe D, Meme D, Mezro G, Lobo R A. Prevention of intrauterine hyperplasia in postmenopausal women with intrauterine progesterone. N Engl J Med 1991; 325: 1811–1821

53. Archer D F, Viniegra-Sibai A, Hsiu J G et al. Endometrial histology, uterine bleeding and metabolic changes in postmenopausal women using a progesterone-releasing intrauterine device and oral conjugated estrogens for hormone replacement therapy. Menopause 1994; 1: 109–116

54. Panay N, Studd J W W, Thomas A et al. Prospective study of menopausal women on subcutaneous oestradiol, switched to the levonorgestrel releasing intrauterine system because of oral progestogen intolerance. Acta Obstet Gynaecol Scand 1997; 76: 56

55. Nilsson C G, Lahteenmaki P, Luukkainen T. Levonorgestrel plasma concentrations and hormone profiles after insertion and after one year of treatment with a levonorgestrel–IUCD. Contraception 1980; 21: 225–233

56. Luukkainen T. Levonorgestrel-releasing IUCD. Br J Fam Plann 1991; 19: 221–224

57. Gambrell R D. Progestogens in estrogen replacement therapy. Clin Obstet Gynecol 1995; 38: 890–901

58. Spellacy W, Buhi W C, Birk S A. Carbohydrate and lipid studies in women using the progesterone intrauterine device for 1 year. Fertil Steril 1979; 31(4): 381–384

59. Haukkamaa M, Stranden P, Jousimies-Somer H et al. Bacterial flora of the cervix in women using different forms of contraception. Am J Obstet Gynecol 1986; 154: 520–524

60. Cheung A P, Wren B G. A cost-effectiveness analysis of hormone replacement therapy. Med J Aust 1992; 156: 312–316

CHAPTER 10

Refractory menorrhagia

M. C. P. Rees

Introduction

Menorrhagia is the main presenting complaint in women referred to gynaecologists. Menorrhagia is a complaint of excessive menstrual bleeding, but in objective terms is a blood loss greater than 80 ml/period. By the age of 43, one in 10 women will have undergone hysterectomy.[1] About 73,000 hysterectomies and 10,000 endometrial ablations were performed in England in 1993/94, of which about two-thirds were undertaken for women presenting with menorrhagia. In the same year 822,000 prescriptions were issued to 345,225 women for this condition.

Refractory menorrhagia: definition

Refractory menorrhagia is the complaint by the woman and her physician that her perceived excessive menstrual blood loss (MBL) is not responding to treatment. Several options have to be considered to account for this.

First, her loss may be so excessive that, unless the treatment produces amenorrhoea, it has been insufficiently controlled. For example, with tranexamic acid where pretreatment blood loss is less than 200 ml/menstruation, 92% of women will have their blood loss reduced to less than 80 ml on therapy.[2,3] However, if blood loss exceeds 250 ml, tranexamic acid is very unlikely to achieve a loss within normal limits. A similar pattern would be expected with prostaglandin (PG) synthetase inhibitors.

Second, she may have a pretreatment blood loss less than 80 ml and the perceived reduction in loss on therapy is not sufficient for her. This was illustrated in a study including women with normal MBL, where therapy with mefenamic acid did not reduce loss and actually increased it.[4] The reasons why women with normal loss complain of menorrhagia is currently being examined in a primary care study in Oxford.

Third, the patient may have unsuspected uterine pathology, such as a submucous fibroid or endometrial polyp, which makes medical treatment ineffective. This has been shown with both gestrinone and PG synthetase inhibitors.[5,6] It is unfortunate that, in many studies, patients in whom treatment has failed are not followed up with hysteroscopy to check for such pathology.

Investigation

Menstrual blood loss estimation

The ideal investigation is actually to measure MBL. This can be undertaken non-invasively using the well-established alkaline haematin method, where sanitary devices are soaked in 5% sodium hydroxide to convert the blood to alkaline haematin, the optical density of which is then measured.[5] It is well established from many studies where subjective and objective assessments have been compared that patients' estimations are unreliable indicators of MBL:[2,8] at present it has been estimated in hospital practice that only 40% of women complaining of menorrhagia have measured losses greater than 80 ml.[9] The level in general practice is currently being examined in a trial in Oxford.

Various visual scoring techniques have been devised; however, they do not provide an objective measure. Recently, variations of the alkaline haematin technique using non-ionic detergent and sodium carbonate have been described.[10] Unfortunately, at present, routine measurement of MBL is not available in clinical practice.

Haemoglobin

As a substitute, a haemoglobin measurement may be helpful, but it is only a guide. Hypochromic microcytic anaemia is suggestive of menorrhagia and, in women of reproductive age, the main source of blood loss is the uterus rather than any organ system (such as the gastrointestinal tract). However, the absence of anaemia does not exclude menorrhagia: losses of 800–1000 ml can occur without anaemia.

Investigation for pathology

In terms of pathology, the commonest cause of refractory menorrhagia is an unsuspected submucous fibroid or endometrial polyp. The best method of diagnosis is hysteroscopy to provide direct visualization of the endometrial cavity; this technique is increasingly being used. A thickened endometrium is suggestive of a polyp or other pathology (hyperplasia, malignancy). Premenopausally, total anteroposterior thickness (both endometrial layers) varies from 4 to 8 mm in the proliferative phase and peaks at 8–16 mm during the secretory phase. Detection of endometrial polyps can be enhanced by instillation of contrast medium into the uterine cavity. However, it must be remembered that although ultrasound cannot replace hysteroscopy, it is a useful adjunct.

Disorders of haemostasis, such as von Willebrand's disease, deficiencies of factors V, VII and X, and idiopathic thrombocytopenic purpura are thought to increase MBL, however, blood loss was not objectively measured in the cases originally reported. When it has been measured, platelet disorders (thrombocytopenia) rather than coagulation disorders have been implicated in menorrhagia. These could be considered as rare causes of refractory menorrhagia and could thus be investigated. There are no data for the effect of anticoagulants on MBL.

Management strategies

Counselling

It is of concern that only 40% of women complaining of menorrhagia actually have objective menorrhagia; thus, counselling would be a better option in women with normal blood loss. This was first shown in a study of 17 women referred for hospital treatment for menorrhagia, in whom blood loss was less than 80 ml. A 3-year follow-up of these women showed that only one woman had opted for hysterectomy: two had taken drug therapy and the remainder had accepted the advice given by the counsellor. This has also been found in other recent studies.[10,12] The effectiveness of reassurance and counselling is not known; it is currently being assessed in primary care in a randomized controlled trial in Oxford.

Medical treatment

The treatment preferred by women with refractory menorrhagia is to be rendered amenorrhoeic. The options to consider are the progesterone/levonorgestrel intra-uterine systems, the combined oral contraceptive pill taken continuously, danazol, gestrinone or gonadotrophin-releasing hormone (GnRH) analogues. Medical therapy is indicated when there is no obvious pelvic abnormality and the woman wishes to retain her fertility. Since menstrual loss, in the absence of pathology, does not change markedly, treatment is long term; thus, the drug regimen chosen must be effective, must have few or mild side effects and must be acceptable to the patient.

Intra-uterine progesterone (or, more especially, levonorgestrel) is successful in reducing MBL. With progesterone released at 125 µg daily (Progestasert), menstrual loss is significantly reduced after 1 month, but the duration of bleeding is somewhat prolonged; 12 months after insertion, menstrual loss is 35% of the pre-insertion blood loss.[13] With the levonorgestrel intra-uterine contraceptive device (IUCD), reductions of MBL of 88% and 96% are found after 6 months and 12 months, respectively.[14] The levonorgestrel intra-uterine system should now be considered to be a serious candidate as an alternative to surgical management for refractory menorrhagia in the absence of pelvic pathology. Counselling about irregular bleeding, which can occur in the first few months after insertion, is essential.

Oestrogen/progestogen

The combined oral contraceptive pill is often used clinically to reduce MBL. In general, the reduction in loss is about 50%. Taken continuously, it will render the woman amenorrhoeic, in the absence of breakthrough bleeding. This should be considered as an option in suitable women.

Danazol

Danazol is an isoxazol derivative of 17α-ethinyl testosterone, which acts on the hypothalamic–pituitary–ovarian axis as well as on the endometrium to produce atrophy. Studies have shown MBL reductions ranging from 50 to 85%, or amenorrhoea.[8,15,16] However, the clinical use of danazol is limited by its androgenic side effects, which include weight gain and skin rashes. The use of danazol is probably best restricted to women awaiting surgery.

Gestrinone

Gestrinone is a 19-nortestosterone derivative that has antiprogestogenic, anti-oestrogenic and androgenic activity. In a placebo-controlled study, gestrinone (2.5 mg) was given twice-weekly for 12 weeks to 19 women with proven menorrhagia: ten women became amenorrhoeic and a marked reduction in MBL was seen in five; placebo had no effect. In three of the non-responders, submucous fibroids were found at subsequent hysterectomy. The therapy was well tolerated, since all women completed the trial.[5] However, the androgenic side effects of gestrinone preclude long-term therapy.

GnRH analogues

GnRH analogues can be used to reduce MBL by pituitary downregulation and subsequent inhibition of ovarian activity, resulting in amenorrhoea. However, the induced hypo-oestrogenic state, with its adverse effects on bone metabolism, limits its use beyond 6 months. When cyclical oestrogen/progestogen hormone replacement therapy (HRT) has been used in conjunction with GnRH analogues, median MBL after 3 months' treatment in the women with objective menorrhagia was 74 ml.[17] This combination is expensive and should not be used as a first-line treatment.

Surgical treatment

Hysterectomy   Hysterectomy can guarantee amenorrhoea and is offered more often to younger women whose families are complete, because many are reluctant to take treatment long term. Although it is 100% effective, hysterectomy is accompanied by significant morbidity (pyrexia, haemorrhage, infection) but, fortunately, a low mortality rate. Estimates of the risk of operative mortality vary from 0.4 to 2 per 1000 women, depending on the definition of operative mortality and type of study. Mortality in women under the age of 50 for hysterectomy for non-malignant conditions has been estimated as 4.2 per 10,000. Short-term morbidity is high, with complication rates of 25% for vaginal and 43% for abdominal hysterectomy; similarly, mortality for vaginal hysterectomy is half that of abdominal hysterectomy. The reason is unclear but may reflect selection of healthier women for the vaginal operation.[6,18]

Concern exists regarding the long-term sequelae, which may include premature onset of ovarian failure even when ovaries are conserved, psychosexual dysfunction, urinary tract and bowel symptoms. In general, hysterectomy has a beneficial effect on mental wellbeing; however, although some studies report increased sexual enjoyment, others report reduced libido.

Most data are available for abdominal or vaginal hysterectomy, rather than laparoscopic hysterectomy. This last approach is under evaluation: for example, the Vaginal Abdominal and Laparoscopic Uterine Extirpation (VALUE) hysterectomy study is currently under way in the United Kingdom.

Endometrial ablative techniques   The ablative methods employed are resection of the endometrium, or ablation of the endometrium by laser, rollerball diathermy, radiofrequency, cryoablation, microwaves and thermal balloons. Like hysterectomy, these treatments should be offered only to women who desire no further children. The endpoints of these treatments differ from that of hysterectomy, since not all women are rendered amenorrhoeic. Success of endometrial ablative techniques has generally been measured in terms of induced amenorrhoea or significantly reduced menstrual flow.[10,18–21] Rates of amenorrhoea vary from 20 to 24% and of reduced flow from 30 to 93%. It has been suggested that endometrial ablative techniques are not suitable where there is significant dysmenorrhoea, although, if combined with laparoscopic uterine nerve ablation (LUNA) performed at the same time, it has been shown to be effective.[22]

Women in whom treatment has failed are variously managed by a repeat procedure or hysterectomy. Reoperation rates vary from 6 to 23%, with higher rates found in studies with longer follow-up. Interestingly, women with genuine menorrhagia are less likely to be dissatisfied with endometrial ablation or to require hysterectomy than women with normal loss.[10] A randomized controlled trial of hysterectomy and endometrial resection with 2-year follow-up shows more improvement of menstrual symptoms and higher rates of satisfaction with hysterectomy.[21]

Conclusions

Refractory menorrhagia is a common problem, but is difficult to manage in the absence of routine availability of MBL measurements. Access to these would result in a more appropriate use of health care resources.

References

1. Kuh D, Stirling S. Socioeconomic variation in admission for diseases of female genital system and breast in a national cohort aged 15–43. Br Med J 1995; 311: 840–843

2. Preston T J, Cameron I T, Adams E J, Smith S K. Comparative study of tranexamic acid and norethisterone in the treatment of ovulatory menorrhagia. Br J Obstet Gynaecol 1995; 102: 401–406

3. Bonnar J, Sheppard B L. Treatment of menorrhagia during menstruation: randomised controlled trial of ethamsylate, mefenamic acid and tranexamic acid. Br Med J 1996; 313: 579–582

4. Fraser I S, Pearse C, Shearman R P et al. Effect of mefenamic acid in patients with a complaint of menorrhagia. Obstet Gynecol 1981; 58: 543–551

5. Turnbull A C, Rees M C P. Gestrinone in the treatment of menorrhagia. Br J Obstet Gynaecol 1990; 97: 713–715

6. Coulter A, Kelland J, Long A et al. The management of menorrhagia. Effective Health Care Bulletin No.9. Leeds: University of Leeds, 1995

7. Hallberg L, Nilsson L. Determination of menstrual blood loss. Scand J Clin Lab Invest 1964; 16: 244–248

8. Chimbira T H, Anderson A B M, Naish C et al. Reduction of menstrual blood loss by danazol in unexplained menorrhagia: lack of effect of placebo. Br J Obstet Gynaecol 1980; 87: 1152–1158

9. Fraser I S, McCarron G, Markham R. A preliminary study of factors influencing the perception of menstrual blood volume. Am J Obstet Gynecol 1984; 149: 788–793

10. Gannon M J, Day P, Hammadieh N, Johnson N. A new method for measuring menstrual blood loss and its use in screening women before endometrial ablation. Br J Obstet Gynaecol 1996; 103: 1029–1033

11. Rees M. Role of menstrual blood loss measurement in management of complaints of excessive menstrual bleeding. Br J Obstet Gynaecol 1991; 98: 327–328

12. Higham J, Reid P. A preliminary investigation of what happens to women complaining of menorrhagia, but whose complaint is not substantiated. J Psychosom Obstet Gynaecol 1995; 16: 211–214

13. Berqvist A, Rybo G. Treatment of menorrhagia with intrauterine release of progesterone. Br J Obstet Gynaecol 1983; 90: 255–258

14. Milsom I, Andersson K, Andersch B, Rybo G. A comparison of flurbiprofen, tranexamic acid, and a levonorgestrel-releasing intrauterine contraceptive device in the treatment of idiopathic menorrhagia. Am J Obstet Gynecol 1991; 164: 879–883

15. Dockeray C J, Sheppard B L, Bonnar J. Comparison between mefenamic acid and danazol in the treatment of established menorrhagia. Br J Obstet Gynaecol 1989; 96: 840–844

16. Fraser I S, McCarron G. Randomised trial of two hormonal and two prostaglandin-inhibiting agents in women with a complaint of menorrhagia. Aust N Z J Obstet Gynaecol 1991; 31: 66–70

17. Thomas E J, Okuda K J, Thomas N M. The combination of depot gonadotrophin releasing hormone agonist and cyclical hormonal replacment therapy for dysfunctional uterine bleeding. Br J Obstet Gynaecol 1991; 98: 1155–1159

18. Vilos G A, Pispidikis J T, Botz C K. Economic evaluation of hysteroscopic endometrial ablation versus vaginal hysterectomy. Obstet Gynecol 1996; 88: 241–245

19. Unger J B, Meeks G R. Hysterectomy after endometrial ablation. Am J Obstet Gynecol 1996; 175: 1432–1436

20. O'Connor H, Magos A. Endometrial resection for the treatment of menorrhagia. N Engl J Med 1996; 335: 151–156

21. Sculpher M J, Dwyer N, Byford S, Stirrat G M. Randomised controlled trial comparing hysterectomy and endometrial resection: effect on health related quality of life and costs two years after surgery. Br J Obstet Gynaecol 1996; 103: 142–149

22. Ewen S P, Sutton C J G. A combined approach for heavy painful periods. Laparoscopic uterine nerve ablation and TCRE. Gynaecol Endosc 1994; 3: 167–168

CHAPTER 11

Menorrhagia and infertility

M. D. Hansotia and K. P. Paghdiwalla

Introduction

Menorrhagia is a symptom denoting excessively heavy menstrual bleeding. It is a complaint that is difficult to verify objectively, even with a detailed history. The presentation of patients to the doctor depends on the issue of tolerance and perception, which varies from one society to another. Menorrhagia is an extremely debilitating condition during the reproductive life of a woman, and occurs in 9–14% of the population. Besides being a social inconvenience, it leads to chronic anaemia from iron deficiency due to the excessive blood loss. Excessive vaginal bleeding, or menorrhagia, is one of the most common presenting symptoms for gynaecological patients. In conjunction with the trauma and travails of infertility, this leads to a set of patients that require the highest level of care and understanding.

According to Short,[1] the reduction of family size, by the extensive use of contraception and sterilization, has resulted in an approximately tenfold increase in the number of periods that women experience during their reproductive life.

Definition

From the population studies done by Hallberg et al.[2] and Cole et al.,[3] menorrhagia is defined as a blood loss of 80 ml or more per period. The percentage contribution of blood to the total menstrual discharge varies from 2 to 82%.[4] The incidence of anaemia increases when the losses exceed 80 ml. The diagnosis is reached from the patient's history alone.

Mechanism of menstruation

Vascular theory

Studies by Markee[5] almost 50 years ago hold true: he showed that vasoconstriction of the spiral arterioles leads to ischaemia and subsequent menstruation.

Haemostatic theory

The endometrium has a high fibrinolytic activity and the menstrual blood does not clot.[6] Menstrual blood contains platelets that fail to aggregate in response to pro-aggregatory agents such as ADP and collagen; it contains no fibrinogen and contains reduced amounts of coagulation factors compared with peripheral blood.[7]

Lysosomal autolysis

The luteal phase of the menstrual cycle shows increased lysosomal activity,[8] which leads to release of autolytic enzymes and degradation of the vessel walls and endometrium.

Regeneration

Regeneration of the endometrium begins within 48 hours of the onset of menstruation.[9] This regeneration helps both in vascular stasis and in achieving control of the blood loss.

Aetiology

This chapter discusses menorrhagia *vis-à-vis* infertile patients; hence, the discussion regarding aetiology and management is restricted to this subgroup of patients (Table 11.1).

Table 11.1 Infertility-associated aetiology of menorrhagia

Systemic disorder	Thyroid dysfunction
	Coagulation disorders
Dysfunctional uterine bleeding	Ovulatory menorrhagia
	Anovulation
	Luteal insufficiency
	Polycystic ovarian disease
Organic pathology	Fibroids
	Adenomyosis
	Cystic endometriosis
	Endometrial polyps
	Endometrial hyperplasia/carcinoma
	Pelvic tuberculosis

Systemic disorder

Thyroid dysfunction

Thyroid dysfunction has long been associated with menstrual irregularities and infertility. In a study by Wilansky and Greisman[10] of 15 hypothyroid women, corrective administration of small doses of thyroxine led to disappearance of the complaint of menorrhagia.

Coagulation disorders

There are limited data concerning the quantity of blood loss in women with coagulation disorders. In a study by Fraser et al.,[11] in which objective measurements were made on 15 women, estimated blood loss was up to 750 or even 1000 ml in some women.

Ahuja et al.[12] reported treating a 13-year-old girl with pubertal menorrhagia, which necessitated multiple blood transfusions. Her coagulation profile confirmed the diagnosis of von Willebrand's disease. The menorrhagia was controlled by cyclical use of oestrogen–progestogen combination drugs. The important clinical implication of this case is that the patient with menorrhagia may have an underlying coagulation disorder, which can successfully be managed by hormonal therapy.

Dysfunctional uterine bleeding (DUB)

The diagnosis of DUB is made by the exclusion of organic disease as a cause of the abnormal menses; the condition accounts for about 80% of cases of menorrhagia. Of these, over 80% will have no abnormality of the hypothalamic–pituitary–ovarian axis, and it is likely that the disorder is the result of local endometrial factors. There appears to be not only a preponderance of vasodilatory prostaglandins in the endometrium of women with menorrhagia but also an excessive increase in fibrinolytic activity within the uterine cavity. Once a diagnosis has been reached with the aid of history, examination, haematological and endocrine investigations, hysteroscopic-guided dilatation and curettage when appropriate, medical treatment is the usual first-line approach. Non-steroidal anti-inflammatory drugs such as mefenamic acid, or antifibrinolytic agents such as tranexamic or epsilon-aminocaproic acids, will reduce blood loss by between 25 and 50%. Medications that suppress ovarian function, such as danazol or gonadotrophin-releasing hormone (GnRH) analogues, are highly effective in lessening, or inhibiting, menstrual loss, but at the expense of side effects and convenience, respectively. The combined contraceptive pill may reduce blood loss by 50% but is not appropriate for older women. Cyclical gestogens such as norethisterone have been widely employed, particularly for the treatment of anovulatory cycles, but their place in the management of ovulatory DUB is less clear.

Ovulatory menorrhagia

It has long been a belief that the majority of cases of menorrhagia are associated with anovulatory cycles. However, Haynes et al.[13] found no difference in the levels of follicle-stimulating hormone (FSH), luteinizing hormone (LH), 17β-oestradiol or progesterone during the cycle, in a study of 27 women with a heavy menstrual loss (> 80 ml), compared with 13 women with a light loss (< 80 ml). In a series by Smith et al.,[14] 50–80% of the endometrial specimens did not show any abnormality.

It is, therefore, suggested that most menstrual bleeding occurs because of progesterone withdrawal from an oestrogen-primed endometrial lining, in both heavy and light bleeders in the presence of regular cycles. Ovulatory DUB, which is most prevalent in parous women between the ages of 20 and 40, is associated with regular cycle intervals and premenstrual molimina.[15] Midcycle and perimenstrual spotting can often be treated with observation only but, depending upon patient and/or physician concerns, periodic hormonal suppression is effective. The management of menorrhagia should include the following: (1) exclusion of pathology in the genital tract; (2) reduction in activity during days of heavy flow; (3) the avoidance of aspirin in the week before and on days of flow; (4) non-steroidal anti-inflammatory drugs; (5) cycle suppression with oral contraceptives, danazol or depot progestin; (6) luteal phase progestin; and (7) surgical intervention.

Anovulatory menorrhagia

Anovulation can occur at any age and is physiological in the first year or two after the menarche and for several years before the menopause. Anovulatory cycles are characteristically irregular and are marked by prolonged episodes of bleeding unassociated with signs or symptoms of ovulation. Specific causes of anovulation, such as hyperprolactinaemia, thyroid disease, androgen excess, anorexia, obesity and excess exercise, can be treated specifically; otherwise, therapy depends upon patient goals. Cycle regulation can be affected by monthly courses of progestin, such as medroxyprogesterone acetate (Provera), 10 mg daily for 10 days each month. Contraception and cycle regulation can both be accomplished with oral contraceptives; fertility, on the other hand, will require ovulation induction. Patients with structural lesions, or those who do not resume normal withdrawal bleeding patterns on hormone therapy, should be subjected to further evaluation and treatment.

Luteal insufficiency

Subtle changes of progesterone synthesis and secretion and its effect on the endometrium have been implicated in the aetiology of menorrhagia, infertility and early pregnancy losses by Di Zerega et al.[16] Abnormalities of the luteal phase have been implicated in 15–25% of cases of ovulatory menorrhagia on the grounds of irregular shedding and ripening, on a histological basis, by Murthy et al.[17] Further research is needed to prove conclusively the relationship between peripheral levels of steroid and their action on the uterine lining.

Polycystic ovarian disease

Polycystic ovarian disease (PCOD) is defined as a state of chronic anovulation, with androgen excess and with or without hirsutism. This extreme form of clinical disease must be differentiated from the polycystic ovarian syndrome (PCO). Farquhar et al.[18] found the prevalence of PCO to be 21% in a general population between the ages of 18 and 45 years; pelvic ultrasonography is used to diagnose this condition. Patients with evidence of hirsutism or hyperandrogenism may need further hormonal assay for FSH, LH, testosterone, dehydroepiandrosterone and 17-hydroxyprogesterone to rule out adrenal hyperplasia or ovarian hyperandrogenism. The clinician should not make the diagnosis of polycystic ovarian syndrome solely on ultrasonic evidence, because small cysts in the ovary are very common.

About 75–85% of women with PCOD ovulate when treated with clomiphene citrate (CC). For those who fail to ovulate with CC, human menopausal gonadotrophin (hMG), human chorionic gonadotrophin (hCG), or pure FSH with and without GnRH analog have been used.[19] This therapy has a substantial risk of hyperstimulation syndrome and multiple gestation, besides the cost considerations. Gjønnaess[20] reported a high ovulation rate after partial ovarian destruction by electrocautery through the laparoscope, and proposed that all women with PCOD undergoing laparoscopy for any indication must undergo bilateral ovarian electrocautery as primary treatment. When infertility is not an issue, PCOD alone is not an indication for laparoscopy.

Heylen et al.[21] reported an argon laser ovarian capsule drilling and vaporization technique for PCOD. Of 44 anovulatory women with PCOD who were treated laparoscopically with the argon laser, 80% were previously resistant to CC therapy. After surgery, spontaneous ovulation occurred in 80% of the women; spontaneous conception occurred in 55% of patients, and another 18% of the women who were previously resistant to CC conceived postoperatively after CC therapy. This gives an overall conception rate of 73% after 18 months (using life-table analysis). Two

Table 11.2 Protocols used for assisted reproduction in patients with polycystic ovarian disease at the authors' fertility clinic

Protocol*	Cycles	Ovulation cycles		Pregnancy cycles	
		No.	%	No.	%
No drugs	20	7	35	1	5
Clomiphene	39	30	76.9	3	7.6
CC/hMG/hCG	33	28	84.8	6	18.1
FSH/hCG	55	45	81.8	10	18.1
FSH/hMG/hCG	15	13	86.6	2	13.3
GnRH (short)	15	12	80	3	20
GnRH (long)	20	18	90	1	5

*CC, clomiphene citrate; FSH, follicle-stimulating hormone; GnRH, gonadotrophin-releasing hormone; hCG, human chorionic gonadotrophin; hMG, human menopausal gonadotrophin.

different drilling techniques were used: these were classical vaporization of the ovarian capsule (22 women), and simple perforation of the ovarian capsule with subcapsular destruction of the ovarian stroma (22 women). No differences in ovulation or pregnancy rates were observed postoperatively between the two techniques. These results suggest that patients with PCOD can be induced to ovulate, and subsequently to conceive, by laparoscopic argon laser treatment. The technique with minimal trauma to the ovarian capsule seems preferable. The occurrence of filmy adhesions postoperatively does not reduce tubal motility and hence does not affect the pregnancy rate.

Table 11.2 lists the various protocols used for assisted reproduction in patients with PCOD, at the authors' fertility clinic.

Organic pathology

Fibroids

Although uterine myomas are extremely common, the majority are asymptomatic and therefore require no treatment. Pelvic ultrasound, hysteroscopy and, infrequently, magnetic resonance imaging are useful in the confirmation of this diagnosis, especially when long-term expectant management is to be used. Many indicators previously recommended for treatment are empiric in nature and have been discarded in modern times. Current standards dictate that prophylactic intervention is seldom warranted.[22]

The definitive treatment of fibroid-related menorrhagia is hysterectomy. Clearly, this operation cannot be undertaken for infertile women. Numerous medical options are available to help an infertile woman with myomas. Benagiano et al.[23] report a study using Zoladex (goserelin acetate) 3.6 mg i.m. once a month for 4 months, in patients with multiple myomata. They demonstrated a decrease in uterine and fibroid volumes of between 37 and 40%, and 44 and 47%, respectively. There was also a decrease in mean blood loss in the treatment group, when they subsequently underwent myomectomy. On stopping treatment, the size invariably reverts to pretreatment levels in about 4–6 months.

Endometrial resection is an alternative to hysterectomy, but for the infertile patient it does not leave a normal cavity for subsequent implantation. Hysteroscopic resection of sessile or pedunculated myomas is justifiable, even in the infertile group of patients, since it leaves behind very little scarring and cavity distortion. Romer[24] reported a series of 20 patients undergoing hysteroscopic myoma resection because of menometrorrhagia. Solitary myoma was diagnosed sonographically, hysteroscopically and histologically. Fourteen patients had been pretreated with GnRH-analogues for 2 or 3 months, whereas in six patients the transcervical resection of myomas was carried out immediately after menstruation. In a follow-up period of 3–18 months, eumenorrhoea could be achieved in 19 patients. In one patient, a second operation for resection of a small myoma was necessary. There were no intra- or postoperative complications. The resection of myomas is a useful organ-retaining option of treatment in patients with submucous myoma and menometrorrhagia.

Smith and Uhlir[25] reported a series of 64 myomectomies describing the indications, technique and efficacy of the procedure. The majority of operations were performed on large multinodular uteri. Indications included enlarging pelvic mass, menorrhagia, anaemia and pregnancy wastage in women who wished to preserve reproductive capability. Although infertility was not the primary indication in any case, 32 patients were nulligravid; only 10 patients were parous and 14 had a history of spontaneous abortion or pregnancy wastage. The average age of the patients was 35.8 years (range 27–47 years). There were no major complications and no patients received blood transfusions. Follow-up revealed three patients with recurrent tumours necessitating repeat procedures. Successful pregnancies have occurred in 40% of those attempting pregnancy. Thus, it appears that successful myomectomy can be performed in most patients regardless of uterine size, thereby preserving reproductive potential.

Adenomyosis

Adenomyosis is a disease of the older age-group of women, its maximum incidence occurring between 35 and 45 years. Hitherto, the only certain diagnosis was made histopathologically on surgically extirpated specimens; however, recently, various sufficiently accurate techniques have been suggested to permit diagnosis of this condition in situ. Brosens et al.,[26] by the use of endovaginal ultrasonography, have described predictive characteristics in the diagnosis of adenomyosis. Endovaginal sonography was performed and the uterine body morphometry and myometrial echogenicity were assessed: this demonstrated a sensitivity of 86%, a specificity of 50%, a positive predictive value of 86%, and a negative predictive value of 77%. McCausland[27] suggests that a routine myometrial biopsy to diagnose adenomyosis should be added to the diagnostic armamentarium during operative hysteroscopy. With these methods it might be possible to delineate the epidemiological characteristics of adenomyosis and to clarify whether it has a pathogenic role in unexplained ovulatory menorrhagia and juvenile dysmenorrhoea. Resectoscopic treatment has been proposed in some mild forms of adenomyosis to avoid hysterectomy (not relevant for women wishing to conceive in the future), whereas it seems improbable that medical treatment can offer any definitive solution. It is yet not fully established whether adenomyosis is really a disease or merely a paraphysiological condition.

Endometriosis

Mahmood et al.[28] investigated menstrual symptoms in relation to pelvic pathology, through a prospective questionnaire-based study. Menstrual symptoms of menorrhagia, irregular menses, and premenstrual spotting were associated with cystic endometriosis or infective pelvic pathology with equal frequency. Deep dyspareunia, pain after intercourse and recurrent pain unrelated to menstruation or coitus is more likely to be associated with endometriosis. Dysmenorrhoea is, of course, the commonest reported symptom in women suffering from endometriosis. Although these symptoms may raise a high index of clinical suspicion for endometriosis, these are not entirely reliable indicators of the disease or its severity. Diagnostic laparoscopy should be considered before institution of treatment in women complaining of pelvic pain and menstrual symptoms.

Surgical treatment is mainly restricted to the laparoscopic approach in infertile couples, except in the most severe cases of pelvic adhesions involving adjacent viscera. The techniques have gradually evolved from drainage alone to fulguration and finally to excision of the endometriomal cyst wall. Drainage alone is associated with a 100% recurrence within 6–9 months, and hence should only be used for palliation to reduce intra-ovarian pressure in patients undergoing ovarian stimulation with gonadotrophins for in vitro fertilization (IVF) or assisted reproduction technique (ART) cycles. As the same can be achieved through the vaginal route under transvaginal ultrasonographic control, without general anaesthesia, laparoscopy should be reserved only for cases in which more advanced fulguration or cystectomy is intended. Dicker[29] studied 41 women with endometriomas who had failed to conceive during the previous IVF–embryo transfer (ET) cycles and who had undergone transvaginal ultrasonic needle-guided aspiration of the endometriomas before the next oöcyte retrieval. A significantly higher number of oöcytes were retrieved and a higher number of embryos were transferred in the aspiration group.

It has been the authors' policy at the fertility clinic to aspirate all ovarian cysts larger than 25 mm, after downregulation with GnRH agonist. This permits better visualization of the follicles and makes the ovaries more accessible for oöcyte retrieval. In a series by Reich,[30] 12 of 20 women (60%) achieved a term pregnancy following a laparoscopic endometriomal cyst excision procedure alone. In the eight cases of women with endometriomas who did not conceive, in six there was a well-documented male infertility factor.

Pelvic tuberculosis

One of the commonest causes of infertility in the Indian subcontinent is pelvic tuberculosis. Although the predominant effect is on the fallopian tubes, a small percentage of women may present with abnormal uterine bleeding as the chief complaint.

In a study by Parikh et al.[31] from the Indian subcontinent, 117 women with a tubal factor were found to have tuberculosis as the cause of tubal blockage: on laparoscopy, 49.5% were found to have simple tubal blockage, 15.3% showed tubovarian masses, and 23.9% had a frozen pelvis. Of 75% who complained of menstrual irregularities, thus indicating endometrial involvement, 25.6% underwent an IVF procedure. The pregnancy rate after IVF–ET was 16.6% per transfer. Marcus et al.[32] assessed the outcome of IVF–ET in cases of tuberculous infertility; they studied the factors associated with success or failure of treatment in ten patients with tuberculous infertility who underwent 22 cycles of IVF and nine of cryopreserved–thawed ET at Bourn Hall Clinic, Cambridge, UK. All patients underwent endometrial assessment by ultrasonography. Four patients had preliminary hysteroscopy, endometrial biopsy, and Doppler uterine blood-flow studies. Six clinical pregnancies resulted in three live births in three patients and one current pregnancy in a fourth patient. There was one ectopic pregnancy and one twin pregnancy that aborted spontaneously at 14 weeks. The patients who had trophic endometrium achieved pregnancy at a rate of 42.9% (six of 14) (per embryo transfer) compared with 0% (none of 14) if the endometrium was atrophic. IVF–ET offers the only realistic treatment for tuberculous infertility. Preliminary assessment of the endometrium is helpful in assessing prognosis in these cases. Gürgan et al.[33–34] reported two patients with pelvic–peritoneal tuberculosis and elevated serum and peritoneal fluid levels of CA-125: the first was a young and infertile woman who had cul-de-sac nodularity and dysmenorrhoea; the other was postmenopausal and presented with weight loss and ascites. While a preoperative diagnosis of endometriosis was made in the former, intraperitoneal malignancy was considered in the latter. The diagnosis of pelvic–peritoneal tuberculosis was reached by laparoscopic-directed biopsy in both patients; serum levels of CA-125 returned to normal limits following antituberculous drug treatment.

Hansotia et al.[35] reported one of the largest series of patients with genital tuberculosis undergoing IVF. They showed significantly lower endometrial thickness in patients with genital tuberculosis — 11.5 mm in the study group compared with 12 mm in the control group ($p = 0.002$), although the clinical pregnancy rates did not differ significantly. Hansotia et al.[34] recommended the use of ultrasound examination for evaluation of the endometrial thickness, as an important screening test in the assessment of patients with genital tuberculosis.

Conclusions

- Menorrhagia, although a gynaecological symptom, is closely linked through its aetiopathogenesis to infertility. Ovulatory dysfunction is a common denominator in the causation of menorrhagia and infertility; hence, its early diagnosis and management form the mainstay of treatment.
- Organic pathological conditions, such as myomas, adenomyosis, endometriosis and pelvic tuberculosis, must be managed conservatively, either surgically or in combination with pharmacological suppression.
- Assisted reproduction will have to form the mainstay of management in the more complex and resistant cases in which previous surgical attempts have failed, or in those that are not treatable, even surgically.
- Management of menorrhagia and infertility will be, of necessity, a multispeciality approach, integrating the expertise of reproductive endocrinologists, endoscopists and IVF specialists.

References

1. Short R V. The evolution of human reproduction. Proc R Soc Lond 1976; 195: 3–24
2. Hallberg L, Hogdahl A M, Nilsson L, Rybo G. Menstrual blood loss, a population study. Acta Obstet Gynecol Scand 1966: 45: 320–351

3. Cole S K, Billewicz W Z, Thomson A M. Sources of variation in menstrual blood loss. J Obstet Gynaecol Br Commw 1971; 78: 933–939

4. Fraser I S, McCarron G, Markham R, Resta T. Blood and total fluid content of menstrual discharge. Obstet Gynecol 1985; 65: 194–198

5. Markee J E. Menstruation in intra-ocular endometrial transplants in the rhesus monkey. Contrib Embryol 1940; 28: 219–308

6. Scommegna A, Vorys N, Givens J R. Menstrual dysfunction. In: Gold J J, Josimovich J B (eds) Gynecologic endocrinology. New York: Harper and Row, 1980: 290–326

7. Hahn L. Composition of menstrual blood. In: Diczfalusy E, Fraser I S, Webb F T C (eds) WHO Symposium on endometrial blood and steroidal contraception. London: Pitman, 1980

8. Wood J C. Lysosomes of the uterus. In: Bishop M W H (ed) Advances in reproductive physiology, No. 6. London: Elek Science, 1973: 221–230

9. Ferenczy A. Studies on the cytodynamics of human endometrial regeneration. I. Scanning electron microscopy. Am J Obstet Gynecol 1976; 124: 64–74

10. Wilansky D L M, Greisman B. Early hypothyroidism in patients with menorrhagia. Am J Obstet Gynecol 1989; 160: 673–677

11. Fraser I S, McCarron G, Markham R et al. Measured menstrual blood loss in women with menorrhagia associated with pelvic disease or coagulation disorder. Obstet Gynecol 1986, 68: 630–633

12. Ahuja R, Kriplani A, Choudhary V P, Takkar D. von Willebrand disease: a rare cause of puberty menorrhagia. Aust N Z J Obstet Gynaecol 1995; 35(3): 337–338

13. Haynes P J, Anderson A B, Turnbull A C. Patterns of menstrual blood loss in menorrhagia. Res Clin Forums 1979; 1(2): 73–78

14. Smith S K, Abel M H, Kelly R W, Baird D T. The synthesis of prostaglandins from persistent proliferative endometrium. J Clin Endocrinol Metab 1982; 55: 284–289

15. Field C S. Dysfunctional uterine bleeding. Prim Care 1988; 15(3): 561–574

16. Di Zerega G S, Hodgen G D. Luteal phase dysfunction infertility: a sequel to aberrant folliculogenesis. Fertil Steril 1981; 35: 489–499

17. Murthy Y S, Arronet G H, Parekh M C. Luteal phase inadequacy. Its significance in infertility. Obstet Gynecol 1970; 36: 758–761

18. Farquhar C M, Birdsall M, Manning P et al. The prevalence of polycystic ovaries on ultrasound scanning in a population of randomly selected women. Aust N Z J Obstet Gynaecol 1994; 34: 67–72

19. Farhi J, Homburg R, Lerner A, Ben-Rafael Z. The choice of treatment for anovulation associated with polycystic ovary syndrome following failure to conceive with clomiphene. Hum Reprod 1993; 8: 1367–1371

20. Gjønnaess H. Ovarian electrocautery in the treatment of women with polycystic ovary syndrome (PCOS): factors affecting the results. Acta Obstet Gynecol Scand 1994; 73: 407–412

21. Heylen S M, Puttemans P J, Brosens I A. Polycystic ovarian disease treated by laparoscopic argon laser capsule drilling: comparison of vaporization versus perforation technique. Hum Reprod 1994; 9(6): 1038–1042

22. Hutchins F L Jr. Uterine fibroids. Diagnosis and indications for treatment. Obstet Gynecol Clin North Am 1995; 22(4): 659–665

23. Benagiano G, Kivinen S T, Fadini R et al. Zoladex (goserelin acetate) and the anemic patient: results of a multicenter fibroid study. Fertil Steril 1996; 66(2): 223–229

24. Romer T. Hysteroscopic myoma resection in hypermenorrhea. Z Arzti Fortbild (Jena) 1996; 90(3): 259–262

25. Smith D C, Uhlir J K. Myomectomy as a reproductive procedure. Am J Obstet Gynecol 1990; 162(6): 1476–1482

26. Brosens J J, de Souza N M, Barker F G et al. Endovaginal ultrasonography in the diagnosis of adenomyosis uteri: identifying the predictive characteristics. Br J Obstet Gynaecol 1995; 102(6): 471–474

27. McCausland A M. Hysteroscopic myometrial biopsy: its use in diagnosing adenomyosis and its clinical application. Am J Obstet Gynecol 1992; 166(6): 1619–1628

28. Mahmood T A, Templeton A A, Thomson L, Fraser C. Menstrual symptoms in women with pelvic endometriosis. Br J Obstet Gynaecol 1991; 98(6); 558–563

29. Dicker D, Goldman J A, Feldberg D et al. Transvaginal ultrasonic needle guided aspiration of endometriotic cysts before ovulation induction for in vitro fertilization. J in Vitro Fert Embryo Transf 1991; 8: 286–289

30. Reich H, McGlynn F J. Treatment of ovarian endometriomas using laparoscopic surgical techniques. J Reprod Med 1986; 31(7): 577–584

31. Parikh F R, Nadkarni S G, Kamat S A et al. Genital tuberculosis — a major pelvic factor causing infertility in Indian women. Fertil Steril 1997; 67(3): 497–500

32. Marcus S F, Rizk B, Fountain S, Brinsden P. Tuberculous infertility and in vitro fertilization. Am J Obstet Gynecol 1994; 171(6): 1593–1596

33. Gürgan T, Urman B, Yarali H. Results of in vitro fertilization and embryo transfer in women with infertility due to genital tuberculosis. Fertil Steril 1996; 65(2): 367–370

34. Sheth S S. Elevated CA 125 in advanced abdominal or pelvic tuberculosis. Int J Gynecol Obstet 1996; 52: 167–171

35. Hansotia M D, Desai S K, Dalal A et al. In vitro fertilization in patients with genital tuberculosis makes a difference. Submitted

CHAPTER 12

Haematological aspects of menorrhagia

S. J. Parekh and S. K. Bichile

Introduction

Haematological disorders causing excessive uterine bleeding may have serious consequences, sometimes requiring emergency blood transfusion support and, more frequently, causing persistent iron-deficiency anaemia, resulting in chronic fatigue and poor performance. Although cessation of menstruation is a complex phenomenon, the haemostatic mechanism has an important role in the process.[1]

The exact frequency of haemostatic disorders causing abnormal uterine bleeding is difficult to assess. Published reports may have bias in the selection of patients and a wide variation in the type of laboratory investigations performed.[2,3] Claessens and Cowell[4] found the incidence of coagulation disorders to be almost 20% among adolescent girls seeking advice for menorrhagia. In America, the incidence of coagulopathies in the gynaecological population is thought to be 5% or higher.[5] Yet the precise diagnosis of haemostatic disorders (particularly von Willebrand's disease [vWD]) often eludes gynaecologists, primarily owing to inadequate evaluation of these disorders.[6–8]

Diagnosis

Haematological disorders that may cause excessive uterine bleeding are listed in Table 12.1. Some women bleed profusely, whereas others do so only when exposed to a haemostatic challenge (such as trauma or surgery). Precise diagnosis needs a systematic clinical and laboratory approach. At the same time, local uterine and pelvic disease must be ruled out and the hypothalamic–pituitary–ovarian axis should also be evaluated.

Clinical history

A careful and detailed history usually provides important initial clues to arouse suspicion of a haematological disorder. It may also help to plan appropriate laboratory investigations in a cost-effective way. The following points, in particular, should be addressed:

1. Is there a history of episodes of epistaxis? (Spontaneous and recurrent epistaxis strongly suggests an underlying haemostatic disorder.)
2. Is there a history of bleeding gums or skin bruising? Did the patient have a haematoma after intramuscular injection? If bleeding is limited to mucocutaneous sites (purpura, epistaxis, bleeding gums), this suggests

Table 12.1 Haematological disorders causing excessive uterine bleeding

Platelet disorders
- Thrombocytopenia

(a) Bone marrow (BM) failure	Aplastic anaemia
	Acute leukaemia
	BM infiltration
	Antineoplastic drugs
(b) Immune thrombocytopenia	Idiopathic thrombocytopenic purpura
	Drugs
	HIV-1
	SLE
(c) Non-immune thrombocytopenia	Thrombotic thrombocytopenic purpura
	Haemolytic uraemic syndrome
	HELLP

- Platelet function abnormalities

(a) Congenital:	Glanzmann's thrombasthenia
	Bernard Soulier syndrome
	Storage pool disease
(b) Acquired:	Drugs — NSAIDs

Von Willebrand's disease
- Congenital
- Acquired

	Hypothyroidism
	Angiodysplasia
	SLE
	Monoclonal gammopathy
	Lymphoproliferative diseases

Coagulation protein abnormalities

- Congenital:	Fibrinogen
	Factor VIII and factor IX
	Factor XI*
	Factor XIII
- Acquired:	Disseminated intravascular coagulation
	Oral anticoagulants
	Heparin
	Liver diseases
	Acquired inhibitors (factor VIII)

Excessive fibrinolysis
- Antiplasmin deficiency
- PAI-1 deficiency

* Most often in Ashkenazi Jews.

HELLP, haemolysis, elevated liver enzymes, low platelets; HIV, human immunodeficiency virus; NSAIDs, non-steroidal anti-inflammatory drugs; PAI, plasminogen activator inhibitor; SLE, systemic lupus erythematosus.

thrombocytopenia, platelet function defects or vWD, whereas a deep haematoma suggests coagulation factor deficiency.

3. Does the patient give a history of excessive and/or prolonged bleeding after tooth extraction, surgery or major trauma?
4. Did the patient require blood transfusions after an otherwise minor surgical procedure or after delivery?
5. Does the patient notice excessive menstrual bleeding after ingestion of drugs such as non-steroidal anti-inflammatory drugs (NSAIDs) or aspirin?
6. Is the patient receiving heparin or oral anticoagulants?
7. Is there a similar history of menorrhagia or mucocutaneous bleeding in a sister, mother or aunt? Does the father have haemophilia or epistaxis or excessive bleeding after tooth extraction or surgery?
8. Is there a history of recurrent spontaneous abortion with or without post-partum haemorrhage?

Although a clinical history serves as the most effective way of arousing suspicion of the presence of a haemostatic disorder, two limitations must be borne in mind:

1. Patients with acquired haemostatic problems may have previously withstood haemostatic challenge normally;
2. Every patient may not have been exposed to haemostatic challenge sufficient to unmask a mild haemostatic problem; excessive uterine bleeding may be the only manifestation.

Physical examination

Physical examination should include careful inspection of the trunk and extremities for purpura and ecchymosis; palpation for enlargement of lymph nodes, spleen and liver; examination of joints; examination of sclera for icterus, and fundoscopic examination for retinal haemorrhages.

Laboratory evaluation

Laboratory investigations should include initial screening tests followed by specific measurements, which confirm and quantify the precise defect.

Initial investigations (Table 12.2)

A complete blood count, including platelet count, reticulocyte count and erythrocyte sedimentation rate (ESR) determination, provide important clues to the diagnosis. The commonest cause of isolated thrombocytopenia is idiopathic thrombocytopenic purpura (ITP), whereas thrombocytopenia associated with leucopenia and anaemia suggests possible bone marrow failure (e.g. aplastic anaemia, acute leukaemia or infiltration of bone marrow). Bone marrow aspiration and core biopsy help to differentiate these conditions. Thrombocytopenia with increased reticulocyte count indicates associated increased haemolysis (e.g. Evans' syndrome, HELLP — see Glossary on p. 152). Thrombocytopenia with markedly increased ESR is encountered in systemic disorders, such as systemic lupus erythematosus (SLE), human immunodeficiency virus (HIV) infection and malignancies. Careful evaluation of the peripheral blood smear is absolutely essential and could be highly informative. Thrombocytopenia with younger

Table 12.2 Screening tests for suspected haemostatic disorders

1. Platelet count
2. Ivy (template) bleeding time
3. Prothrombin time
4. Activated partial thromboplastin time
5. Thrombin time

platelets (larger than normal) indicates increased peripheral destruction (e.g. ITP) rather than decreased production (e.g. marrow failure). Very large platelets are found in the Bernard Soulier syndrome. Absence of platelet clump formation in a directly prepared peripheral blood smear is characteristic of Glanzmann's thrombasthenia. Thrombocytopenia with fragmentation of erythrocytes is suggestive of microangiopathic haemolytic anaemia (see Glossary on p. 152).

Coagulation screening tests, such as prothrombin time (PT), activated partial thromboplastin time (aPTT) and thrombin time (TT), serve as screening tests for detection of coagulation factor deficiencies. However, meticulous quality control is required: each laboratory should determine its own normal range of values; the results obtained on patients' plasma must be compared with normal control values and expressed as a ratio.

PT is a measure of deficiency of factors II, V, VII and X. Isolated prolongation of PT suggests factor VII deficiency, liver disease or warfarin ingestion (extrinsic pathway). aPTT is a measure of deficiency of factors VIII, IX, XI and XII (intrinsic pathway) as well as II, V and X (common pathway). Factor XII deficiency, however, is not associated with clinical bleeding and factor XI deficiency is most frequently seen in Ashkenazi Jews. Simultaneous prolongation of both PT and aPTT indicates multiple factor deficiencies, such as disseminated intravascular coagulation (DIC), liver disease, or the use of oral anticoagulants. TT is a measure of fibrinogen function and is prolonged in afibrinogenaemia, dysfibrinogenaemia and the presence of heparin.

The alterations in screening tests observed in various haemostatic disorders are listed in Table 12.3. Normal screening tests almost exclude significant coagulation protein defects except factor XIII deficiency and abnormalities of the fibrinolytic system (α_2-antiplasmin deficiency and plasminogen activator inhibitor [PAI–1] deficiency). If the clinical history is strongly suggestive of a haemostatic disorder and results of all screening tests are normal, then investigations for factor XIII deficiency (urea stability test) and fibrinolytic system (euglobin clot lysis assay and tests for α_2-antiplasmin and PAI–1) are carried out. A scheme for investigations of haemostatic disorders is given in Figure 12.1.

Diagnosis of von Willebrand's disease
Von Willebrand's disease is the most common hereditary bleeding disorder, yet it is often unrecognized and may be particularly severe among adolescent women when oestrogen stimulation of the endometrium produces a highly vascular endothelial lining.[8] Von Willebrand factor (vWF) plays an important role in haemostasis by acting as a bridge between platelets and injured vascular endothelium. It circulates in the plasma as a complex with factor VIII (VIIIC–vWF) and also protects factor

Table 12.3 Results of screening tests in haemostatic disorders*

Disorder	Platelet count	Bleeding time	Prothrombin time	Partial thromboplastin time
Vascular disorder	N	↑	N	N
Thrombocytopenia	↓	↑	N	N
Platelet function defect	N	↑	N	N
Coagulation disorder	N	N**	↑ or N	↑ or N

N, Normal; ↓, reduced; ↑, increased.

* Patients with a history strongly suggestive of haemostatic disorder and having all above tests normal, warrant tests for factor XIII deficiency, α_2-antiplasmin deficiency and PAI–1 deficiency.

** Except in von Willebrand's disease.

Figure 12.1 Scheme for investigation of haemostatic disorders.

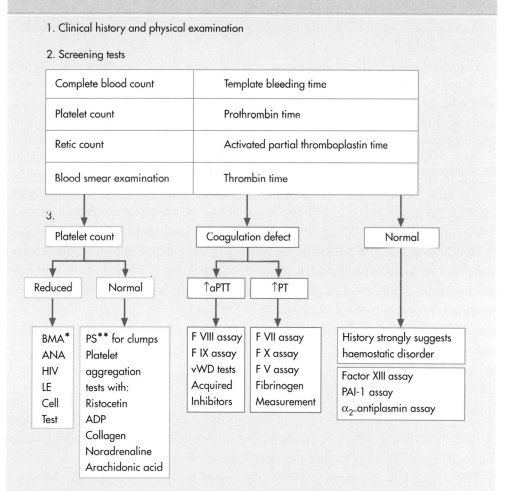

ANA, antinuclear antibodies; BMA, bone marrow aspiration; F, factor; HIV, human immunodeficiency virus; LE, lupus erythematosus; PS, peripheral blood smear; vWD, von Willebrand's disease.

VIII from proteolytic degradation. Thus, in the absence of vWF, the factor VIIIC activity may also be low.

The laboratory diagnosis of vWD is complex. The various laboratory features are as follows:

- Prolonged Ivy (template) bleeding time
- Prolonged aPTT
- Decreased factor VIIC level
- Decreased vWF antigen (ELISA, immunoelectrophoresis)
- Decreased vWF level (ristocetin cofactor assay)
- Abnormal multimeric analysis of vWF protein [sodium dodecyl sulphate (SDS) agarose gel electrophoresis]
- Abnormal platelet aggregation tests with ristocetin.

vWD is a very heterogeneous disease, usually with autosomal dominant inheritance, and several types of vWD are described.[9–12] It should be noted that initial screening tests (BT and aPTT) may be normal in the mild variety of vWD.

Among vWD patients, 80% are of type I, with subnormal levels of structurally and functionally normal vWF; in type II vWD, patients have structurally and functionally abnormal vWF, and type III vWF is characterized by total absence of vWF at storage sites.[12]

The subtypes of vWD can be differentiated by multimeric analysis of the patient's vWF, using SDS gel electrophoresis. The multimers are stained with radiolabelled antibodies and visualized by autoradiography.[12] Type I vWD has normal multimeric structure present in plasma and platelets (all bands present), whereas type II is characterized by absence of high-molecular-weight multimers. Type II vWD is further divided into subtypes IIA, IIB and IIC, based on multimer analysis on platelet surface and in plasma separately.

Alternatively, crossed immunoelectrophoresis may be used to distinguish variants. Further distinction may also be made by platelet aggregation studies, using different concentrations of ristocetin: in type I vWD, platelet aggregation is absent at all concentrations of ristocetin; in type IIB, platelet aggregation occurs even at very low concentrations of ristocetin (hyperaggregability of platelets).

The distinction between the various types of vWD has direct therapeutic implications. Desmopressin acetate (DDAVP) is of benefit in type I disease and mild type IIA (DDAVP releases vWF from endothelial cells), whereas in type IIB it is contraindicated; in type III disease it is ineffective.[13]

Diagnosis of acquired inhibitors of coagulation

Acquired inhibitors of coagulation are defined as substances in the blood that directly inhibit the clot-promoting ability of coagulation factors.[14] They can occur as alloantibodies (e.g. antibodies induced against factor VIII in patients with haemophilia) or as spontaneously developing autoantibodies.

The commonest acquired inhibitor is against factor VIII and may have an autoimmune pathogenesis. However, acquired inhibitors against other factors can occur. Spontaneous inhibitors are clinically suspected in women who develop sudden appearance of bleeding with prolonged aPTT (and normal platelet count), particularly during the post-partum period.[15] The diagnosis of inhibitors is confirmed when the prolonged aPTT does not get corrected to normal when the test is repeated on a 50/50 mixture of the patient's plasma with control plasma. A more prevalent disorder is the antiphospholipid antibody syndrome (including 'lupus' anticoagulant). Paradoxically, this autoantibody leads to thrombosis, recurrent abortions and foetal loss.

Diagnosis of thrombocytopenia

The various conditions producing thrombocytopenia are listed in Table 12.1, the commonest being ITP. In adults, it presents with the insidious onset of mucous membrane bleeding or easy bruisability. The bone marrow examination reveals increased number of megakaryocytes and this finding helps to differentiate ITP from other disorders such as bone marrow suppression or acute leukaemia. Sometimes, ITP is a manifestation of other more serious systemic disorders, such as lupus erythematosus, HIV or lymphoproliferative disorders and tests such as those for HIV antibodies and antinuclear antibodies must be carried out.

Diagnosis of platelet function abnormalities

Platelet function abnormalities are suspected in those patients who have clinical manifestations suggestive of platelet deficiency (purpuric lesions, mucous membrane bleeding) but have a normal platelet count. Various qualitative platelet disorders causing menorrhagia are listed in Table 12.4. These disorders are common in parts of South India and their diagnosis is suspected with a history of consanguinity and autosomal recessive inheritance. Glanzmann's thrombasthenia (absence of the glycoprotein IIb/IIIa receptor) and the Bernard Soulier syndrome (absence of the Ib/IX receptor) cause persistent and intractable menorrhagia. Platelet aggregation studies on the patient's platelet-rich plasma are carried out with various agonists (ADP, adrenaline, collagen, ristocetin and arachidonic acid). On the other hand, the commonest acquired platelet-function defects are secondary to drugs, particularly NSAIDs such as aspirin, ibuprofen and naproxen, which inhibit platelet thromboxane A2 synthesis.

Diagnosis of disorders of the fibrinolytic system

The fibrinolytic system causes degradation of fibrin by plasmin (the inactive precursor form is plasminogen). The principal activator of plasminogen in vivo is the enzyme tissue plasminogen activator (tPA). The system is inhibited by α_2-

Table 12.4 Platelet function disorders and aggregation studies

Disorder	Agonists used for aggregation studies of diagnostic significance
Glanzmann's thrombasthenia	ADP, adrenaline, collagen, arachidonic acid
Bernard Soulier syndrome	Ristocetin
von Willebrand's disease	Ristocetin
Storage pool disease	ADP, adrenaline, collagen

ADP, adenosine diphosphate.

antiplasmin (which directly inhibits plasmin) and PAI-1. Congenital deficiencies of α_2-antiplasmin are known to cause menorrhagia.[16] Initial screening tests are inadequate to detect these defects and specific assays for α_2-antiplasmin and PAI-1 must be performed.

Management

The management of menorrhagia depends upon the underlying cause. In some patients (e.g. those with immune thrombocytopenia or acquired anticoagulants), the treatments available may yield rewarding results, whereas, in others (e.g. those with Glanzmann's thrombasthenia), no permanent cure can be offered. In such patients, treatment with hormones, danazol, ethamsylate or antifibrinolytic agents (tranexamic acid) may be of temporary benefit. Recent reports indicate that locally enhanced fibrinolysis plays a role even in essential menorrhagia,[17] and antifibrinolytic agents such as Cyklokapron (tranexamic acid) may be effective in reducing menstrual blood flow. The majority of patients with recurrent menorrhagia have chronic iron-deficiency anaemia and need oral iron therapy for prolonged periods. Occasionally, women with acute or massive menstrual blood loss may require emergency blood transfusion.

Von Willebrand's disease

The 80% of patients with vWD who have type I disease are best managed with DDAVP, administered as a concentrated nasal spray (1.5 mg/ml). Each spray delivers 150 µg (0.1 ml) DDAVP,[18] and produces a rapid increase in the level of vWF and factor VIII, with peak concentrations reached at 2 hours. A single dose of 150–300 µg is effective for up to 24–48 h and a repeat dose is not advisable before 48 h because replenishment of stores of endogenous vWF takes about 48 h. A distinct advantage of the nasal spray of DDAVP is that it can be self-administered and used in the home or workplace; however, it cannot be used in patients with nasal congestion and atrophic rhinitis. Intravenous desmopressin is used in these situations and before surgery and invasive procedures.

DDAVP is not effective in type III vWD and is contraindicated in type IIB vWD because it may cause thrombocytopenia due to hyperaggregation of platelets. Side effects of DDAVP include nausea, vomiting, headache, abdominal cramps and occasional allergic reactions. Long-term use of DDAVP may cause hyponatraemia, owing to its antidiuretic effect, and such patients are advised to restrict their water intake.

Women with severe vWD may need administration of blood products to control bleeding. Fresh-frozen plasma and cryoprecipitate are rich sources of vWF, however, the risks of transfusion-associated infectious diseases (HIV, hepatitis B and C) and immunomodulation are of major concern. Commercial intermediate-purity factor VIII preparations (Haemate P, Centeon) have all the multimers of vWF and are therapeutically effective. These preparations have an advantage in that they are heat treated and chemically treated for virus inactivation. Factor VIII of very high purity is not a good source of vWF and should not be used.

Platelet disorders

Oral prednisolone (1–2 mg/kg) is the first-line treatment for ITP and is initially effective in 60% of women. However, long-term use of steroids has a drawback of serious side effects and 40% of adults do not obtain a permanent response. Failure of a trial of oral prednisolone for 3 months or more warrants consideration of splenectomy. Intravenous immunoglobulin (IvIG), administered at a daily dose of 400 mg/kg/day, for 5 days as infusion, may rapidly increase the platelet count and may be considered for women who bleed profusely and need an urgent increase in the platelet count. It is effective in controlling the bleeding; however, it is very expensive and the action is short lived; repeated courses of IvIG may be needed. In approximately 5% of patients, splenectomy has failed and they may need long-term immunosuppressive therapy (azathioprine) or short courses of pulse high dose i.v. methyl prednisolone.

Hereditary platelet function disorders
Glanzmann's thrombasthenia and the Bernard Soulier syndrome can produce severe, recurrent and sometimes life-threatening menorrhagia requiring transfusions of platelet concentrates to control bleeding and packed red blood cells (RBC) to correct anaemia. These patients rapidly develop alloantibodies against glycoprotein IIb/IIIa and Ib/IX respectively, which makes them refractory to subsequent platelet transfusion. There is no cure.

Acquired factor VIII inhibitors (antibodies)
Women with acquired factor VIII antibodies are treated with infusions of porcine factor VIII concentrate (Hyate C, Speywood Pharmaceuticals) or activated factor IX complex (Autoplex T, Baxter). Infusion of recombinant factor VIIa (Novo Nordisk) is also effective. Oral prednisolone given for 4 weeks may be effective in suppressing acquired inhibitors.[15] Some patients may need IvIG infusions.

Glossary

AFLP (acute fatty liver of pregnancy) Virtually all patients have a prolonged prothrombin time, hypofibrinogenaemia, thrombocytopenia and DIC. Maternal bleeding may be uncontrollable and liver failure may be progressive and life threatening.

Angiodysplasia This is degenerative dilatation of the small blood vessels resulting in recurrent bleeding without any defect in the blood coagulation factors. Can be demonstrated by angiography.

APS (antiphospholipid syndrome) This is common in young women with a history of recurrent foetal loss and thrombotic complications. Also known as lupus anticoagulant syndrome or anticardiolipin antibody syndrome. Some patients may have thrombocytopenia.

Bernard Soulier syndrome This is a bleeding disorder, characterized by thrombocytopenia, giant platelets and autosomal recessive inheritance (defect in platelet membrane glycoprotein Ib/IX receptor). Consanguinity is common.

DIC (disseminated intravascular coagulation) This is also known as consumption coagulopathy. It is a haemorrhagic syndrome following uncontrolled activation of clotting factors and fibrinolytic enzymes. Fibrin is deposited in the intravascular system and tissue necrosis is common. This is an important complication of pregnancy.

Evans' syndrome This is characterized by a combination of autoimmune haemolytic anaemia and autoimmune thrombocytopenic purpura; the direct Coombs' test is usually positive and gives a clue to the diagnosis.

Glanzmann's thrombasthenia This is a haemorrhagic diathesis of autosomal recessive inheritance characterized by a prolonged bleeding time, defective clot retraction, normal platelet count but functional abnormality of platelets (defect in platelet membrane glycoprotein IIb–IIIa receptor). Consanguinity is common.

HELLP (haemolysis, elevated liver enzymes, low platelets) Of patients with pre-eclampsia, 5% develop this syndrome. Immediate delivery is recommended, if feasible, under cover of platelet transfusion support.

HUS (haemolytic uraemic syndrome)/TTP (thrombotic thrombocytopenic purpura) This is haemolytic anaemia and thrombocytopenia occurring with acute renal failure, neurological complications and hepatocellular dysfunction. HUS usually occurs in children; TTP is the identical disease in adults. Microangiopathic red cell and platelet destruction is related to intravascular fibrin deposition in multiple organs.

Idiopathic thrombocytopenic purpura (ITP) This is an autoimmune disorder characterized by ecchymoses and bleeding from mucous membranes and extremely low platelet counts. Menorrhagia may be severe and persistent. Platelets are being destroyed by antiplatelet antibodies.

Lymphoproliferative diseases This is a group of disorders due to proliferation of a clone of lymphoid cells (detected by morphological evaluation of the peripheral blood, bone marrow or lymph node biopsy), e.g. malignant lymphoma.

MAHA (micro-angiopathic haemolytic anaemia) This is haemolysis due to narrowing or obstruction of small blood vessels, causing fragmentation of red blood cells and destruction of platelets. During pregnancy, several syndromes are observed, e.g. pre-eclampsia, HELLP, HUS, TTP, SLE, APS, AFLP.

Monoclonal gammopathy This group of disorders is due to proliferation of a clone of lymphoid or plasma cells (detected by serum or urine electrophoresis). The monoclonal immunoglobulin production is usually due to myeloma or lymphoma.

SLE (systemic lupus erythematosus) This is an inflammatory connective tissue disease, frequently presenting with fever, joint pains, erythematous skin lesions, pleurisy, glomerular lesions, anaemia, a positive LE cell test and serum antinuclear antibodies. It is quite common in young women.

Storage pool disease This hereditary disorder of platelet function is due to abnormalities of platelet granules and can be diagnosed by platelet aggregation studies and by electron microscopic examination of platelets.

References

1. Ewenstein B M. The pathophysiology of bleeding disorders presenting as abnormal uterine bleeding. Am J Obstet Gynecol 1996; 75: 770–777

2. Mukherjee J, Roy Chaudhuri N N. A review of 70 cases of puberty menorrhagia. J Obstet Gynaecol India 1986; 36: 121–125

3. Radha R, Shah S, Vaidya P. Adolescent menorrhagia. J Obstet Gynaecol India 1992; 42: 686

4. Claessens E A, Cowell C A. Acute adolescent menorrhagia. Am J Obstet Gynecol 1981; 139: 277–280

5. Brenner P F. Proceedings of symposium: 'Women with bleeding disorders and role of the obstetrician and gynaecologist'. 43rd Annual meeting Am Coll Obstet Gynecol. Am J Obstet Gynecol 1996; 175: 761–762

6. Rick M E. Diagnosis and management of Von Willebrand's syndrome. Med Clin North Am 1994; 78: 609–623

7. McDonagh J, Kacmorek E, Hee Lee M. Fibrinogen and factor XIII, biology and disorders of fibrin formation and cross linking. In: Handin R I, Stosell T P, Lux S E (eds) Blood: principles and practice of hematology. Philadelphia: Lippincott, 1994: 1219–1259

8. Wathern P I, Henderson M C, Witz C A. Abnormal uterine bleeding. Med Clin North Am 1995; 79: 329–344

9. Saddler J E, Matsushi K T, Dorg Z et al. Molecular mechanism and classification of vWD. Thromb Haemost 1995; 74; 161–166

10. Conti M, Mari D, Conti E et al. Pregnancy in women with different types of von Willebrand disease. Obstet Gynecol 1986; 68: 282–285

11. Ruggeri Z M. Pathogenesis and classification of von Willebrand's disease. Hemostasis 1994; 24: 265–275

12. Ruggeri Z M, Zimmermann T S. Variant von Willebrand's disease characterisation of two subtypes by analysis of multimeric composition of Factor VIII von Willebrand Factor in plasma and platelets. J Clin Invest 1980; 65: 1318–1325

13. Logan L J. Treatment of von Willebrand disease. Semin Thromb Hemost 1992; 6: 1079

14. Exner T. Diagnostic methodologies for circulating anticoagulants. Thromb Haemost 1995; 74: 338–344

15. Hauser I, Schneider B, Lechner K. Postpartum Factor VIII inhibitors: a review of the literature with special reference to the value of steroids and immunosuppressive treatment. Thromb Haemost 1995; 73: 1–5

16. Miles L A, Plav E F, Donelly K J et al. A bleeding disorder due to deficiency of alpha 2 antiplasmin. Blood 1982; 39: 1246–1251

17. Gleeson N, Deritt M, Sheppard B L, Bonnar J. Endometrial fibrinolytic enzyme in women with normal menstruation and dysfunctional uterine bleeding. Br J Obstet Gynaecol 1993; 100: 768–771

18. Rose E H, Aledott L M. Nasal spray DDAVP for mild hemophilia and vWD. Ann Intern Med 1991; 114: 563–568

CHAPTER 13

Endometrial resection and long-term follow-up

A. Pooley and C. J. G. Sutton

Introduction

Transcervical resection of the endometrium (TCRE) was first described, in 1983, by DeCherney and Polan, who had used a urological resectoscope to remove the endometrium of women with intractable bleeding who were unfit for major surgery owing to blood dyscrasia or extreme anaesthetic risk.[1] Some impressive results were obtained, with amenorrhoea achieved, and the technique began to be considered as a viable alternative to hysterectomy in the treatment of menorrhagia. Subsequent reports of high levels of success and patient satisfaction led to an exponential increase in the use of endometrial resection and related techniques during the early 1990s. A survey in August 1990 reported that 36 British centres had performed more than 4000 endometrial ablation procedures, of which 70% had been performed using resection.[2] During the year from April 1993, more than 10,000 procedures were performed in England and Wales alone, with 75% of all gynaecological units offering this service.[3]

This substantial change in the management of menorrhagia has taken place in the absence of good prospective research to establish the safety and long-term efficacy of these techniques. The early publications largely described the personal series of experts in operative hysteroscopy and reported excellent outcomes, although frequently with follow-up intervals of months rather than years.[4] Subsequent reports began to emerge describing increasing late failure rates of between 9 and 22%, and the need to resort to hysterectomy in many cases. It was suggested that the failure rate might be as high as 10% per annum,[5] with a report from one health region in England suggesting that the introduction of endometrial ablation had led to an increase in the use of surgery for menorrhagia with no reduction in the rate of hysterectomy.[6] The opportunity has been lost to mount a large prospective long-term assessment of these techniques, now that they are so widely practised (and requested by patients). It is necessary, therefore, to rely on the long-term results of large series, subjected to appropriate analysis, to establish the true worth of these techniques. Endometrial resection, often combined with rollerball ablation of the cornua and uterine fundus, is the most widely practised technique for endometrial destruction, and is familiar to most gynaecologists. A description is given below of the main variations in practice, and some of the potential pitfalls.

Patient selection

When counselling a patient about the possibility of undergoing an endometrial resection, a realistic account must be provided of the likely outcome for that individual. There is now sufficient evidence to enable description of certain groups of women for whom endometrial ablation is less likely to provide long-term relief from menorrhagia, including younger women and those with a markedly enlarged or multiple fibroid uterus. The endometrium has remarkable powers of regeneration, which appears more vigorous in younger women. Women aged under 45 must be made aware that they have a higher chance of failure than those aged over 45.

Endometrial resection is suitable for women with one or more submucous fibroids, but fibroids with a substantial intramural portion can be difficult to treat, especially when greater than 20 mm in diameter. Higher complication and failure rates can be expected when attempting endometrial resection combined with resection of uterine fibroids, the main risks being perforation, bleeding and excessive fluid intravasation. There is no recognized upper limit of size of uterus for which endometrial resection is appropriate, but success is much less likely if the uterine cavity is substantially enlarged beyond 12 cm.

One advantage that endometrial resection has over all ablative techniques is that all the resected material is available for histological examination. Cases have been described where a focus of adenocarcinoma has been discovered in the tissue obtained at endometrial resection, when a preoperative endometrial biopsy showed no abnormality.[7] It is still wise to have the result of an endometrial biopsy beforehand, as retrograde peritoneal seeding of adenocarcinomatous cells during hysteroscopy has been described.[8] Endometrial ablation is contraindicated in the presence of endometrial cellular atypia or adenomatous hyperplasia, but not if simple or cystic glandular hyperplasia without atypia is the only abnormality. Women with menorrhagia frequently present with other associated symptoms, which may not be improved by endometrial ablation. Premenstrual pelvic pain may indicate the presence of endometriosis, which can be sought for, and treated by operative laparoscopy at the same time as the endometrial resection. Menstrual pain is frequently proportional to the volume of blood lost, and will be improved by the reduction in flow following TCRE, especially the characteristic cramping pains associated with the passage of large clots (clot colic). Severe dysmenorrhoea, either primary or associated with endometriotic implants on or within the uterosacral ligaments (secondary dysmenorrhoea), can often be helped by laparoscopic uterine nerve ablation[9,10] or presacral neurectomy,[11] performed at the same time. Symptoms of the premenstrual syndrome are unlikely to be directly affected by endometrial resection, but the absence of menorrhagia may lead to a more general improvement in well-being at this time.

Endometrial ablation is not suitable for women who harbour any thoughts of having a further pregnancy. Successful pregnancy is possible, but there is a high chance of serious problems, including growth retardation due to poor placentation, placenta accreta, and the need for caesarean hysterectomy.[9,12] Women who have not been sterilized prior to surgery should be offered concomitant laparoscopic tubal ligation, and those who decline must be advised of the need to use reliable contraception at all times thereafter.

Endometrial preparation

With all forms of endometrial ablation, the intention is to destroy or remove all layers of the endometrium, preventing any regeneration. The endometrial thickness varies during the menstrual cycle, from 3 mm just after menses to 12 mm or more in the late luteal phase. Ensuring that all procedures are performed in the immediate postmenstrual phase can be logistically difficult, and most practitioners use some form of pharmacological endometrial preparation. This provides significant advantages, including increased safety due to an optimal view of the endometrial cavity, a reduced volume of tissue to be removed, reduced operating time, and reduced complications, with less fluid intravasation and bleeding.

The pharmacological options available for endometrial preparation include danazol, progestogens, or an analogue of gonadotrophin hormone-releasing hormone (GnRH) given by injection or nasal spray. The use of GnRH analogues appears to provide the most effective and reliable endometrial thinning, and is the most acceptable to patients.[13] Danazol must be given with care to patients receiving anticoagulant treatment, as it potentiates the effects of warfarin. Progestogens must be given at high dose for longer periods, and produce the least reliable results.

Equipment

When operative hysteroscopy was first performed, the equipment was borrowed from urological colleagues. There are now many variations in design of operating hysteroscopes and, consequently, many varying techniques. The ideal hysteroscope for endometrial resection should be circular in cross-section and have separate inflow and outflow channels, which is essential for good vision. The fenestrations for outflow should be as near the tip as possible, so that outflow is maintained even when operating close to the internal cervical os.

The hysteroscope must have a degree of sideview, with 30 degrees providing the greatest safety, but a less panoramic view of the cavity than provided by a 12-degree hysteroscope. An 8 mm cutting loop will cut to a depth of 4 mm, which is the depth required to ensure probable removal of the basal layers of the endometrium when pretreated. A 6 mm loop will cut a trough 3 mm deep, which will provide greater safety for the less experienced but may increase the chance that residual viable endometrium will be left behind, although the authors have found the results to be virtually identical.[14] Typically, the loop is angled at 60–90 degrees to the shaft, but some surgeons use a forward-angled loop to treat the cornua and fundus of the uterus. Most operating hysteroscopes have a spring-controlled passive return action such that, at rest, the cutting loop is housed within the shaft of the instrument and has to be actively revealed for use.

Procedure

Endometrial ablation is now widely practised under regional or local anaesthesia, with or without intravenous sedation.[15] The small (but not insignificant) chance of major complication means that this should be performed either in a fully equipped operating theatre or within easy reach of such facilities. It is essential to have adequate monitoring, the minimum of which should be continuous electrocardiography and pulse oximetry. A single intravenous dose of a broad-spectrum antibiotic such as Augmentin (amoxycillin with clavulanic acid;

Beecham Research, Welwyn Garden City, UK) is recommended as prophylaxis against the small chance of infective complication.

The patient should be placed in the lithotomy position, but head-down tilt should be used with caution, as this may produce a negative pressure in the uterine venous plexus, with the potential for air embolus if air is allowed to enter the uterine cavity once resection has begun. The surgeon may sit or stand, but must have an unobstructed view of the video monitor. Video monitoring is essential both for an adequate view and also for teaching purposes. If the field of view is obscured for any reason, the procedure should be halted until adequate vision is restored. The use of concomitant laparoscopy should be considered in circumstances where an increased risk of perforation exists, such as repeat procedures, during resection of large or deep-seated fibroids, and when operating in the presence of congenital uterine malformation. The use of abdominal ultrasonography has been described to give added control during endometrial resection.[16]

The fluid for uterine distension must be non-ionic for electrosurgical procedures. The two most commonly used solutions are 1.5% glycine and 4% sorbitol, the latter being more expensive but not having the toxic nitrogenous and ammoniacal breakdown products of glycine. The pressure of fluid within the uterine cavity should be the minimum necessary for adequate distension and view. The fluid can be instilled using a specific constant-pressure variable-flow device, but adequate distension can be achieved using gravity, with the bag of fluid suspended one metre above the patient. This corresponds to a pressure of approximately 75 mmHg and requires the use of wide-bore tubing to connect the bag to the resectoscope. Pressures of 50–80 mmHg are usually adequate, but greater pressures, up to 100 mmHg, can be used for short periods if arterial bleeding is compromising good vision, with the risk of increased fluid intravasation.

Fluid intravasation is inevitable, with the total volume being proportional to the fluid pressure within the uterus and the duration of the procedure. One way to minimize this is to remove the resectoscope with each strip of resected material. This reduces the time of uterine distension and maintains optimum visualization of the cavity. With this technique, and a gravity feed system, the authors have not encountered a case of fluid overload, after more than 1200 cases. It is essential to monitor inflow and outflow volumes strictly, which is best achieved by giving a member of theatre staff the sole task of monitoring the fluid status. A standard 3 litre bag of 1.5% glycine may show variations of as much as 10% in the actual volume contained within it. The upper limit for safe absorption of 1.5% glycine is generally accepted as 1.5 litres, and the procedure should be stopped if this point is reached, even if the operation is incomplete. Other monitoring methods have been described, including breath ethanol analysis and serum measurements of sodium or glycine; however, none of these gives the immediate warning of overload provided by simple volumetric analysis. Overload is most likely to occur during complicated prolonged operations, especially when endometrial resection is combined with the resection of submucous fibroids. A sudden rise in the fluid deficit should lead one to suspect that the uterus has sustained a perforation.

The power setting used during endometrial resection should be the minimum necessary to allow efficient surgery. If the setting is too low, the loop will not pass through the tissues without snagging. The higher the setting, the greater will be the chance of arcing within the instrument, and of capacitive heating along the wire.

There is no one setting that can be recommended because diathermy machines vary in design and calibration. The most commonly used settings are 80–120 W of cutting current, with 50–100 W for coagulation, with a degree of blended current. The current should never be engaged when the instrument is not in contact with the tissues, which invites the risk of arcing within the barrel of the resectoscope.

It is useful to adopt a routine when performing endometrial resection, the exact sequence of which is not important. It is the authors' practice to begin by treating the cornua and fundus of the uterus with the rollerball, and then to resect the uterine walls in a methodical fashion, beginning posteriorly in the midline. It should be remembered that the uterine wall varies in thickness, from 18–20 mm at its thickest to a minimum of as little as 4 mm at the cornua. There will be a zone of necrosis beyond the cutting loop or rollerball, the depth of which will depend on the power used and the speed of passage across the tissues. The loop or rollerball should never be allowed to remain stationary while the power is connected, especially at the cornua, and the current should always be applied with the electrode coming towards the operator. The rollerball can be used, after resection is complete, to ensure haemostasis. Some surgeons treat the whole of the resected cavity a second time, either with repeat resection, or with rollerball coagulation. One observational study appears to show that best results are obtained by laparoscopically controlled resection, followed by rollerball coagulation, repeat resection to the cornua and, finally, laparoscopic unipolar coagulation of the cornual regions of the uterus.[17]

Follow-up

Patients should be advised about the likely duration of postoperative vaginal bleeding and discharge, which can last up to 4 weeks. The majority will continue to experience some menstrual blood loss, which will (it is hoped) be light or minimal, but occasionally the first periods are still heavy. Follow-up in the outpatient clinic should be at 6 months, by which time intra-uterine scarring and synechia formation will have taken place, when it will be possible to establish the early success of the procedure. Subsequent visits will permit the surgeon to monitor the longer-term success rates but are not of clinical value, unless the patient has developed problems. It is likely that even women who achieve amenorrhoea after endometrial ablation will have small islands of viable endometrium trapped in scar tissue. All women who have any degree of regular menstrual loss after the procedure clearly have residual endometrium; it is essential, therefore, that any hormone replacement therapy given subsequently should include a progestogen to prevent the development of endometrial hyperplasia and dysplasia. There are now several case reports of endometrial adenocarcinoma presenting after previous endometrial ablation.[18] In most cases the presenting complaint was of abnormal uterine bleeding in a similar fashion to the usual presentation. Women should be advised to report to their surgeon or family doctor if they have abnormal or postmenopausal bleeding — as all women should.

Long-term follow-up

The ultimate place of endometrial resection and related techniques in the field of gynaecological surgery will depend largely on their long-term success or failure. Several endpoints can be used to define success or otherwise. Patient satisfaction is frequently used in comparative studies of hysterectomy versus endometrial ablation, with most studies showing no significant difference in satisfaction rates,[19,20] even up to three years.[21] There are usually non-significant trends in favour of hysterectomy, which is not surprising, given that only hysterectomy guarantees a cure from the presenting complaint of excessive menstruation. If one makes the assumption that, in the absence of endometrial ablation, all patients would have had a hysterectomy, then long-term avoidance of hysterectomy is a valid measure of success. In practice, some women will opt for a minor procedure such as endometrial resection, but would not feel that their symptoms justify major surgery such as hysterectomy. However, using survival from hysterectomy as the endpoint enables life-table analysis to be performed on the survival data. This is the only valid form of analysis for such data, as it takes account of the patients lost to follow-up, and enables prospective patients to be given an accurate account of their likely chances of success. It is also necessary to have data covering at least 5 years of follow-up. Most of the published series have follow-up of 3 years or less, and some of less than a year. It is clear that there are a significant number of cases of late recurrence of menorrhagia occurring 2 or 3 years after endometrial ablation. Below, the long-term life-table analysis of a large series of cases of endometrial resection, with up to 5 years follow-up, is described.[22]

Endometrial resection has been performed in the authors' institution in Guildford since August of 1988, according to the practice described above. At the end of 1992 a total of 399 procedures had been performed. An audit of these cases was conducted at the end of 1994, allowing a minimum of 2 years follow-up of all cases, and up to 6 years for some. Hospital computer records were examined to identify all subsequent hospital gynaecological episodes after the initial 6-month outpatient visit. A detailed questionnaire was sent to all patients who had had no further contact with the hospital services, asking about their menstrual status and any gynaecological history since their discharge from the hospital clinic.

The procedures were performed at two sites, with 158 on one site performed exclusively by the senior surgeon, and 241 performed on a second site, of which 114 were performed at least in part by one of nine registrars or research fellows training in the department. Failure of medical therapy was documented in 187 (47%) of patients, and 97.7% of patients received endometrial suppression preoperatively. Intra-operative findings included 112 (28%) patients with significant fibroids, and 142 (36%) whose uterine cavity was more than 7 cm in length.

There were 28 cases of intra-operative or early postoperative complication, a rate of 7%, which is similar to that in another large series of endometrial resections,[23] and lower than those in several other series.[20,24] The complications included one case of failure to dilate the cervix, 14 cases of early bleeding treated by intra-uterine balloon tamponade, and 12 (3%) cases of uterine perforation. In total there were six cases of hysterectomy performed intra-operatively, or in the early postoperative period. There were no cases of fluid overload, which the authors attribute to their use of a gravity feed system for distension, removing the resectoscope with each strip of tissue and avoiding the performance of overlong procedures. Repeat endometrial resection was performed on 28 patients (7%) to treat the recurrence of symptoms; half of these patients were subsequently satisfied, and half had a hysterectomy at a later date. After follow-up of between 2 and 6 years, a total of 78 patients (19.5%) had had a hysterectomy; the most common indications were recurrent bleeding symptoms, the development of pelvic pain, or a combination of the two. Of this group, 51% were found to have pathological findings at surgery, including fibroids, adenomyosis, haematometra and endometriosis. Seven women had a hysterectomy for incidental reasons including uterovaginal prolapse, premenstrual syndrome, enlarging fibroids and ovarian carcinoma. In total, 23.7% of patients had some form of gynaecological surgery after 2–6 years of follow-up, which is similar to the findings of another similar survey.[23] Although the need for further surgery after endometrial ablation is seen as a failing of these procedures, it must be remembered that further surgery is not unusual after hysterectomy.[20,25]

Using time of surgery as the entry point, and time of hysterectomy as the exit point, it is possible to perform life-table analysis, thereby adjusting for those patients lost to follow-up. Table 13.1 shows that the highest interval hysterectomy rate was 12.1% during the first 12 months after surgery, falling substantially after the second completed year of follow-up; 96% of all hysterectomies were performed in the first 3 years after the initial surgery. One other study includes such a large number of patients with life-table analysis of long-term follow-up;[23] this study of 525 patients showed a cumulative hysterectomy rate of 9% at 5 years, with 98% of hysterectomies performed within 3 years of the endometrial resection.

Separate life-table curves were calculated for those patients aged under 45 and for those aged 45 and over, which could be compared using Mantel's test. The cumulative hysterectomy rate at 5 years was 15% for those aged 45 and over, compared with 30.9% for those aged under 45, which was statistically significant (Mantel's test = 76.78, $p < 0.01$). This shows that, in the authors' hands, a woman aged under 45 having an endometrial resection is twice as likely to have a hysterectomy in the next 5 years as a woman aged over 45. This does not mean that endometrial resection should not be offered to younger women, but the authors are obliged to give an accurate account of likely outcomes.

A similar comparison of life-table curves shows that the group operated upon by the senior surgeon had a cumulative hysterectomy rate at 5 years of 12.6% compared with 32.8% for those operated upon by a group including surgeons in training, which was also statistically significant (Mantel's test = 60.59, $p < 0.01$). None of the nine junior surgeons had performed more than ten endometrial resections, which must account at least in part for the lower chance of long-term

Table 13.1 Life-table analysis for hysterectomy after endometrial resection

Year	A	B	C	D	E	F	G	H
0–1	399	88	355	43	0.121	0.879	0.121	0.879
1–2	268	8	264	27	0.102	0.898	0.211	0.789
2–3	233	63	201.5	5	0.025	0.975	0.231	0.769
3–4	165	74	128	3	0.023	0.977	0.249	0.751
4–5	88	69	53.5	0	0	1.0	0.249	0.751

Column values: A, number of patients entering interval; B, patients lost to follow-up in interval; C, adjusted denominator; D, number having hysterectomy in interval; E, interval hysterectomy rate; F, interval survival from hysterectomy rate; G, cumulative hysterectomy rate; H, cumulative survival from hysterectomy rate.

success in these patients. This series of procedures was performed before the development of realistic laboratory simulation of resection, with which to gain initial familiarity with the technique. It is now possible for junior surgeons to spend the early part of their 'learning curve' in the training laboratory, and to attain a degree of skill before their first attempt at endometrial resection on a patient.

Conclusions

It is clear that endometrial resection offers women with menorrhagia a significant chance of long-term resolution of their symptoms at the cost of a minor day-case procedure that need not even involve general anaesthesia. It is important to be aware of the small risk of serious complication and, equally, to educate the patient about these risks. These risks can be minimized, and success rates optimized, by good training and by strict adherence to accepted practices. Endometrial resection is appropriate for women with menorrhagia for whom medical therapy is unsuccessful, poorly tolerated or contraindicated. The patient should be motivated to avoid hysterectomy and to accept the limitations and chances of success that the procedure has to offer. The authors are confident that endometrial resection is a genuine alternative to hysterectomy, with a high chance of long-term success and patient satisfaction, especially when performed by an experienced surgeon on women aged over 45 years.

References

1. DeCherney A H, Polan M L. Hysteroscopic management of intrauterine lesions and intractable uterine bleeding. Obstet Gynecol 1983; 6: 392–397

2. Macdonald R, Phipps J, Singer A. Endometrial ablation: a safe procedure. Gynaecol Endosc 1992; 1: 7–9

3. Marsh M, Overton C, McPherson K. MISTLETOE update. London: Royal College of Obstetricians and Gynaecologists Medical Audit Unit (pamphlet). 1994

4. Magos A L, Baumann R, Lockwood G M et al. Experience with the first 250 endometrial resections for menorrhagia. Lancet 1991; 337: 1074–1078

5. Lewis B V. Guidelines for endometrial ablation. Br J Obstet Gynaecol 1994; 101: 470–473

6. Bridgeman S A. Trends in endometrial ablation and hysterectomy for dysfunctional uterine bleeding, in Mersey region. Gynaecol Endosc 1996; 5: 5–8

7. Colafranceschi M, Bettocchi S, Mencaglia L et al. Missed detection of uterine carcinoma before endometrial resection: a report of three cases. Gynecol Oncol 1996; 62(2): 298–300

8. Romano S, Shimoni Y, Muralee D et al. Retrograde seeding of endometrial carcinoma during hysteroscopy. Gynecol Oncol 1992; 44: 116–118

9. Ewen S P, Sutton C J G. A combined approach to heavy painful periods. Laparoscopic uterine nerve ablation and TCRE. Gynaecol Endosc 1994; 3: 167–168

10. Sutton C J G. Laparoscopic treatment of dysmenorrhoea. In: Sutton C J G, Diamond M (eds) Endoscopic surgery for gynecologists. Chapter 25. 2nd Edition. London: Saunders, 1998: 249–260

11. Biggerstaff III E D, Foster S N. Laparoscopic surgery for dysmenorrhoea: uterine nerve ablation and pre-sacral neurectomy. In: Sutton C J G (ed) Gynecological endoscopic surgery. London: Chapman and Hall, 1997; 63–84

12. Whitelaw N L, Sutton C J G. Pregnancy following endometrial ablation. Gynaecol Endosc 1993; 1: 129–132

13. Sutton C J G, Ewen S P. Thinning the endometrium prior to ablation: is it worthwhile? Br J Obstet Gynaecol 1994; 101 (suppl): 10–12

14. Sutton C J G, Ewen S P. Complications of endometrial resection: is the smaller loop safer? Gynaecol Endosc 1993; 2: 103–104

15. Ferry J, Rankin L. Transcervical resection of the endometrium using intracervical block only. A review of 278 procedures. Aust N Z J Obstet Gynaecol 1994; 34: 457–461

16. Letterie G S, Kramer D J. Intraoperative ultrasound guidance for intrauterine endoscopic surgery. Fertil Steril 1994; 62(3): 654–656

17. Browne D S. Endometrial resection — a comparison of techniques. Aust N Z J Obstet Gynaecol 1996; 36(4): 448–452

18. Copperman A B, DeCherney A H, Olive D L. A case of endometrial cancer following endometrial ablation for dysfunctional uterine bleeding. Obstet Gynecol 1993; 82(4 Pt 2 suppl): 640–642

19. Gannon M J, Holt E M, Fairbank J et al. A randomized trial comparing endometrial resection and abdominal hysterectomy for the treatment of menorrhagia. Br Med J 1991; 303: 1362–1364

20. Pinion S B, Parkin D E, Abramovich A N et al. Randomized trial of hysterectomy, endometrial laser ablation, and transcervical resection for dysfunctional uterine bleeding. Br Med J 1994; 309: 979–983

21. Pooley A S, Ewen S P, Sutton S J G. Does transcervical resection of the endometrium really avoid a hysterectomy: life-table analysis of a large series. J Am Assoc Gynecol Laparosc 1998; 5(3): 229–235

22. O'Connor H, Magos A L. Endometrial resection for menorrhagia: evaluation of the results at 5 years. N Engl J Med 1996; 335: 151–156

23. Dwyer N, Hutton J, Stirrat G M. Randomized controlled trial comparing endometrial resection with abdominal hysterectomy for the surgical treatment of menorrhagia. Br J Obstet Gynaecol 1993; 100: 237–243

24. Grant J M, Hussein I Y. An audit of abdominal hysterectomy over a decade in a district hospital. Br J Obstet Gynaecol 1984; 91: 73–77

25. O'Connor H, Broadbent J A, Magos A L et al. Medical Research Council randomized trial of endometrial resection versus hysterectomy in the management of menorrhagia. Lancet 1997; 349: 897–901

CHAPTER 14

Fibroids and menorrhagia: the role of myolysis

D. R. Phillips

Introduction

Leiomyomas, the most common solid pelvic tumours, occur in 25–30% of women during their reproductive years. Approximately 20–50% of these women experience symptoms that require treatment, with the most common complaints being excessive and/or prolonged menses, intermenstrual bleeding, pelvic pressure and the appreciation of a pelvic mass.[1]

Determining the appropriate treatment of uterine leiomyomas involves assessing not only the size, location and growth rate of the tumours but also the symptoms and coexisting pelvic pathology as well as the age, reproductive status and desires of the patient. Therapy is warranted if a leiomyoma and its associated symptoms interfere with her health, the ability to bear a viable child, and/or the quality of her life. Before the development of operative endoscopy, symptomatic leiomyomas were successfully managed by transabdominal myomectomy or hysterectomy. Even though these procedures were invasive and morbid, they were the only surgical remedies available.

Currently, transcervical endometrial ablation or resection (TEMR), an outpatient procedure in which the endometrium is destroyed or removed, can be an effective alternative to hysterectomy for women with intractable menorrhagia. Any existing submucous leiomyomata can also be concomitantly resected. Although total amenorrhoea is achieved in 36–84% of cases of endometrial ablation or resection, depending upon the technique used,[2–8] and success rates of 76–100%[2–5,9–12] have been reported after resection of submucous leiomyomas, operative hysteroscopy does not routinely treat intramural and subserosal leiomyomata. The presence of an intramural leiomyoma (and possibly even a subserosal one) can substantially contribute to the symptoms of abnormal uterine bleeding; therefore, these lesions also should be evaluated for surgical treatment.

Laparoscopic myolysis (leiomyoma [myoma] coagulation) was developed in Germany in 1986[13] and was first reported in the literature and first performed in the United States in 1990.[14] It involves using either a neodymium:yttrium aluminium garnet (Nd:YAG) laser bare fibre,[14–21] a monopolar needle[22] or bipolar coagulation needles,[14–18,20,21] hyperthermia electrode (diathermy),[23] or, recently, hypothermia probe (cryomyolysis)[24] to destroy the stroma and vascular supply of the targeted intramural or subserosal leiomyoma, resulting in significant shrinkage or even disappearance of the leiomyoma and resolution of its former associated symptoms.

Selection of patients

Usually, the candidate for myolysis is the perimenopausal woman with subserosal and/or intramural leiomyomata, with or without submucosal leiomyomas, presenting with one or more of the following symptoms: menorrhagia; intermenstrual bleeding; pelvic pressure; pain, or the appreciation of a pelvic mass. She has the required inclusion criteria for hysterectomy, but wants to avoid this procedure or abdominal myomectomy. In most cases, a laparoscopic myomectomy would be time-consuming, technically difficult, or unnecessary for pathological evaluation. Occasionally, a woman with similar symptoms who is infertile or who wishes to retain her capacity to bear a child may also be a candidate. However, it should be emphasized that the long-term results of conception, success of carrying to term, and appropriate mode of delivery have not been studied sufficiently and the subsequent pregnancy risk is not yet known.

The diagnosis of uterine leiomyoma is usually made by abdominopelvic examination: location and size of the leiomyoma are determined by ultrasonography, hysteroscopy, sonohysterography, and/or occasionally by magnetic resonance imaging (MRI). Endometrial sampling is required to determine if endometrial cancer or a precursor lesion is present, which would be a contraindication to conservative pelvic surgery.

Before myolysis, depot leuprolide acetate (Lupron, Tap Pharmaceuticals, Inc., Deerfield, IL, USA) or a comparable gonadotrophin-releasing hormone (GnRH) agonist regimen is usually administered in three monthly treatments of 3.75 mg each. Two groups of women should not be considered candidates for myolysis: these are (1) those who remain symptomatic after 3 months of this GnRH agonist pretreatment, even if there is significant shrinkage in uterine and leiomyoma volumes, and (2) those whose total uterine volume (TUV) has not been reduced by at least 25% after GnRH agonist therapy, because of the remote possibility that a leiomyosarcoma may be present.

Pelvic and vaginal ultrasonography should be performed preoperatively before and after GnRH agonist pretreatment and between 3 and 6 months. Measurements of the volume of the uterus and of each leiomyoma are calculated using the prolate ellipse equation: volume = $(0.523) (D_1) (D_2) (D_3)$, where D_1, D_2, and D_3 represent the three largest diameters (length, transverse, and anteroposterior).[25]

Technique

Immediately before myolysis, women with chronic menorrhagia undergo concomitant transcervical endometrial ablation or resection (TEMR), if childbearing is not a consideration, and resection of any existing submucous leiomyomata (TSR). To reduce blood loss and fluid absorption and to facilitate dilation of the cervix,[26,27] 20 ml vasopressin (0.05 U/ml) is used intracervically.

Following the hysteroscopic portion of the surgery, a uterine mobilizer is placed on the cervix to optimize the position of the uterus for the laparoscopic surgery. During laparoscopy, if any pedunculated subserosal leiomyoma is present it is removed by desiccation of its base with bipolar coagulation and then excision with scissors, knife or unipolar electrode. At the completion of myolysis, the intact or morcellated leiomyoma may be delivered either from one of the laparoscopic ports or through a culdotomy incision.

Laparoscopic leiomyoma coagulation is most commonly performed using either

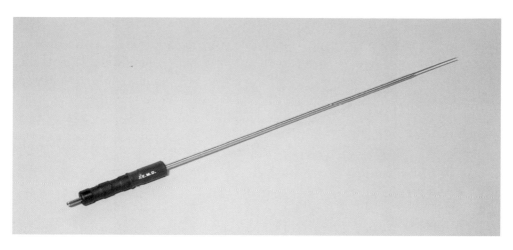

Figure 14.1 Bipolar coagulation needles (32 cm long, with two parallel needles 5 cm long). (J.E.M.D. Medical 1-800-233-3670.)

the Nd:YAG laser bare fibre or bipolar coagulation needles. Because of the fragility of the bare fibre and the inferior haemostatic effect that it produces, a bipolar coagulation technique is now exclusively used by this author. This method uses a bipolar coagulation instrument 32 cm long (J.E.M.D. Medical, Hicksville, NY; Fig. 14.1) connected to an electrosurgical generator. The active electrodes are two parallel needles 5 cm long.

The proper placement of the ancillary ports and the stabilization of the uterus are of paramount importance. At least two ports should be developed in the lower-right and lower-left abdominal regions, lateral to the deep epigastric blood vessels and sufficiently cephalad so that the leiomyoma(s) can be approached perpendicularly. The coagulation instrument is passed through one of these ports; 70 W of power is used. The uterus is usually stabilized by directly anchoring the leiomyoma or uterus with a 5 or 10 mm myoma drill (WISAP, Sauerlach, Germany), a corkscrew-grasping device delivered through either a 5 or 10 mm lower abdominal port. Occasionally, if applying high-flow suction and irrigation is warranted to facilitate the procedure, a third 5 mm trocar is placed suprapubically. Alternatively, a 10 mm bipolar coagulation needle instrument with irrigation and suction can be used, usually obviating the need for a third 5 mm puncture site.

A dilute vasopressin solution (5–20 ml; 0.05 U/ml) is transabdominally administered with an 18-gauge needle to just beneath the serosal surface of the uterus overlying the leiomyoma. The bipolar needles are used to perforate subserous or intramural leiomyomas systematically in increments of 5–10 mm that extend across the serosal surface to the base, forming parallel cylinders of desiccated, denatured tissue. To maximize the coagulation effect to the leiomyoma, all passes are performed slowly (8–15 mm/s) and are directed perpendicularly to the serosal surface to minimize the force necessary for entry (Fig. 14.2). An effort is made to reduce the coagulation of the uterine serosal surfaces by applying energy after the electrodes have pierced approximately 2–5 mm below the surface and by discontinuing the energy just prior to removing the needles when the pass has been completed. At the endpoint of the procedure, almost the entire leiomyoma surface is pale and blanched.

A modification of this laparoscopic technique is used in those patients who wish

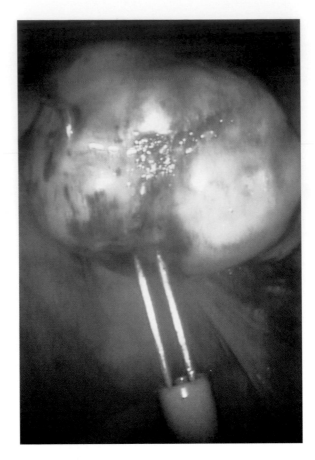

Figure 14.2 Perforation of a leiomyoma with bipolar needles.

to bear a child: instead of the entire leiomyoma being perforated with the bipolar coagulation needles, only the circumference of the base of the leiomyoma is perforated every 5 mm in an attempt to destroy the blood supply to the lesion while minimizing the damage to the overlying serosal surface.

Results

From February 1992 to the end of March 1995, the author's studies with myolysis involved 167 women with a mean age of 44.7 years. The TUV decreased from 620 cm³ prior to leuprolide medication to 297 cm³, 1 month after the third dose and immediately before surgery (Table 14.1).

Of the 52 women with chronic menorrhagia, 50 underwent TEMR; 22 women who had submucous myomas also had those lesions concomitantly resected (TSR). Two other patients who wanted to preserve their fertility underwent TSR without TEMR.

Complications

None of the women had any intra-operative complications; they all were discharged from the ambulatory surgery unit within a mean of 5.1 hours after surgery was completed. Eight patients (3.6%) complained of transient pyrexia up to a maximum of 102.8 °F for a mean of 7.5 days postoperatively, with minimal elevations of estimated sedimentation rates and white blood cell counts and without pelvic or abdominal discomfort (Table 14.2). They were placed on

Table 14.1 Uterine leiomyomata measurements*

Measurement	Surgery	Time period			
		Premedication	Post-leuprolide	3–6 months postoperative	7–12 months postoperative
TUV	Myolysis	637 ± 35.7; 105–2002	291 ± 11.9; 87–1133	121 ± 7.8; 6–601	139 ± 8.0; 6–605
	Myolysis with TEMR and/or TSR	582 ± 25.1; 126–2116	311 ± 13.6; 84–989	99 ± 6.4; 9–588	113 ± 6.9; 6–590
	Total	620 ± 28.4; 110–2312	297 ± 13.0; 78–1011	114 ± 6.5; 6–601	131 ± 7.2; 6–605
LLD	Myolysis	6.7 ± 0.2; 2.6–12.4	5.4 ± 0.2; 2.3–11.9	2.6 ± 0.1; 0–5.6	2.9 ± 0.2; 0–5.9
	Myolysis with TEMR and/or TSR	6.5 ± 0.2; 2.7–11.3	5.3 ± 0.2; 2.4–10.8	2.6 ± 0.1; 0–5.8	2.8 ± 0.2; 0–6.0
	Total	6.6 ± 0.2; 2.6–13.4	5.4 ± 0.2; 2.3–11.7	2.6 ± 0.1; 0–5.8	2.9 ± 0.2; 0–6.1
TLV	Myolysis	198 ± 13.9; 9–602	83 ± 4.5; 7–367	26 ± 2.4; 0–168	31 ± 2.5; 0–177
	Myolysis with TEMR and/or TSR	181 ± 10.9; 7–577	84 ± 4.5; 5–361	23 ± 2.2; 0–167	27 ± 2.3; 0–179
	Total	193 ± 11.5; 6–602	83 ± 4.6; 4–367	25 ± 2.3; 0–171	30 ± 2.4; 0–183

* Based on 115 women having myolysis and 52 women having myolysis with TEMR and/or TSR. All volumes are expressed in terms of mean ± SEM; range, cm^3; all diameters in cm. The two surgery groups, myolysis and myolysis with TEMR and/or TSR, showed no statistically significant differences ($p > 0.05$).

TUV, total uterine volume; LLD, longest leiomyoma diameter; TLV, total leiomyoma volume; TEMR, transcervical resection of endomyometrium; TSR, transcervical resection of submucous leiomyoma.

antibiotics and analgesics and responded well to this conservative therapy.

One woman who underwent laparoscopic laser myolysis without hysteroscopic surgery developed symptoms of acute leiomyoma degeneration one day postoperatively. She responded well to oral antibiotics, analgesics and bedrest, and became asymptomatic 5 days postoperatively. Two women developed a suprapubic abdominal wall haematoma which limited ambulation for 2–3 weeks. They responded well to conservative therapy and resumed normal activities within 3 weeks.

Table 14.2 Complications

Complication	Myolysis, no. (%)	Myolysis with TEMR and/ or TSR, no. (%)	Total no. (%)	Statistical significance, p
Transient pyrexia	4 (3.5)	4 (7.7)	8 (4.8)	0.21
Myoma degeneration	1 (0.9)	0	1 (0.6)	0.69
Abdominal wall haematoma	0	2 (3.8)	2 (1.2)	0.10
Urinary tract infection	2 (1.7)	1 (1.9)	3 (1.8)	0.68
Total	7 (6.1)	7 (13.5)	14 (8.4)	0.10

Based on 115 women initially having myolysis and 52 having myolysis with TEMR and/or TSR.

Data did not reach the level of significance.

TEMR, transcervical endometrial resection; TSR, transcervical resection of submucous leiomyoma.

Reoperation

Postoperatively, eight women (3.6%) complained that one or more of the following symptoms had recurred: pain, pressure or menorrhagia. Although a repeat conservative endoscopic procedure or medical therapy was offered, only the two patients complaining of menorrhagia chose repeat TEMR at 7 and 9 months postoperatively (Table 14.3). One of the patients who had a repeat procedure subsequently became hypo-amenorrhoeic; the other continued to have symptoms and ultimately chose to have a laparoscopically assisted vaginal hysterectomy 5 months after the repeat hysteroscopic procedure. During the laparoscopic procedure, no pelvic adhesions were noted. Pathological review of the myometrium revealed severe diffuse adenomyosis with multifocal areas of microcysts containing chocolate-brown fluid, predominantly at the area of serosal defects.

A 37-year-old woman underwent laser myolysis of a posterior fundal intramural leiomyoma (4.5 cm) that was undetectable clinically or by ultrasound 3 months postoperatively. However, 15 months after surgery she suddenly developed lower abdominal pressure and appreciation of a rapidly growing abdominal mass. MRI revealed a predominantly low-density pelvic mass (14 cm) with multiple foci of hyperintensity. The patient underwent a total abdominal hysterectomy as there was a possibility of leiomyosarcoma: a filmy adhesion 5 mm wide was noted that extended from the site of the previous myolysis to the anterior abdominal wall; pathology revealed a benign leiomyoma.

Three of five women chose hysterectomy, and the other two chose a repeat myolysis, for recurrent symptoms of pelvic pressure and pain from 7 to 27 months postoperatively (Table 14.3). One hysterectomy was performed laparoscopically and two vaginally. During the laparoscopically assisted vaginal hysterectomy, thick adhesions were noted on the posterior wall of the uterus between the site of the previous myolysis, the large bowel, and the anterior abdominal wall. Pathological evaluation of the three uteri revealed diffuse adenomyosis and leiomyomata in all specimens. None of the extirpated uteri from the five women who had hysterectomy or the two uteri examined during the repeat myolysis showed evidence of regrowth of leiomyomata at the site of previous myolysis surgery. The

Table 14.3 Subsequent gynaecological surgery performed after 6 months

Initial surgery	TEMR no. (%)	Repeat myolysis no. (%)	Hysterectomy no. (%)	Total no. (%)
Myolysis		1 (0.6)	*1 (0.6)	2 (1.2)
Myolysis with TSR and/or TEMR	**2 (1.2)	1 (0.6)	*5 (3.0)	8 (4.8)
Total	2 (1.2)	2 (1.2)	6 (3.6)	10 (6.0)

Based on a follow-up of 36.0 ± 1.2 (mean ± SEM; range 18–54) months of 115 women initially having myolysis and 52 having myolysis with TEMR and/or TSR.

TEMR, transcervical resection of endomyometrium; TSR, transcervical resection of submucous leiomyoma.

* This difference was significant ($p = 0.01$).

** One patient had repeat TEMR and then a subsequent hysterectomy.

patients who underwent repeat myolysis have remained asymptomatic to this date.

Amenorrhoea, hypomenorrhoea, and eumenorrhoea were considered satisfactory menstrual results after TEMR, and eumenorrhoea is a satisfactory menstrual result after TSR. After 6 months of surgery, satisfactory results were achieved in 50 of the 52 women (96.2%). Hysteroscopic procedures added a mean of 29.4 minutes to the total operating time, which was determined from when the resectoscope was inserted to when the resection was completed. There were no intra-operative or postoperative complications arising from this portion of the surgery.

TUV decreased very significantly from 620 cm³ prior to leuprolide medication to 131 cm³, 7–12 months postoperatively (Table 14.1). Of the 19 women who had second-look laparoscopy 6 months after surgery, 14 showed no adhesions at the myolysis sites (Fig. 14.3). The other five women had thick and thin avascular adhesions extending from the bowel to some of the uterine serosal surgical sites; they were asymptomatic.

The two women who wanted to retain their childbearing options underwent myolysis and TSR: one woman conceived 7 months postoperatively; the other, 8 months postoperatively. They both had uneventful pregnancies and vaginal deliveries of healthy male infants weighing 2796 and 3211 g, respectively.

Discussion

The ability of myolysis to resolve symptomatic leiomyomas has been confirmed by many investigators.[13–23] The first report to discuss the use of a Nd:YAG laser bare fibre to perforate leiomyomata as large as 10 cm in diameter described the perforation of the leiomyoma every 5 mm to produce contiguous cylinders of denatured and devascularized stroma.[14] Women were pretreated for 3–6 months with depot leuprolide acetate, which reduced leiomyoma volumes by 40–60%. Within 6–9 months postoperatively, the diameters of the leiomyomas continued to decrease by approximately 50–70%. There was no regrowth of leiomyomas during a 12-month follow-up period, and no subsequent hysterectomies or abdominal surgeries were performed on the 75 patients studied.

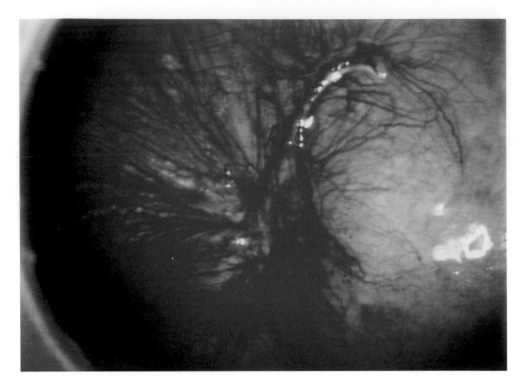

Figure 14.3 Elective second-look laparoscopy 6 months postoperatively after myolysis, showing the radial pattern of superficial blood vessels.

The same investigator later reported an expansion to a series of 300 myolysis cases (150 performed using a Nd:YAG laser and an equal number performed using bipolar coagulation), 6 months postoperatively. There was leiomyoma shrinkage of 30–50% beyond the effect of the depot leuprolide.[15–18] There were no cases of myoma regeneration; therefore, no patient required a repeat procedure or hysterectomy for this reason. One patient, however, developed a pelvic abscess and subsequently underwent hysterectomy. Another patient developed bacteraemia and responded well to intensive antibiotic therapy. Six patients developed myoma degeneration but responded well to conservative therapy.

The issue of whether to offer myolysis to women wishing to bear a child is controversial. Although studies of women whose leiomyomas have been destroyed by various methods are limited, they have clearly demonstrated that conception and viable pregnancies are attainable after myolysis.[22,23,28] However, the extent to which the integrity and tensile strength of the uterine walls remain intact after myolysis has not been ascertained. Recently, two women who conceived within 3 months of myolysis, experienced spontaneous uterine rupture, one at 32 weeks and the other at term during labour.[29] The first case resulted in death of the foetus, which was delivered by a hysterotomy; in the second case a healthy infant was delivered during an emergency caesarean section and the uterine rupture was repaired uneventfully; both women had routine postoperative courses. Furthermore, it was reported[30] that a spontaneous rupture of a gravid uterus occurred at 26 weeks gestation. The patient, who had complained of primary infertility and pelvic pain, underwent bipolar myolysis of an intramural fundal leiomyoma (3 cm); she conceived on her third cycle of clomiphene citrate. Emergency laparotomy for severe abdominal pain suggestive of intra-abdominal haemorrhage revealed a rupture in the fundal area. Although the uterine repair and the mother's postoperative course were uneventful, the infant died after 27 weeks of intensive care from multiple disorders related to prematurity and anaemia. Until the data, including long-term follow-up, become available from randomized studies, only after careful consideration of its advantages and disadvantages should myolysis should be offered to women who wish to bear a child.

Conclusions

For the perimenopausal woman who wishes to retain her uterus, myolysis — a technically easy procedure to perform with minimal complication rates — provides symptomatic relief by markedly reducing the sizes of the subserosal and intramural leiomyomas as well as the size of the uterus. Patients with chronic menorrhagia can undergo concomitant TEMR, TSR, or both. Until further studies are concluded, myolysis should be performed selectively and cautiously in women contemplating pregnancy.

References

1. Buttram V C Jr, Reiter R C. Uterine leiomyomata: etiology, symptomatology, and management. Fertil Steril 1981; 36: 433–445

2. Phillips D R. Endomyometrial resection of menopausal women with annoying uterine bleeding on estrogen replacement therapy. J Am Assoc Gynecol Laparosc 1995; 2: 389–393

3. Phillips D R, Nathanson H G, Meltzer S M et al. Transcervical electrosurgical resection of submucous leiomyomas for chronic menorrhagia. J Am Assoc Gynecol Laparosc 1995; 2: 147 153

4. Wortman M, Daggett A. Hysteroscopic endomyometrial resection: a new technique for the treatment of menorrhagia. Obstet Gynecol 1994; 83: 295–298

5. Phillips D R. A comparison of endometrial ablation using the Nd:YAG laser or electrosurgical techniques. J Am Assoc Gynecol Laparosc 1994; 1: 235–239

6. Vancaille T G. Electrocoagulation of the endometrium with the ball-end resectoscope. Obstet Gynecol 1989; 74: 425–427

7. Garry R, Erian J, Grouchmal S A. A multi-centre collaborative study into the treatment of menorrhagia by Nd:YAG laser ablation of the endometrium. Br J Obstet Gynaecol 1991; 98: 357–362

8. Loffer F D. Hysteroscopic endometrial ablation with the Nd:YAG laser using a non-touch technique. Obstet Gynecol 1987; 69: 679–682

9. Neuwirth R S. Hysteroscopic management of symptomatic uterine fibroids. Am J Obstet Gynecol 1978; 131: 91–94

10. DeCherney A, Diamond M P, Eavy G, Polan M L. Endometrial ablation for intractable uterine bleeding: Hysteroscopic resection. Obstet Gynecol 1987; 70: 668–670

11. Derman S G, Rehnstrom J, Neuwirth R S. The long-term effectiveness of hysteroscopic treatment of menorrhagia and leiomyomas. Obstet Gynecol 1991; 77: 591–594

12. Corson S L, Brooks P G. Resectoscopic myomectomy. Fertil Steril 1991; 55: 1041–1044

13. Gallinat A, Leuken R P. Addendum — Current trends in the therapy of myomata. In: Leuken R P, Gallinat A (eds) Endoscopic surgery in gynecology. Berlin: Demeter Verlag, 1993: 69–71

14. Goldfarb H A. Nd:YAG laser laparoscopic coagulation of symptomatic myomas. J Reprod Med 1992; 36: 636–638

15. Goldfarb H A. Removing uterine fibroids laparoscopically. Contemp Ob/Gyn 1994; 39: 50–72

16. Goldfarb H A. Bipolar laparoscopic needles for myoma coagulation. J Am Assoc Gynecol Laparosc 1995; 2: 175–179

17. Goldfarb H A. Laparoscopic coagulation of myoma (myolysis). In: Hutchins F L, Greenberg M D (eds) Obstet Gynecol Clin North Am. Uterine fibroids. Philadelphia: Saunders, 1995: 807–819

18. Goldfarb H A. Laparoscopic coagulation of myoma (myolysis). In: Tolandi T (ed) Infertil Reprod Med Clin North Am. Uterine myomas. Philadelphia: Saunders, 1996: 129–141

19. Nisolle M, Smets M, Malvaux V et al. Laparoscopic myolysis with the Nd:YAG laser. J Gynecol Surg 1993; 9: 95–99

20. Phillips D R. Laparoscopic leiomyoma coagulation (myolysis). Gynaecol Endosc 1995; 4: 5–12

21. Phillips D R, Nathanson H G, Milim S J et al. Experience with laparoscopic leiomyoma coagulation (myolysis) and concomitant operative hysteroscopy: a three-year follow-up of 167 cases. J Am Assoc Gynecol Laparosc 1997; 4: 425–433

22. Wood C, Maher P, Hill D. Myoma reduction by electrocautery. Gynaecol Endosc 1994; 3: 163–165

23. Chapman R. Treatment of uterine myomas by interstitial hyperthermia. Gynaecol Endosc 1993; 2: 227–234

24. Zreik T G, Rutherford T J, Palter S F et al. Cryomyolysis: a new procedure for the conservative treatment of uterine fibroids. J Am Assoc Gynecol Laparosc 1998; 5: 33–38

25. Goldstein S R, Horii S C, Snyder J R et al. Estimation of nongravid uterine volume based on a nomogram of gravid uterine volume: its value in gynecological abnormalities. Obstet Gynecol 1988; 72: 86–90

26. Phillips D R, Nathanson H G, Milim S J et al. The effect of dilute vasopressin solution on blood loss during operative hysteroscopy: a randomized controlled trial. Obstet Gynecol 1996; 88: 761–766

27. Phillips D R, Nathanson H G, Milim S J et al. The effect of dilute vasopressin solution on cervical dilatation: a randomized controlled trial. Obstet Gynecol 1997; 89: 507–511

28. Donnez J, Gillerot S, Bourgonjon D et al. Neodymium:YAG laser hysteroscopy in large submucous fibroids. Fertil Steril 1990; 54: 999–1003

29. Vilos G A, Daly L J, Tse B M. Pregnancy outcome after laparoscopic electromyolysis. J Am Assoc Gynecol Laparosc 1998; 5: 289–292

30. Arcangeli S, Pasquarette M M. Gravid uterine rupture after myolysis. Obstet Gynecol 1997; 89: 857

CHAPTER 15

Embolization of myomata

B. McLucas

Introduction

Embolization of pelvic vessels to treat acute pelvic haemorrhage is an established procedure within gynaecology and obstetrics. Perhaps the longest history of efficacy is noted in cases of haemorrhage associated with pelvic malignancy, when surgery is either impossible or must be postponed until radiation or further evaluation is necessary.[1] In the treatment of post-partum haemorrhage, embolization has a success rate of close to 100%,[2] compared with the (at best) 50% success of either hypogastric artery ligation[3] or uterine artery ligation.[4] Several different occlusion techniques are available, including coils, or particles of a permanent or temporary nature. The choice of the occlusion method will be determined by the nature of the disease and desire for function within the structure being embolized.

Leiomyomata are the most common benign tumours in both sexes. Approximately 40% of women over 40 years of age suffer from myomata of the uterus (fibroids).[5] At the Hôpital Lariboisière in Paris, France, Ravina and his co-workers followed patients who were initially referred for temporizing embolization prior to definitive surgery, either myomectomy or hysterectomy.[6] These patients were, in many cases, able to avoid surgical intervention altogether after initial embolization when the myomata shrank after arterial embolization. Ravina then began to study the effects of embolic therapy as a stand-alone alternative to surgery. His initial work detailing therapy for 16 patients was reported in 1995 in the *Lancet*.[7] Among others,[8] the present author's group at the University of California, Los Angeles (UCLA), has been able to duplicate the results of the French team.[9,10]

Patients and methods

Patient characteristics

This chapter outlines the results of the author's first 25 patients given embolic therapy, who were seen over a period from 1 January 1996 to 30 May 1997 at UCLA. All patients have been followed for more than 6 months after embolization. Patients who were candidates for embolization were surgical candidates; all suffered from pelvic haemorrhage. Five women were perimenopausal or menopausal; the others were ovulatory. Eight patients were noted to have additional gynaecological problems at pre-embolization laparoscopy; six had adhesions from prior pelvic surgery, two had endometriosis, categorized as American Fertility Society grade moderate or above. All patients had multiple myomata documented on pelvic examination and ultrasound.

Every patient had previously undergone invasive procedures for control of symptoms including myomectomy (ten patients), myoma lysis (three patients) and endometrial ablation (five patients). All patients were screened by hysteroscopy performed under local anaesthesia to exclude a malignant cause for their symptoms. In addition, patients underwent laparoscopy under general anaesthesia during which needle biopsy of the largest myoma was performed and adnexal pathology was noted. Prior to embolization, ultrasound examination of the pelvis included measurement of the total uterine volume and of the diameter of the largest myoma, and Doppler flow studies of the uterine arteries. Laboratory studies included complete blood count, coagulation panel, and tests of renal function and follicle-stimulating hormone levels.

No patient was found to have any condition that would make her vulnerable to haemorrhagic, ischaemic or infectious complications of embolization such as coagulopathies, salpingitis, diabetes mellitus or vasculitis. All patients were offered hysterectomy; the risks and benefits of the embolization procedure were described by both a gynaecologist and an interventional radiologist. At the time of writing, the author's team is offering embolization to patients who wish to bear children; however, for the group reported here, patients were cautioned against future pregnancies until more could be learned about the long-term results of the procedure.

Technique

The patient's right groin was 'prepped' and draped and the right femoral artery was punctured under local anaesthesia with a 4 or 5 Fr catheter and a glide catheter. The contralateral (left) common iliac, internal iliac, and anterior division were catheterized in sequence. Using digital subtraction arteriography, the uterine artery was selected. In five patients a 0.018 Tracker microcatheter was needed for entry of the uterine artery; all catheterizations were aided by digital road-mapping. Once the left uterine artery had been entered, it was embolized with 500–700 µm polyvinyl alcohol particles (PVA), except one patient who received 300–500 µm PVA. The endpoint of embolization is cessation of blood flow. Figures 15.1 and 15.2 show the right uterine artery outlined by contrast, prior to (Fig. 15.1) and after (Fig. 15.2) embolization.

After stasis in the left uterine artery, a Waltman loop technique was used to enter the ipsilateral right internal iliac artery. Similar subselective catheterization and free-flow embolization was performed on the right side. The length of the procedure varied between 45 and 90 minutes (average 75 minutes). After removal of the catheter and wire, haemostasis was effected by direct compression for 15 minutes. Patients were confined to bedrest for 6 hours following embolization to prevent bleeding from the arterial puncture site. In 50% of the author's patients, overnight observation was required for pain control.

Analgesia

In the initial group of ten patients, an anaesthesiologist provided general anaesthesia for all save one patient who received conscious sedation (fentanyl and midazolam). Subsequent patients have all been managed by this latter method without difficulty. Patients embolized under sedation also received local anaesthesia at the right femoral puncture site. None of the sedated patients needed conversion

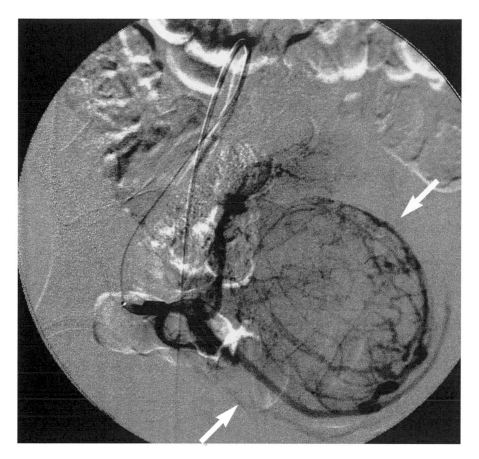

Figure 15.1 The right uterine artery, outlined by contrast, prior to embolization; arrows outline myoma.

to general anaesthesia. Five patients received 100 mg lignocaine (lidocaine) injected directly into the uterine artery for periprocedural analgesia. All patients received 60 mg ketorolac in the post anaesthesia care unit, eight intravenously and two intramuscularly. The total post-procedural analgesia and subsequent pain levels of patients were recorded.

Clinical follow-up
Measures of success were patients' responses to a telephone questionnaire administered 5 months after embolization. Also followed were ultrasound examinations at 6 weeks and 6 months after embolization, which included measurements of total uterine volume and myoma diameter, as well as Doppler flow studies of the uterine arteries.

Results
Angiographic findings
Hypervascular uterine masses with bilateral blood supply were demonstrated in six patients; masses with unilateral blood supply could be seen in two patients, and three patients showed diffuse vascularity without obvious mass. One of the early patients with unilateral distortion of the blood supply underwent unilateral embolization; in all the other patients bilateral procedures were performed.

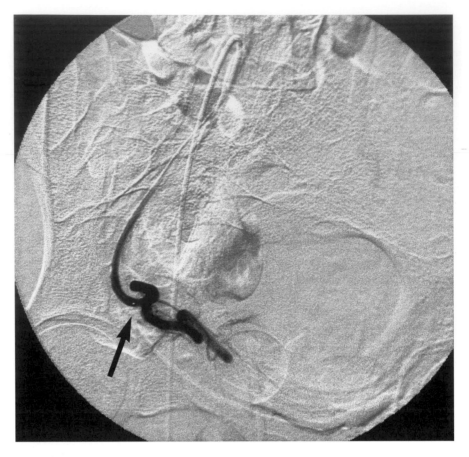

Figure 15.2 The right uterine artery, outlined by contrast, following embolization: arrow shows the catheter tip.

Clinical results

No complications were encountered, either in the procedure room or in the postanaesthesia suite. One patient has had incomplete follow-up. Twenty-four patients completed the questionnaire and underwent follow-up ultrasound examination. One patient experienced post-procedural fever and leucocytosis (to 22,000) 3 weeks after embolization. Initially she was successfully treated with antibiotics intravenously; she then returned to the hospital, where a computed tomogram revealed a pelvic abscess. This patient underwent a total abdominal hysterectomy, during which purulent material was seen.

Ultrasound changes

All patients underwent ultrasound examination prior to embolization, which demonstrated myomatous change. Prior to embolization, average uterine dimensions were $9.8 \times 5.8 \times 7.3$ cm (calculated volume 224 ± 99 cm^3), whereas after the procedure the dimensions were $8.7 \times 4.6 \times 5.9$ cm (calculated volume 127 ± 48 cm^3). The average reduction in uterine volume was 40%, with a range of 22–61% (Fig. 15.3). Similar decreases in myoma volumes were observed, as the sonograms on one patient (taken before the procedure and compared with those taken 6 weeks and 6 months after the procedure) revealed (Figs. 15.4a–c). The one patient who underwent unilateral embolization, and who failed to demonstrate relief of symptoms, none the less showed a 34% reduction in uterine volume.

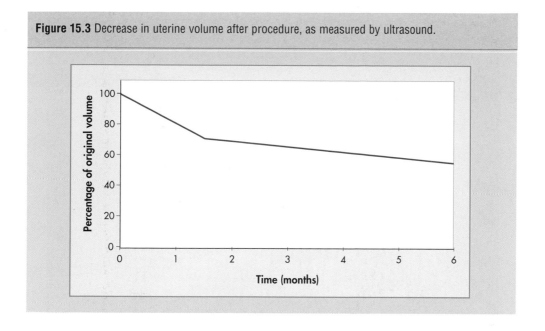

Figure 15.3 Decrease in uterine volume after procedure, as measured by ultrasound.

Morbidity

In patients undergoing conscious sedation, no intra-operative complaints of pain were noted. In the recovery room following embolization, seven patients reported pain: four rated the pain as mild, one described moderate cramping, and two recorded pain as severe. Four of the five women who received intra-arterial lignocaine during the procedure experienced pain, including all three women with moderate or severe pain. This injection practice is no longer part of the embolization protocol. Only two patients required intravenous morphine or hydromorphone in recovery; the remainder were managed with oral ketorolac. No patient required a patient-controlled anaesthesia pump. All but five patients were discharged on the day of the embolization procedure; those five patients required overnight admission for pain control. Two patients experienced crampy pain 1–2 weeks after embolization, which was alleviated by oral medication alone.

Three patients complained of post-procedural fever; one patient with a fever ultimately underwent hysterectomy. All patients stated that they were satisfied with the procedure and would undergo it again if symptoms recurred.

Discussion

Transcatheter embolization of uterine arteries is not a new procedure in either gynaecology or obstetrics. The author, among others, has urged physicians to consider this as an initial therapy for patients with acute bleeding.[1] Doppler ultrasound has demonstrated a decrease in uterine artery flow in patients suffering from myomata who were treated with gonadotrophin-releasing hormone agonists; the rationale for devascularization was therefore established. Initial work on embolization was performed by Ravina and his group in Paris, France. A multicentre study of 31 patients found that embolization significantly reduced blood loss when performed as an adjunct to surgical myomectomy.[6] Several patients who were given embolization so that they could donate autologous blood, did not require surgery at all. This prompted Ravina to study the effect of embolization as an alternative to myomectomy or hysterectomy.[11] His group found that 88% of 16

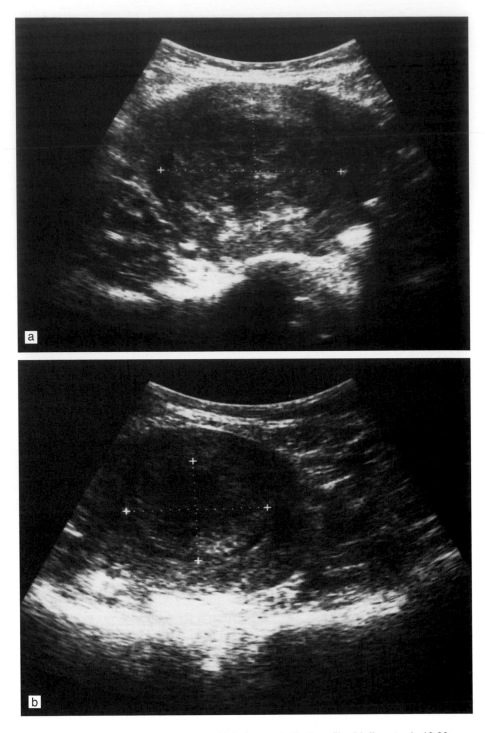

Figure 15.4 Reduction in volume of myoma: (a) before embolization, fibroid diameter is 12.33 cm; (b) 6 weeks after embolization, ultrasound shows shrinkage to 7.35 cm.

patients suffering from menorrhagia related to myomata demonstrated symptomatic improvement, and in 70% a decrease in tumour volume was recorded.

In all the patients in the present author's study population, both hormonal and surgical therapies had failed, compared with failure in only three of Ravina's population who had undergone prior myomectomy. The results obtained by the author have supported Ravina's findings: every patient undergoing embolization

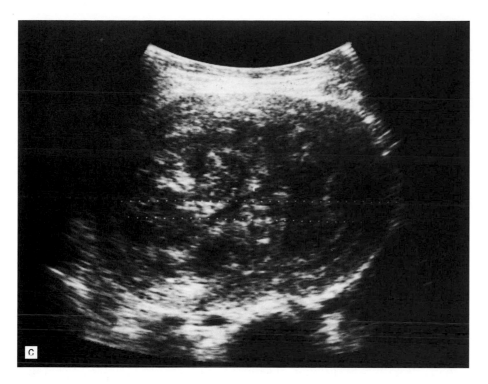

Figure 15.4 (continued) Reduction in volume of myoma: (c) 6 months after embolization, ultrasound of the same fibroid shows shrinkage to 5.33 cm.

reported a decrease in menorrhagia, similar to the 88% reported by Ravina. Sonographic reductions in total uterine volume and individual myoma reduction were also consistent with Ravina's results. Ultrasound and clinical results did not necessarily match, however, since decrease in uterine volumes did not predict the patient in whom embolization failed. Nevertheless, the three patients who reported the best results did show very large reductions in uterine size.

A difference between the author's group and that of Ravina was his choice of a smaller 300 µm PVA particle, compared with the author's 500 µm range; several of the differences between the results in the author's patients and those of Ravina may be explained by this difference in particle size. With regard to efficacy, 70% of the patients in Ravina's group experienced complete resolution of symptoms, compared with only 30% of the author's patients. However, the post-procedural pain experienced by Ravina's patients was greater, reflecting greater ischaemia with smaller particles. The one patient who was embolized with 300 µm particles in the present author's series had severe, prolonged pain; furthermore, the results of her embolization were no better than those of others embolized with the 500 µm PVA particles.

The author's patient undergoing unilateral embolization demonstrates the validity of pathological studies demonstrating the anastomoses between left and right uterine arteries in myomas.[2] Other studies have reported failure when only one artery was embolized.[11]

Antibiotic therapy before the procedure, when the arterial bed is still open, is now routine following the development of an abscess in one patient without obvious predisposing factors. Fever after embolization is a commonly reported side effect,[12] so it is noteworthy that few of the author's patients complained of fever.

Any report of delayed temperature elevation should therefore be vigorously evaluated.

The initial procedures were performed under general anaesthesia; however, as experience was gained, the author's team changed to conscious sedation. No patients experienced discomfort during this method of analgesia. The patients in whom intravenous lignocaine was used may have experienced vasodilatation, which seeded particles more distally in the vascular bed, causing greater ischaemia. As the results did not improve with this technique, it has been abandoned.

Conclusions

Transcatheter embolization of the uterine arteries is a promising new method for treatment of symptomatic myomata. Patients undergoing bilateral embolization may be informed of the likelihood of symptom relief as well as reduction in uterine size and individual myoma dimensions. The author's team now have follow-up data representing more than 18 months in many patients without any regrowth of myomas. Other studies have reported a 15% second-surgery rate after myomectomy.[13] It is possible that the embolization technique offers better overall results than myomectomy. Certainly, the risks to the patient from embolization are less than those of traditional myomectomy, with its known morbidity of haemorrhage, adhesion formation and infection.

Patients wishing to bear children will be studied next for embolization. Ravina[14] recently reported a follow-up of a larger group of patients, four of whom became pregnant and carried to term without complication; one of these patients delivered term twins!

References

1. Vedantham S, Goodwin S C, McLucas B, Mohr G. Uterine artery embolization: an underused method of controlling pelvic hemorrhage. Am J Obstet Gynecol 1997; 176: 938–948

2. Mitty H A, Sterling K M, Alvarez A, Gendler R. Obstetric hemorrhage: prophylactic and emergency arterial catheterization and embolotherapy. Radiology 1993; 188: 183–187

3. Clark S L, Phelan J P, Yeh S Y et al. Hypogastric artery ligation for obstetric hemorrhage. Obstet Gynecol 1985; 66: 353–356

4. O'Leary J A. Uterine artery ligation in the control of postcesarean hemorrhage. J Reprod Med 1995; 40(3): 189–193

5. Rosai J. Ackerman's Surgical pathology. St Louis: Mosby, 1989: 1083–1087

6. Ravina J H, Bouret J M, Fried D et al. Value of preoperative embolization of uterine fibroma: report of a multicenter series of 31 cases. Contracept Fertil Sexual 1995; 23(1): 45–49

7. Ravina J A, Herbreteau D, Ciraru-Vigneron N et al. Arterial embolisation to treat uterine myomata. Lancet 1995; 346: 671–672

8. Bradley E A, Reidy J F, Forman R G et al. Transcatheter uterine artery embolisation to treat large uterine fibroids. Br J Obstet Gynaecol 1998; 105: 235–240

9. McLucas B, Goodwin S, Vedantham S. Embolic therapy for myomata. Min Invas Ther Allied Technol 1996; 5: 336–338

10. Goodwin S G, Vedantham S, McLucas B et al. Preliminary experience with uterine artery embolisation for uterine fibroids. JVIR 1997; 8: 517–526

11. Gilbert W M, Moore T R, Resnik R et al. Angiographic embolization in the management of hemorrhagic complications of pregnancy. Am J Obstet Gynecol 1992; 166: 493–497

12. Chung J W, Park J H, Han J K et al. Hepatic tumors: predisposing factors for complications of transcatheter oily chemoembolization. Radiology 1996; 198: 33–40

13. Buttram V, Reiter R. Uterine leiomyomata: etiology, symptomatology, and management. Fertil Steril 1981; 36: 433–445

14. Ravina, J H, Bouret J M, Ciraru-Vigneron N et al. Recourse to particular arterial embolization in the treatment of some uterine leiomyoma. Bull Acad Natl Med (Paris) 1997; 181: 233–243

CHAPTER 16

Bilateral uterine artery embolization for fibroids

W. J. Walker

Introduction

Most women with fibroids are asymptomatic but an estimated 20–50% of patients have symptoms such as pelvic pain, pelvic pressure, abnormal uterine bleeding, urinary frequency or compressive bowel symptoms.[1] A review of the literature indicates that approximately 30% of patients with myomas experience menorrhagia;[1] in addition, 41% of pregnancies associated with myomas end in abortion[2] (as shown by the preoperative abortion rates in patients undergoing myomectomy).

In the United States in 1990, a total of 592,000 hysterectomies were carried out,[3] and approximately 150,000 hysterectomies are carried out each year for fibroids.[4] In the United Kingdom, from 1993 to 1995, a total of 72,362 hysterectomies were performed in the National Health Service alone.[5] According to Vessey et al.[6] from the United Kingdom, fibroids were the commonest cause of hysterectomy and it was estimated that 20% of women in their study would have had a hysterectomy by the age of 55.[6]

Hysterectomy has a mortality rate of 1–2/1000,[7] a 3/1000 rate of life-threatening events in low-risk groups (Collaborative Review of Sterilization [CREST] study) and a rate of serious complications of at least 30%, excluding both haemorrhage requiring transfusion and urinary retention.[3] The cost of hysterectomy to the National Health Service in the United Kingdom is approximately £70 million/year;[5] thus, in appropriate patients an effective alternative to hysterectomy, with a lower complication rate and lower cost (particularly when such factors as hospital stay and convalescence are taken into account), is desirable, and bilateral uterine artery embolization may be such an alternative.

Pre-interventional assessment and referral

It is essential that patients are properly investigated prior to the procedure, and this investigation should be carried out by a gynaecologist. At the University of California at Los Angeles (UCLA) it is common practice to perform laparoscopy to look for other diseases such as endometriosis, to exclude pathology of the fallopian tubes and generally to check for other disease in the pelvis; a hysteroscopy and biopsy of the endometrium is carried out to exclude endometrial carcinoma. In the United Kingdom, all the author's patients have been seen by a gynaecologist and evaluated, and most have been offered hysterectomy as the only option. Prior to the procedure the patient has an ultrasound or MRI scan (the author prefers an MRI

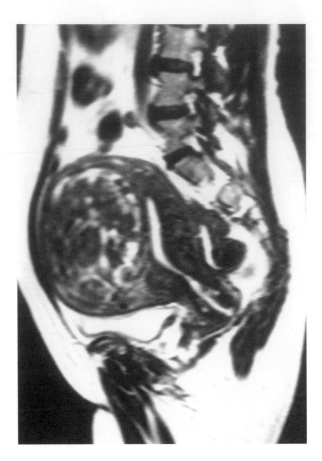

Figure 16.1 A sagittal T2-weighted image showing a large full-thickness interstitial fibroid displacing the endometrial cavity posteriorly.

scan, where possible) (Fig. 16.1). The latter investigation is extremely useful and more accurate than ultrasound: fibroids are more precisely delineated, measured and assessed by this method. In addition, the endometrium is shown clearly on MRI, even though it is considerably distorted and appears obliterated on ultrasound. The endometrium itself, and the junctional zone, can be assessed particularly to exclude adenomyosis. Very often, with large fibroid masses, it is difficult on ultrasound (either transvaginally or transabdominally) to visualize the ovaries, whereas with MRI any ovarian pathology is clearly shown (Fig. 16.2); additionally, non-gynaecological pathology in the pelvis may be visualized.

The patient then discusses the procedure with the radiologist, with particular reference to complications. The aim of the procedure is discussed in terms of fibroid shrinkage and effect on symptoms. The patient signs a specially constructed consent form in which possible complications are tabulated, including the possibility that the procedure might make her sterile. In the author's opinion, the latter is important as the effect of this procedure on fertility is not yet known (see page 192). All patients have a full blood count prior to the procedure, particular attention being paid to the white count and assessment of the hormone profile, haemoglobin and iron stores.

Patients are followed up at 6 weeks, 3 months, 6 months, 12 months and so on. If they have had an MRI prior to the procedure, this investigation is performed again at 6 months in order to determine accurately the degree of shrinkage and

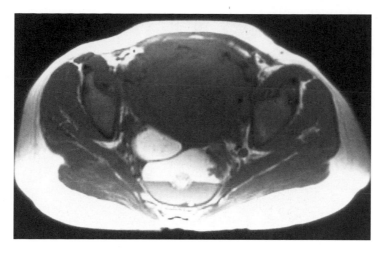

Figure 16.2 A huge fibroid mass with an incidentally discovered large ovarian dermoid obscured on ultrasound by large fibroids.

exclude any occult complications; otherwise, patients have follow-up ultrasound examinations. They receive a questionnaire each visit and have repeat blood tests, the same profile being measured.

Technique

At the Royal Surrey County Hospital (RSCH) in Guildford, the author's team started to practise fibroid embolization in 1996 and subsequently has treated over 80 patients. The technique employed differs little in form from that of the McLucas group at the University of California, Los Angeles (UCLA) (see Chapter 15), except that the author's team commonly enters the uterine artery with a 4 Fr cobra catheter rather than a microcatheter. The microcatheter is then usually introduced through the cobra into the uterine artery and passed approximately halfway along the vessel before the cobra catheter is removed. It is very important to relieve any spasm that may have occurred in the artery, as the object of the procedure is to infuse as many particles as possible into the leash of vessels in the peripheral pseudocapsule. To relieve spasm, the author uses a glyceryl trinitrate (GTN) patch on the patient's forehead and gives 15 mg papaverine slowly, intra-arterially. At UCLA the particle size that has been used in most patients is 500–700 µm, whereas, at RSCH, particles of diameter 150–250, 250–355 and 355–500 µm have been used in all but two cases. In the author's opinion, the smaller particles produce a greater shrinkage (see later), albeit at the expense of increased postoperative pain and possibly an increased risk of complication. Prior to the procedure, patients are given a Voltarol (diclofenac) suppository (100 mg) and after the procedure a patient-controlled anaesthesia (PCA) pump containing morphine (60 mg) and droperidol (6 mg). Most patients begin to develop pain towards the end of the embolization procedure; for this reason, the author sedates patients during the procedure with a mixture of fentanyl, Hypnovel (midazolam) and Maxolon (metoclopramide), so that they are asleep by the end of the procedure. The PCA pump is then set up and they are returned to the ward. Patients usually spend two nights in hospital and are advised to take a week off work. The average case takes approximately 90 minutes, range 40 minutes to 3 hours. The average effective radiation dose to the patient is

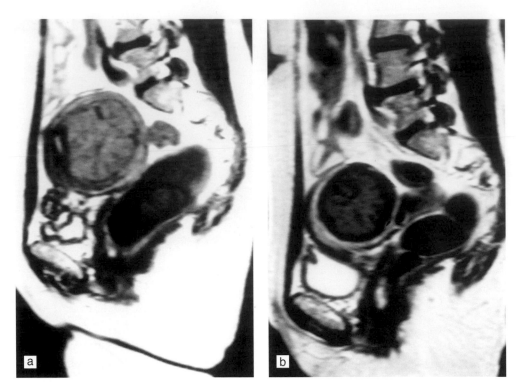

Figure 16.3 T2-weighted MRI scans: (a) pre-embolization; (b) postembolization.

25 mSv. This is equivalent to approximately 3½ times the mean dose associated with a barium enema, although, in recent cases, improvement in technique has lowered this dose. Every attempt is then made to reduce screening time, which is approximately one-third of the total procedure time. Unfortunately, the origin of the uterine artery is very variable and in some cases it can be extremely difficult to catheterize, resulting in long screening times in a small number of cases. In four patients, the attempt to catheterize both uterine arteries at one session failed: in three of these patients, the uterine artery was catheterized at a second session; in the fourth patient a second catheterization was not attempted as the patient's symptoms resolved and she did not wish to undergo a second procedure.

Following the procedure, all patients experience pain in the first 12–24 hours; some — particularly those with larger fibroids — experience bouts of cramping pain over the next 2–3 weeks and may bleed. A few patients may develop a chronic discharge lasting over several months and some, with submucous fibroids, may pass fibroid material vaginally.

Results of fibroid embolization

At the time of writing, 86 of the author's patients have undergone embolization for fibroids. In 57 patients for whom data are available for follow-up of 3 months or more, the average reduction in fibroid volume has been 64% (Fig. 16.3); so far, there has been no regrowth of fibroids. In a few patients with submucous fibroids, resolution has been 100%; in 93% of menorrhagic patients for whom questionnaire data is available their period problems have resolved. All patients with completed questionnaires have been satisfied with the procedure and would recommend it to others. Compression syndrome has been relieved in virtually all: pain has been relieved in 85%, urinary symptoms in 85%, pressure in 92% and swelling in 77%.

Patients returned to work (on average) within 13 days; however, 32% had to consult their general practitioner, mainly for pain relief.

Complications of fibroid embolization

In the UCLA series, one patient developed an infection within the uterus, resulting in hysterectomy (see Chapter 15). In the French series, one patient developed massive necrosis of a subserous fibroid at 8 days postembolization, resulting in intestinal occlusion, hysterectomy and intestinal resection. The French team also had one case of partial dissection of the uterine artery (with no sequelae) and six cases of amenorrhoea — two temporary and four associated with the menopause.[8] In the present author's series there have been two serious complications, both of which were infections leading to hysterectomy. Both patients had large fibroid masses for which hysterectomy only had been offered. The embolization procedures were uneventful, particles of 150–250 μm being used. One patient, who was 34, with a 10-year history of rheumatoid arthritis, developed increasing pain and pyrexia over a 3½ month period. Her white count was never elevated, except in the last phase of her illness. The definitive investigation was an MRI scan that revealed pus in the uterine cavity and perforation of the uterine fundus by an infarcted fibroid (Fig. 16.4); the organism was *Escherichia coli*. A second, 39-year-old, patient developed a high pyrexia, markedly raised white count above 20,000 and rigors, 3 weeks after the procedure. At hysterectomy she was found to have a large tubovarian abscess, previously demonstrated on a CT scan (Fig. 16.5); histology confirmed a tubovarian abscess with pre-existing endometriotic disease of the tube but no infection in the fibroid itself. Very importantly, particles of PVA were found in the ovarian arteries, confirming the fact that uterine artery embolization can cause particulate material to enter the ovarian vessels.

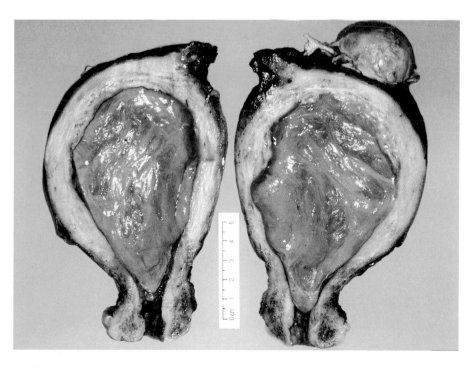

Figure 16.4 An operative specimen of transected uterus showing infarcted fibroid and fundal perforation.

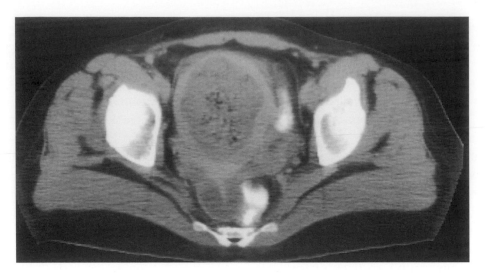

Figure 16.5 A CT scan showing a tubovarian abscess and gas in an infarcted fibroid (note that histological examination showed no evidence of infection in the fibroid).

Four patients developed amenorrhoea: two were perimenopausal (one 53 and the other 54 years of age) and in the other two the amenorrhoea was transient only. One patient developed haemorrhage (or, perhaps a very heavy period) resulting in a fall in haemoglobin concentration from 100 to 54 g/l and requiring blood transfusion.

In addition to the above, three patients have required readmission for suspected infection. Two of these patients were treated with antibiotics and the third received no treatment despite a white count of > 18,000. None appeared sick or had rigors or increasing pain. The author now recognizes this as postembolization syndrome. A CT scan may show gas in the fibroid, but this is not necessarily an indication of infection (Fig. 16.6).

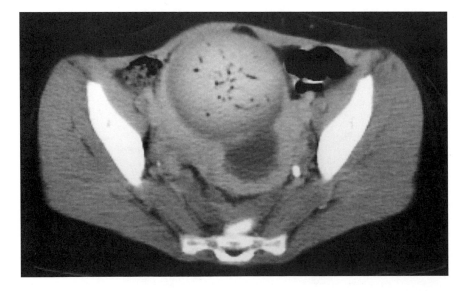

Figure 16.6 A CT scan in a patient with suspected infection previously treated with oral antibiotics from their GP and showing gas in the fibroid. The patient made a full recovery and was not admitted to hospital.

Complications of fibroid embolization are not insignificant: there is probably a 1–3% risk of serious complication leading to hysterectomy. This, however, compares well with the higher serious-complication rate of both myomectomy and hysterectomy. As yet, in at least 600 patients undergoing embolization in the United Kingdom, no patient has died as a result of embolization.

One theoretical complication of fibroid embolization is inadvertent embolization of particles into other pelvic vessels. As yet, no such complications have been observed. This may be because there is a very rich collateral supply in the pelvis. However, embolization of branches of the internal iliac arteries has led to complications such as bladder necrosis,[9] sciatic nerve damage[10] and avascular necrosis of the femoral head.[11] There are also possible complications related to angiography. However, with modern equipment (such as small catheters and sheaths), such complications (which include local thrombosis of the puncture site, false aneurysm formation, and embolization) are very rare: in the thousands of diagnostic arteriograms carried out by the author, no such complications have occurred.

Some have objected to uterine artery embolization on the grounds that a uterine sarcoma may be missed whereas, with hysterectomy, a histological diagnosis would be made and, in addition, a curative operation performed. In the reality of medical practice, this is illusory: uterine sarcoma is extremely rare (incidence less than 0.2%).[5] It was thought that rapid growth in a fibroid was an indication for hysterectomy, on the grounds that this may indicate a sarcoma; this has been shown to be erroneous.[12] In reality, the incidence of uterine sarcoma is less than the incidence of death from hysterectomy, which is 1–2/1000.[7] If there is a clinical suspicion of uterine sarcoma, then ultrasound-guided transabdominal or transvaginal gun biopsy can be carried out for reassurance of the physician or the patient. In addition, it should be remembered that, in the United Kingdom, it is not uncommon for patients to wait 18 months for a routine operation on fibroids — with obvious consequences for the patient with an undetected uterine sarcoma.

Objective of fibroid embolization

In the 40% of women who have fibroids, most of these fibroids do not require treatment. It is common for a radiologist carrying out ultrasound scans in elderly women to find (even large) fibroids that have been asymptomatic throughout life. Furthermore, contrary to popular belief, many fibroids do not shrink after the menopause and they retain their hypervascularity; hence the effect of hormone replacement therapy, even years after the menopause, of causing some fibroids to grow further. As fibroids are not life threatening, the philosophy behind embolization is simply to remove the symptoms of the fibroids, to prevent further growth of the treated fibroids and (it is hoped) to prevent the growth of new fibroids. With regard to the latter, it is possible that the injected particles pass to small hypervascular foci (which would subsequently grow) and infarct these as well; however, as yet this premise is unproven. The degree of shrinkage of the fibroids is, to a certain extent, irrelevant unless the procedure is carried out specifically for cosmetic reasons; what counts is the elimination of symptoms to the patient's satisfaction. Nevertheless, embolization does produce a shrinkage, the reported reduction in fibroid volume depending on the series (UCLA 40%; RSCH 64%; Paris 70%).[13,14]

Fertility

The effect of fibroid embolization on fertility is unknown. So far, there has been no evidence that fertile patients have become infertile following pelvic embolization, and pregnancies have occurred after embolization for gynaecological bleeding,[15,16] cervical ectopic pregnancy[17] and treatment of arteriovenous malformation.[18] However, most embolizations in benign disease in patients of childbearing age have utilized Gelfoam pledgets. These are cubes, usually approximately 1 mm in diameter, which, when injected through a catheter, lodge in the precapillary and pre-arteriolar vessels. Usually, they fragment and are dissipated over a period of days or weeks; flow in the vessel is then re-established. Particles, whether of polyvinyl alcohol (PVA) or Gelfoam powder, or liquid polymers such as isobutyl 2-cyanoacrylate, cause a much more distal block affecting the capillaries and arterials; thus ischaemia would be more likely to be due to the prevention of intramural collateralization. However, in the case of fibroid embolization the normal myometrium very rapidly revascularizes within days, as shown on colour duplex ultrasound examinations. Collateralization is obviously very rapid from vessels such as the ovarian and vaginal arteries, despite occlusion by fine particles. It is believed that these particles preferentially pass to the hypervascular pseudocapsule around fibroids, causing a relative sparing of the 'normal' myometrium. The author has had occasion to embolize a patient with an entirely normal uterus; she had a complex gynaecological history and von Willebrand's disease. On the 6-week follow-up colour duplex ultrasound scan her uterus appeared entirely normal and was normally vascularized.

In the French experience of 76 patients, four patients became pregnant: one miscarried (patient 40 years old); a second patient with AIDS miscarried as a result of infection; the third patient had a successful caesarean section at 35 weeks; the fourth patient had a normal delivery with no complications.[8] Thus, pregnancy is possible after embolization. Certainly, in some cases of patients with small fibroids, resolution on follow-up ultrasound has been 100% in the author's hands with an ultrasonically normal-looking endometrium at 3 months. It is possible that, in these cases, fertility may be improved by embolization, but this is as yet unverified. Most fibroid embolization procedures, however, in the author's experience, have been carried out in patients with large complex interstitial and submucous fibroid masses. Pedunculated subserous fibroids are not usually treated by embolization as there is a risk of them sloughing off into the peritoneal cavity. It is unfortunate that accurate figures for the improvement in fertility in patients with such large complex fibroid masses undergoing myomectomy are lacking; in such cases, myomectomy is often discussed and often abandoned. At the author's institution, however, embolization is not offered routinely for patients whose primary concern is the preservation of fertility: such patients are advised to try to obtain a realistic assessment of the success of a myomectomy in their particular case. Such an assessment by a gynaecologist would be greatly helped by an MRI scan, which shows the exact geography of the fibroid or fibroids in relation to the uterus; however, very few gynaecologists employ this powerful pelvic imaging modality. If fertility is not the patient's primary concern but is a minor issue and the predominant reason for requesting embolization is to eliminate fibroid symptoms, and if, in addition, myomectomy is likely to fail, then the author is prepared to offer this therapy.

Combined procedures

The role of combined procedures has not yet been evaluated. In the author's experience, in one patient with a fibroid mass the size of a term pregnancy, embolization was carried out in order to shrink the fibroid mass prior to hysterectomy, which was performed 3 months later. By that time the fibroid mass had shrunk to the size of a 20-week pregnancy and the uterus was removed through a small transverse incision. It is possible that combining fibroid embolization to prevent further growth of fibroids (or, possibly, the development of new fibroids) with laser endometriectomy and hysteroscopic removal of submucous fibroids may provide an optimal result.

Conclusions

The experience of the teams at UCLA, RSCH and Paris would suggest that uterine artery embolization is effective in shrinking fibroids and reducing or eliminating the symptoms. It is not, however, without complications and the effect on fertility is unknown. More data on long-term follow-up and to elucidate the optimal technique of embolization are needed. In particular, it is necessary to know whether the use of small particles increases the risk of complications and whether it is due to an additional effect of smaller particles on the 'normal' uterine myometrium. So far, however, uterine artery embolization appears to hold promise as an effective alternative to hysterectomy and possibly, in some cases, myomectomy. The complication rate is low and there is a markedly reduced hospital stay and convalescence period, with a potential significant reduction in cost to the health service and morbidity to the patient.

References

1. Wallach E E, Vu K K. Myomata uteria and infertility. Obstet Gynecol Clin North Am 1995; 11(4): 791–799

2. Buttram V C, Reiter R C. Uterine leiomyomata: etiology, symptomatology, and management. Fertil Steril 1981; 36(4): 433–455

3. Wilcox L S, Koonin L M, Pokras R et al. Hysterectomy in the United States 1988–1990. Obstet Gynecol 1994; 83: 549–555

4. Wallach E E. Myomectomy. In: Thompson J D, Rock J A (eds) Te Linde's Operative gynecology, 7th edn. Philadelphia: Lippincott, 1992: 647–662

5. Davies A, Magos A L. Indications and alternatives to hysterectomy. Baillieres Clin Obstet Gynaecol 1997; 11(1): 61–75

6. Vessey M P, Villard-Mackintosh L, McPherson K et al. The epidemiology of hysterectomy: findings in a large cohort study. Br J Obstet Gynaecol 1992; 99: 402–407

7. Martin L, Benson R C. Preoperative and postoperative care. In: Pernoll M L, Benson R C (eds) Current obstetrics and gynecologic diagnosis and treatment, 6th edn. New York: Appleton and Lange, 1987: 798

8. Ravina J H, Bouret J M, Ciraru-Vigneron N et al. Particulate arterial embolization: a new treatment for uterine leiomyomata-related hemorrhage. Presse Med 1998; 27(7): 299

9. Braf Z F, Koorty W W Jr. Gangrene of bladder. Complication of hypogastric artery embolisation. Urology 1977; 9: 670–671

10. Hare W S C, Holland C J. Paresis following internal iliac embolization. Radiology 1983; 146: 47–51

11. Obaro R O, Sniderman K W. Avascular necrosis of the femoral head as a complication of complex embolization for severe pelvic haemorrhage. Br J Radiol 1995; 68: 920–922

12. Parker W H, Fu Y S, Berek J S. Uterine sarcoma in patients operated on for presumed leiomyoma and rapidly growing leiomyoma. Obstet Gynecol 1994; 83(3): 414–418

13. Goodwin S C, Vedantham S, McLucas B et al. Preliminary experience with uterine artery embolization for uterine fibroids. JVIR 1997; 8(4): 517–526

14. Ravina J H, Bouret J M, Ciraru-Vigneron N et al. Recourse to particular arterial embolization in the treatment of some leiomyoma. Bull Acad Natl Med (Paris) 1997; 181(2): 233–246

15. Greenwood L H, Glickman M G, Schwartz P E et al. Obstetric and nonmalignant gynecologic bleeding; treatment with angiographic embolization. Radiology 1987; 164: 155–159

16. Abbas F M, Currie J L, Mitchell S et al. Selective vascular embolization in benign gynecologic conditions. J Reprod Med 1994; 39: 492–496

17. Frates M C, Benson C B, Doubilet P M et al. Cervical ectopic pregnancy: results of conservative treatment. Radiology 1994; 191: 773–775

18. Poppe W, Van Assche F A, Wilms G et al. Pregnancy after transcatheter embolization of a uterine arteriovenous malformation. Am J Obstet Gynecol 1987; 156: 1179–1180

CHAPTER 17

Role of photodynamic therapy

M. J. Gannon, M. R. Stringer and S. B. Brown

Introduction

The ideal endometrial ablation procedure should completely and reliably destroy the entire endometrium while avoiding damage to the myometrium and to other organs. The methods that are currently available do not permit such precise targeting — there is a trade-off between complete endometrial ablation and damage to adjacent organs.

Photodynamic therapy (PDT) was initially developed for the treatment of malignant tumours.[1] PDT utilizes the selective retention of the photosensitizer and its ability to elicit an efficient photodynamic reaction upon activation with penetrating visible light. The first step in treatment is the administration of a photosensitizing drug, which accumulates in the target tissue. Cells that are sensitized in this way can be destroyed by light at an appropriate wavelength, typically generated by a laser and delivered through an optical fibre.

Development of PDT

The photodynamic effect of light-absorbing chemicals was recognized as far back as 1900, and numerous examples have been reported for a wide range of photosensitizers. Endogenous fluorescence from haemolytic bacterial infection of cancers led to the study of porphyrins as photosensitizers. The first use of haematoporphyrin derivative (HPD) to highlight breast cancer was reported by Lipson in 1961.[2] Dougherty later demonstrated eradication of a transplanted mouse mammary tumour using HPD activated by red light from a filtered xenon arc-lamp and he went on to pioneer the development of PDT for cancer treatment.[1] PDT took a major step forward with American Food and Drug Administration (FDA) approval for therapeutic use of the photosensitizer Photofrin II (QLT Photo-Therapeutics Inc., Vancouver, Canada) in December 1995.

Current use of PDT

The use of PDT ranges from the treatment of carcinoma in situ to that of inoperable cancers. PDT is being developed for superficial bladder cancer, as it may provide a greater degree of selectivity than other treatments currently applied to these cases.[1] Superficial skin cancer can be managed by PDT, which is the treatment of choice in certain centres.[3] Advanced tumours of the lung, oesophagus, and head and neck have also shown promising responses.[1]

Photosensitizers

Initial clinical studies were carried out using HPD, which is a complex mixture of monomeric porphyrins and oligomeric porphyrin esters and ethers. A more efficient photosensitizer was obtained by partial removal of the monomers, which do not become localized in tumour tissue, to yield Photofrin II, a semi-purified proprietary preparation of HPD. Photofrin II has specificity for many types of malignant tissue, although it also accumulates in the liver, spleen, kidneys and skin. Photosensitizer accumulation in the skin leads to photosensitization that lasts for up to 6 weeks. During that time, there is a risk of undesirable phototoxic reactions, restricting the wider use of Photofrin II in human subjects.[4] An alternative approach uses natural 5-aminolaevulinic acid (ALA) to produce protoporphyrin IX (PpIX), a precursor of haem in most body cells. Administration of excess ALA leads to accumulation of PpIX, which acts as an endogenous photosensitizer. There is also continuing research into improving the original photosensitizers: currently at least six new second-generation photosensitizing drugs are undergoing phase I and phase II clinical trials.

Photodynamic endometrial ablation

The first attempt at photodynamic endometrial ablation was carried out on ovariectomized rats. The photosensitizer dihaematoporphyrin ether (DHE) was found to have a preferential uptake in the endometrial layer of the oestrogen-primed rat uterus[5]. In a further study, ovariectomized rats were subjected to PDT endometrial ablation.[6] Three hours after DHE injection the right uterine horn was exposed by laparotomy and received photoradiation to the uterine surface using 628 nm light from a gold-vapour laser. Uteri were removed 72 hours later and the PDT-treated right horn was compared histologically with the untreated left horn: examination showed selective coagulation necrosis of the entire endometrium and the inner part of the circular muscle layer of the muscularis in the treated group only.

The next reported study of PDT endometrial ablation was on rabbits which, like rats, have a double uterus, providing a convenient treatment and control uterine horn in each animal. Bhatta and colleagues[7] showed that Photofrin II was taken up and retained preferentially by the endometrium, with the greatest concentration observed in the stroma. Laser light was delivered using an optical fibre with a diffusing tip inserted in the rabbit uterus. When the uterus was examined at 5 and 10 days after treatment, endometrial necrosis was confirmed and related to the dose of Photofrin II. Despite the rabbit's relatively thin myometrium there was no full-thickness uterine destruction.

5-Aminolaevulinic acid

The natural photosensitizer protoporphyrin IX (PpIX) is formed by most living cells in the enzymatic pathway for haem synthesis. The formation of ALA is the first, committed step in the formation of haem. The ultimate step is the conversion of PpIX to haem and this is thought to be a rate-limiting step in the pathway. An exogenously delivered excess of ALA leads to the accumulation of PpIX and thus provides a method for natural photosensitization. The half-life of ALA is approximately 30 minutes and it is completely metabolized within 24 hours, thus avoiding the problem of prolonged skin sensitivity. Kennedy and Pottier[4] studied the distribution of ALA-induced PpIX in normal tissues and found that fluorescence occurred primarily in surface and glandular epithelium of the skin and the lining of hollow organs. Photosensitizer did not tend to accumulate in muscle and connective tissue. This selective uptake in vascular, proliferative tissues could be used to target certain tissues, such as the endometrium, for destruction. Systemic ALA administration has been shown to induce a fivefold greater PpIX fluorescence in rabbit endometrium than in myometrium or stroma.[8]

Light delivery

Red light at a wavelength of 630 nm is usually chosen to perform PDT. This is a longer wavelength than that of the intense absorption band of haemoglobin and therefore penetrates tissue to a greater depth than short-wavelength blue or green light. A penetration of 4–5 mm is sufficient to reach the deepest endometrial glands while leaving a good safety margin of surrounding myometrium. At present only large, complex laser systems are capable of delivering sufficient power (up to about 1 W) for effective treatment at 630 nm. These consist of a primary pumping laser such as an argon-ion or a copper-vapour laser coupled to a separate, tunable dye laser.

The delivery of light from source to treatment site is achieved using a flexible optical fibre. Laser light can be coupled into a fibre less than 1 mm in diameter and transmitted over a distance of several metres with an efficiency of about 70%. For intra-uterine treatment the fibre can easily be delivered through a hysteroscope or within a purpose-made catheter.

Mechanism of action

The three elements required for successful PDT are photosensitizer, light and molecular oxygen. The primary component responsible for cytotoxicity is the activated molecular oxygen species termed singlet oxygen ($^1O_2$). When light of sufficient energy is absorbed by the sensitizer it triggers the release of singlet oxygen, possibly along with other highly reactive intermediates, such as free radicals. The result is an irreversible oxidization of essential cellular components. The destruction of crucial cell membranes, organelles and vasculature leads to cell necrosis.

Developmental experiments

Topical administration has been investigated as a means of minimizing photosensitizer-induced skin sensitivity.[9] Rats were randomized to receive intravenous, intraperitoneal or intra-uterine Photofrin II, and the uterine porphyrin levels were determined. Intra-uterine administration provided the best uptake and distribution within the uterus, at lower drug doses.

The powerful photosensitizer benzoporphyrin derivative (BPD), when instilled into the uterine cavity of rabbits, was shown to accumulate in higher concentration in the epithelial structures of the endometrium than in the stroma and myometrium.[10] The effect of PDT was assessed by examining uteri at 1 and 4 weeks after treatment. Substantial, persistent endometrial destruction was generally observed, although there were regional variations in re-epithelialization.

In a study at Leeds,[11] intra-uterine polyhaematoporphyrin (PHP), which is indistinguishable from Photofrin II, was administered to volunteers before hysterectomy: PHP was selectively taken up by the endometrium.

Intra-uterine ALA for PDT

Intra-uterine administration of ALA in rats induced selective endometrial fluorescence. Exposure of the treated uteri to light produced endometrial ablation.[12] There was preservation of some glandular elements after treatment, yet no regeneration of endometrium was evident at 10 days. The functional effect was confirmed by comparing pregnancy implantation in treated and untreated uterine horns. Those treated by means of ALA PDT showed a profoundly decreased rate of implantation, as well as the absence of functioning endometrium.[13] This study suggests that, although complete endometrial destruction was not immediate, photo-ablation of the endometrium was achieved by direct tissue destruction combined with the effect of local toxicity from photo-ablated tissue.

A similar study confirmed that successful ablation of the rat endometrium could be carried out using intra-uterine ALA PDT.[14] In this study rabbits were also treated. The larger rabbit uterine horn required multiple, segmental irradiation, which resulted in uneven light dosimetry; this may have accounted for variations in re-epithelialization that were found 7 days after irradiation.

Pharmacokinetics of ALA

The study by Wyss et al.[14] of ALA PDT in rats and rabbits was designed to explore the pharmacokinetics and effective distribution of intra-uterine ALA. Peak endometrial fluorescence, and hence PpIX conversion, was observed at 3 hours in both animal models. No significant dose-dependent fluctuations were observed in glandular, stromal and myometrial fluorescence when the ALA concentration was increased from 100 to 400 mg/ml. However, glandular uptake was significantly higher than that of the other structures, regardless of drug concentration. Although the solution of ALA was highly acidic and potentially toxic, buffering to pH 5.5 did not affect the fluorescence levels. Histological appearances of the uteri were similar at 3 and 7 days, showing destruction of glandular epithelium with moderate stromal scarring.

ALA in primates

A study of endometrial PpIX fluorescence was performed on monkeys, in which ALA was administered either via a needle into the uterine fundus, transcervically or by intravenous injection.[15] Hysterectomy was performed after 3 hours. Uterine fluorescence microscopy and spectrofluorophotometry showed selective accumulation of PpIX in endometrium and not in myometrium. Peak fluorescence occurred 4–5 hours after injection and decreased gradually to less than 20% of peak value at 8 hours.

Monkeys were shown to tolerate large doses of ALA without ill effect.[15] Intravenous ALA was given in dosages up to 250 mg/kg, which is 50-fold greater than that required to induce endometrial photosensitization when given directly into the uterus. The only abnormality detected was a trend toward increased serum aspartate aminotransferase at 24 hours, which had returned to pre-ALA levels at 1 week.

First clinical studies

The safety of a large dose of ALA was assessed in a study of the pathogenesis of acute porphyria in humans.[16] Porphyric attacks are accompanied by urinary

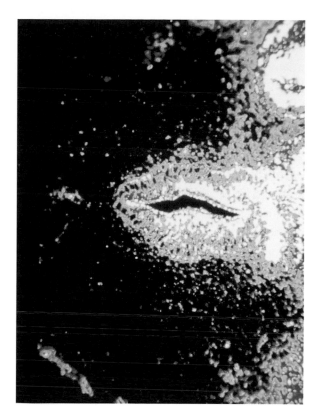

Figure 17.1 Fluorescence microscopy shows an endometrial gland in a 5-aminolaevulinic acid (ALA)-treated uterus. In the authors' study,[17] endometrial glands of the functional and basal layers exhibited similar levels of protoporphyrin IX (PpIX) fluorescence. Most, but not all, glands in the ALA-treated uteri exhibited ALA-induced PpIX fluorescence. PpIX fluorescence was detected to a lesser extent in the stroma and was not observed in the myometrium. No relationship between the ALA dose or duration of treatment and the pattern of PpIX fluorescence was detected.

excretion of ALA, which has led to the belief that ALA is responsible for the neuronal toxicity of porphyria. High ALA excretion also occurs in symptomless patients and experiments have failed to reproduce the proposed effect. The study was designed to simulate the plasma concentration of ALA seen during acute attacks of porphyria. Sustained elevation of ALA was produced in a human volunteer by an oral loading dose of ALA followed by nasogastric instillation over 4 days; the total dose of ALA was 5.8 g. No symptoms or pathophysiological changes were detected in a battery of assays, including serum aspartate aminotransferase levels. Temporary skin sensitivity due to ALA has been described only after a very large systemic dose.

Human endometrial photosensitization

The authors are investigating the use of ALA PDT of the endometrium in model systems and in a series of patients (Fig. 17.1).[17] In all of this work, the ALA is administered directly into the uterine cavity to reduce any possibility of systemic photosensitization. In a series of experiments in uteri perfused ex vivo, ALA was introduced into the cavity and protoporphyrin formation was measured in the endometrium, the underlying myometrium and the perfusate; ALA transfer into the perfusate was also measured. This work demonstrated that protoporphyrin formation in the endometrium was approximately tenfold that in the underlying myometrium and that systemic photosensitization would be unlikely to result from transfer of administered ALA from the uterus into the circulation. Similar results were found in studies carried out in vivo, where ALA was administered to patients scheduled for hysterectomy.

Laser system

In the authors' clinical studies, the optical parameters required for effective treatment were estimated from previous clinical practice for the PDT of hollow organs such as the oesophagus and the bladder. Studies were carried out on a post-hysterectomy uterus to characterize the distribution of light and to predict an adequate treatment time.[18] A light-delivery system was constructed using a balloon catheter with the end replaced by a shaped latex balloon (Fig. 17.2). A fibre modification was designed to emit light over a cylindrical terminal section approximately 2 cm in length.

In the authors' clinical studies a core silica fibre (600 µm) is introduced through the modified catheter to lie within a customized intra-uterine balloon. A solution of Intralipid is then injected into the balloon to scatter light. The combination of cylindrical diffuser and scattering medium ensures that the fluence rate at the balloon surface is evenly distributed. The 630 nm light is generated by a copper-vapour pumped-dye laser, with up to 1 W focused into the fibre. A prescribed light dose of 50 J/cm² is delivered at a rate of 30 mW/cm², with two catheter placements ensuring treatment of the entire endometrial surface in less than half an hour.

Figure 17.2 Diagram of the intra-uterine balloon laser delivery system for photodynamic therapy.

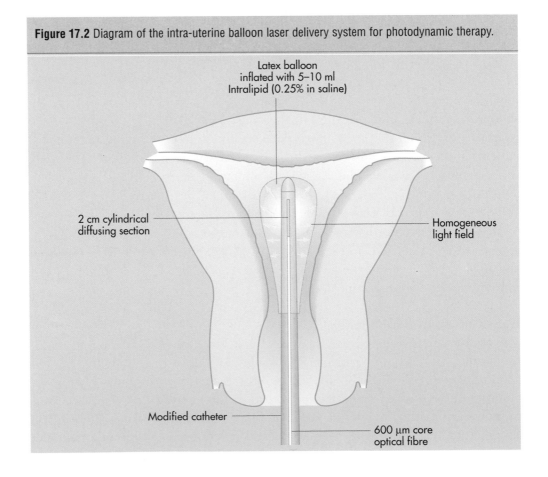

Latex balloon
inflated with 5–10 ml
Intralipid (0.25% in saline)

2 cm cylindrical
diffusing section

Homogeneous
light field

Modified catheter

600 µm core
optical fibre

Photodynamic endometrial ablation

Using their specially designed light-delivery system, the authors are now treating patients with intra-uterine ALA followed by laser light. One-year follow-up is available on the first two series of patients. The first five patients showed a reduction in measured menstrual blood loss (MBL);[19] this was not sufficient to relieve symptoms and all went on to have alternative surgical treatment. Various treatment parameters were modified for the second group of five women: apart from one failure due to fibroids, the remainder showed a reduction in MBL. Complete symptomatic relief was obtained in two women, who did not require further treatment.[20]

The future of PDT

Successful human endometrial ablation depends on the critical interaction of several complex, interrelated factors: these include endometrial thickness, which determines penetration of drugs and light, and endometrial vascularity, which provides tissue oxygenation. The optimum photosensitizer may vary for different indications, as may the dose, route and method of delivery. The ideal parameters of light delivery must be defined, including the treatment wavelength, fluence rate and light dose.

Endometrial regeneration

The acute inflammation and cell death of menstruation is rapidly followed by regrowth of epithelium, which may be complete within about 48 hours. Comparable regeneration is seen only in haematopoietic, intestinal and epidermal tissues. The growth capacity is based on essential endometrial tissue mechanisms that are independent of the hormonal influences of the reproductive system. The origin of renewed endometrium has been variously attributed to undifferentiated stem cells, residual endometrial epithelium, stromal fibroblasts and endothelial cells of ruptured capillaries.[21] Each of these candidate cell lines shares a common location in the layer immediately deep to the superficial endometrium. Prevention of endometrial regeneration has concentrated on obliteration of this layer, which extends to a depth of about 3 mm. None of the methods of endometrial ablation that are now in use can guarantee permanent complete endometrial obliteration.

Targeted destruction

Is the lack of success due to incomplete destruction of regenerative cells or is there a hitherto unknown mechanism of endometrial regrowth? The former is more likely and the solution may lie in precise marking of the tissue for destruction. PDT has the unique facility of targeting the endometrium with a photosensitizer. Although, in theory, this could enable treatment to reach the entire population of endometrial cells, in the authors' experiments an incomplete uptake throughout the endometrium was seen on fluorescence microscopy. Nevertheless, the ratio of photosensitizer uptake has been shown by the authors and by many other workers clearly to favour the endometrium over the myometrium.

Current research includes experiments to enhance photosensitizer uptake throughout the endometrium. Promoters of photosensitizer uptake and modifications to the photosensitizers to aid uptake are being evaluated. Priming of the endometrium by pretreatment with oestrogen has been advocated: this may increase ALA uptake by promoting endometrial proliferation.[9] The penetration-enhancing agent Azone has been added to Photofrin II to enhance uptake and ALA esters are being tried as a means of improving penetration of this drug.

Light delivery

A more uniform light distribution is achieved by distention of the uterine cavity. Fluids such as Hyskon have been used, and the authors have designed an intra-uterine balloon system. An alternative could be the insertion of three or more cylindrical diffusing fibres into an undistended cavity, similar to the insertion of an intra-uterine device; this could be carried out without excessive discomfort or pain.[22]

Current laser systems are associated with high capital and maintenance costs, and this is a limiting factor in the widespread application of PDT. Simpler, more compact and less expensive sources such as diode lasers and filtered arc lamps are now being developed for use in PDT.

Conclusions

The ultimate goal of a simple, outpatient method of endometrial ablation that does not require anaesthesia is being widely pursued. Recent developments, including novel photosensitizers and optical systems, may allow a breakthrough in the role of photodynamic therapy for the treatment of women with menorrhagia.

References

1. Dougherty T J. Photodynamic therapy (PDT) of malignant tumours. Crit Rev Oncol Hematol 1984; 2: 83–116

2. Lipson R L, Baldes E J, Olsen A M. The use of derivative of haematoporphyrin in tumor detection. J Natl Cancer Inst 1961; 26: 1–11

3. Cairnduff F, Stringer M R, Hudson E J et al. Superficial photodynamic therapy with topical 5-aminolaevulinic acid for superficial primary and secondary skin cancer. Br J Cancer 1994; 69: 605–608

4. Kennedy J G, Pottier R H. Endogenous protoporphyrin IX, a clinically useful photosensitizer for photodynamic therapy. J Photochem Photobiol B: Biol 1992; 14: 275–292

5. Schneider D F, Schellhas H F, Wesseler T A et al. Haematoporphyrin derivative uptake in uteri of estrogen-treated ovariectomized rats. Colposc Gynecol Laser Surg 1988; 4: 67–72

6. Schneider D F, Schellhas H F, Wesseler T A, Moulton B C. Endometrial ablation by DHE photoradiation therapy in estrogen-treated ovariectomized rats. Colposc Gynecol Laser Surg 1988; 4: 73–77

7. Bhatta N, Anderson R R, Flotte T et al. Endometrial ablation by means of photodynamic therapy with photofrin II. Am J Obstet Gynecol 1992; 167: 1856–1863

8. Judd M D, Bedwell J, MacRobert A J. Comparison of the distribution of phthalocyanine and ALA-induced porphyrin sensitisers within the rabbit uterus. Lasers Med Sci 1992; 7: 203–211

9. Chapman J A, Tadir Y, Tromberg B J et al. Effect of administration route and estrogen manipulation on endometrial uptake of Photofrin porfimer sodium. Am J Obstet Gynecol 1993; 168: 685–692

10. Wyss P, Tadir Y, Tromberg B J et al. Benzoporphyrin derivative (BPD): a potent photosensitizer for photodynamic destruction of the rabbit endometrium. Obstet Gynecol 1994; 84: 409–414

11. Griffith-Jones M, Lilford R J. 1993, St. James' University Hospital, Leeds, UK. Unpublished results

12. Yang J Z, Van Vugt D A, Kennedy J C, Reid R L. Intrauterine 5-aminolevulinic acid induces selective fluorescence and photodynamic ablation of the rat endometrium. Photochem Photobiol 1993; 57: 803–807

13. Yang J Z, Van Vugt D A, Kennedy J C, Reid R L. Evidence of lasting functional destruction of the rat endometrium after 5-aminolevulinic acid-induced photodynamic ablation: prevention of implantation. Am J Obstet Gynecol 1993; 168: 995–1001

14. Wyss P, Tromberg B J, Wyss M T et al. Photodynamic destruction of endometrial tissue with topical 5-aminolevulinic acid in rats and rabbits. Am J Obstet Gynecol 1994; 171: 1176–1183

15. Yang J Z, Van Vugt D A, Roy B N et al. Intrauterine 5-aminolaevulinic acid induces selective endometrial fluorescence in the rhesus and cynomolgus monkey. J Soc Gynecol Invest 1996; 3: 152–157

16. Mustajoki P, Timonen K, Gorchein A et al. Sustained high plasma 5-aminolaevulinic acid concentration in a volunteer: no porphyric symptoms. Eur J Clin Invest 1992; 22: 407–411

17. Gannon M J, Johnson N, Roberts D J H et al. Photosensitization of the endometrium with topical 5-aminolevulinic acid. Am J Obstet Gynecol 1995; 173: 1826–1828

18. Stringer M R, Hudson E J, Dunkley C P et al. Light delivery schemes for uterine photodynamic therapy. In: Jori G, Moan J, Star W M (eds) Photodynamic therapy of cancer. Proc SPIE 1994; 2078: 41–49

19. Gannon M J, Day P, Hammadieh N, Johnson N. A new method for measuring menstrual blood loss and its use in screening women before endometrial ablation. Br J Obstet Gynaecol 1996; 103: 1029–1033

20. Gannon M J, Vernon D I, Holroyd J A et al. PDT of the endometrium using ALA. Proc SPIE 1997; 2972: 2–13

21. Wyss P, Steiner R, Liaw L H et al. Regeneration processes in rabbit endometrium: a photodynamic therapy model. Hum Reprod 1996; 11: 1992–1997

22. Fehr M K, Madsen S J, Svaasand L O et al. Intrauterine light delivery for photodynamic therapy of the human endometrium. Hum Reprod 1995; 10: 3067–3072

CHAPTER 18

Action in the event of malignant histology

J. M. Monaghan

Introduction

An awareness of malignant histology or a diagnosis of cancer may be generated in the following circumstances:

1. During the preliminary investigation of menorrhagia, such as on a Pipelle sample or following curettage of the endometrial cavity or endocervix.
2. Following treatment of the menorrhagia, usually as an incidental finding after hysterectomy.
3. If it is the practice of the clinician to open the uterus following hysterectomy, when a malignant tumour of the corpus may be identified.

Menorrhagia occurs over a wide age range throughout the menstrual life of women and is now extending into the time when women take hormone replacement therapy. This time-scale overlaps the time patterns for the development of cancers of the cervix and uterine body.

Malignant histology found during diagnosis

As part of the process of identifying the cause of menorrhagia, tissue is removed from the uterine cavity and a histological assessment is made. The tissue that is removed is usually endometrium; however it is not unusual for elements of polyps, fibroids and endocervical tissue to be included in the specimen. Therefore, the following tumour types may be identified (Table 18.1).

Cervical intra-epithelial neoplasia (CIN) and cervical glandular intra-epithelial neoplasia (CGIN)
It is not uncommon for fragments of CIN and CGIN to be found in Pipelle samples and curettage specimens.

Action The patient should be referred for expert colposcopy so that the ecto- and endocervix can be assessed. Cervical cytology should be brought up to date using either a standard spatula or a spatula combined with a brush if the squamocolumnar junction lies within the endocervical canal. Colposcopy will allow the clinician to identify the transformation zone and any significant changes. A large loop excision of the transformation zone (LLETZ) will be best to determine the true histology

Table 18.1 Types of tumour of the uterus or cervix that may be identified during investigation or treatment of menorrhagia

- Cervical intra-epithelial neoplasia (CIN)
- Cervical glandular intra-epithelial neoplasia (CGIN)
- Squamous carcinoma of the cervix
- Adenocarcinoma of the cervix
- Atypical hyperplasias of the endometrium
- Cystic hyperplasia of the endometrium
- Adenocarcinoma of the endometrium
- Adenosquamous carcinoma of the endometrium
- Squamous carcinoma of the endometrium
- Sarcoma of the corpus, usually arising in polyps
- Choriocarcinoma

and, in good hands, will clear the lesion completely. Appropriate review should be organized for treated CIN or CGIN.

Squamous carcinoma and adenocarcinoma of the cervix
These cancers occur in the same age-band of women who develop menorrhagia. Their symptomatology is usually of abnormal bleeding and altered menstrual flow; these cancers should be, therefore, at the forefront of the clinician's mind as a possible diagnosis.

The reporting pathologist will usually report the presence of small fragments of cancer but will be unable to determine the true size and depth of infiltration accurately.

Action It is vital that the patient is seen by an expert colposcopist or gynaecological oncologist so that the true extent of the cancer can be determined. It is not uncommon for cancers of this type to lie entirely or mainly within the endocervical canal, especially in older women. The colposcopist will need to delineate the extent of the disease on colposcopic and clinical examination (staging), and to perform an adequate biopsy, which is best done by taking either a large wedge or cone biopsy or by using the LLETZ technique.[1] The pathologist can then not only give an accurate typing and grading of the tumour but also measure the cancer and thus perform histological staging of the stage Ial, stage Ia2 and microscopic stage Ib1 tumours.[2] This vital information will then allow the clinician to determine accurately the most appropriate way of treating the patient to achieve maximum cure rates with minimal therapeutic side effects and morbidity.

The treatment in a modern gynaecological cancer centre (GCC) will be tailored to the disease and to the patient's personal requirements.

Cystic hyperplasia of the endometrium
This condition is most commonly associated with a metropathic pattern of bleeding, although menorrhagia may be mistaken for it.

Action Although the condition has a low risk of malignancy (approximately 10–15%) and may be reversed using progestogens, many patients are not comfortable living with this low but significant risk. Therefore, it is felt that for patients approaching the menopause, removal of the uterus is the most appropriate action, together with removal of the ovaries where the patient agrees.

Atypical hyperplasias of the endometrium

The nomenclature of hyperplasias of the endometrium continues to confuse. If the hyperplasias with atypia are looked upon as having true malignant potential which increases as the atypia moves from mild to severe, then the clinician can impart an increasing sense of the risk to the patient.

Action Where atypia is mild, an expectant policy can be used — on the understanding that the patient is reviewed for any alteration in menstruation or change in ultrasound assessment of the endometrial thickness. For the patient who is close to the menopause, a simple vaginal or laparoscopy-assisted vaginal hysterectomy is ideal management.

Adenocarcinoma of the endometrium, adenosquamous carcinoma of the endometrium and squamous carcinoma of the endometrium

Approximately 25% of cancers of the corpus will occur in premenopausal women and may be identified during standard diagnostic manoeuvres in the investigation of menorrhagia.

These three conditions should, ideally, have been identified at hysteroscopy and the tissue for diagnosis removed by curettage. The hysteroscopist should have identified the site of the tumour or suspicious area. This information allows the clinician to begin the staging process and determine the most appropriate form of hysterectomy. In some centres, ultrasound or MRI will add some information as to site and depth of infiltration of the tumour.

At present, most cancers of the corpus are managed by general gynaecologists, but the results of therapy are not impressive. It is now thought to be essential that all cancers should be managed by clinicians with a major interest and skill in their care. Such patients should be referred for therapy that will include not only hysterectomy and bilateral salpingo-oöphorectomy but also pelvic washing and node assessment. In current best practice the use of minimal access surgery (MAS) techniques is becoming the norm.[3]

Sarcoma of the corpus, usually arising in polyps

A diagnosis of sarcoma is very unwelcome as this fickle tumour is associated with poor long-term survival. Although the tumour may appear to be well confined to the uterus, its propensity for haematological spread results in all-too-frequent distant metastases that are almost impossible to cure.

Action The mainstay of management is to remove the uterus and, if appropriate, the ovaries and tubes. There seems to be little advantage in removing lymph nodes, except where they are clinically suspect. At present there are no tumour markers of any value, and chemotherapy and radiotherapy offer only palliation rather than the prospect of cure.

Choriocarcinoma
A history of recent pregnancy is most likely, so that a good history would lead the clinician towards this diagnosis. However, there may be a gap of up to 5 years between the pregnancy and the identification of the tumour, although it is relatively rare for the interval to be longer than 2 years.

Action   If this rare cancer is diagnosed, immediate contact with the supraregional centre is essential for guidance on further management.

Malignant histology found following treatment
It is not uncommon for a cancer of the uterus or cervix to be identified inadvertently following hysterectomy. The series of histological patterns shown in Table 18.1 may be found; in addition, some other disconcerting and unwanted histological types may be reported. Although this is often the result of incomplete primary assessment, it can happen in the best-regulated circumstances.

Squamous carcinoma or adenocarcinoma of the cervix
In years gone by, and even today in those countries where cervical cytological surveillance is embryonic, the finding of a cancer of the cervix in a hysterectomy specimen has occurred on approximately 0.5–1% of occasions. Such a finding presents difficult management decisions.

Action
The choices available depend to a large extent on the size of the cancer identified and the margins of normal tissue surrounding it.
Microcarcinoma   Following the identification of microcarcinoma, the following actions may be taken:

- Where the cancer has been measured and is staged as stage Ia1, no further action is necessary except for continuing cytological surveillance, as the risk of nodal metastases is less than 1%.
- Where the cancer is staged as stage Ia2 (i.e. not invading deeper than 5 mm, and 7 mm wide) then the risk of node metastases is small but significant (3–5%). Consideration should be given to the use of an MAS technique involving laparoscopic removal of pelvic lymph nodes, with further action depending upon findings.

True invasive cancer   The identification of true invasive cancer, where the cancer is staged as Ib1 (i.e. where invasion is greater than 5 × 7 mm but no diameter is > 40 mm), necessitates further therapy. The risk of node metastases is of the order of 5–15% and there is a significant risk of local recurrence due to inadequate surgical margins. These risks are increased with poorly differentiated tumours.
The following actions may be taken:

- Radiation therapy across the whole pelvis at a standard postoperative dose with a central boost to the upper vagina is a realistic option.
- Further surgery in the form of radical parametrectomy and pelvic lymphadenectomy has been suggested but is not, in the author's view,

technically satisfactory; however, it should avoid the need for radiation following surgery.

- Laparoscopic pelvic lymphadenectomy followed by a local limited radiotherapy treatment to the upper vagina is now the author's treatment of choice for this difficult problem.

Adenocarcinoma of the endometrium

The identification of an adenocarcinoma of the uterus following hysterectomy for menorrhagia is relatively common. The cancers are usually small and superficial. However, elements of information required for management decisions are usually missing:

1. Peritoneal washings will not have been carried out, so that staging cannot be fully recorded.
2. The lymph nodes will usually not have been palpated, removed or sampled in the pelvis or para-aortic region, further restricting information needed for determining future management.

Nevertheless, the pathologist will be able to type and grade the tumour and to determine the depth of myometrial invasion; these are the most important determinants of prognosis and indicators for further management.

Action If the cancer is poorly differentiated and/or has invaded the outer half of the myometrium, addition of a course of external beam irradiation to the pelvis should be considered. It is not generally thought to be necessary to give vault irradiation at this time. In the opinion of most oncologists, vault irradiation should be preserved for that small percentage of patients who develop vault recurrences, thus saving some 90% of patients from the risk of radiation complications.

If the tumour is extensive, further assessment in the form of chest X-ray and possible CT or MRI assessment of nodes may be helpful. At present there are no tumour markers available to assist with long-term review.

The use of progestogens is of no value, with the possible exception of those cases in which lung metastases are demonstrable.

Sarcomatous change in fibroids

Probably, the most difficult management situation is when a hysterectomy has been performed to treat menorrhagia in the presence of fibroids, and both the clinician and patient are shocked to find that the fibroids are the site of sarcomatous change.

An even greater concern is the very rare circumstance where sarcomatous change is found in a fibroid removed at myomectomy. In these circumstances there is added pressure to preserve the uterus.

Action It is important to obtain a comprehensive histology report detailing the tissue types and mitotic activity: these two elements have an immense bearing on future management. Premenopausal patients with a low mitotic count (less than five mitoses per ten high-power field), less atypia and the tumour arising within a fibroid tend to have a very good prognosis. Where there is a high mitotic count (more than ten mitoses per ten HP field), 5-year survival falls to very low figures of 10–20%.

The following tissue types may be detected on histological examination:

* Leiomyosarcomas
* Endometrial stromal sarcomas (low- and high-grade stromal sarcomas)
* Mixed müllerian tumours.

Other, rarer, types include rhabdomyosarcomas, which are referred to as sarcoma botryoides in young children.

Reference to a GCC is important. Where the sarcoma has been identified following myomectomy and the patient wishes to preserve her uterus, there are virtually no series reported and no trials of management on which to base advice. Individual reports have shown that the most frequent action is to reoperate and remove the uterus, although long-term survival has been seen with conservative management.[4] Patients with good prognostic factors should be chosen for this approach.

For the post-hysterectomy patient, reference to a GCC will generate the advice to perform a chest X-ray and then to refer the patient for admission to a trial of adjunctive chemotherapy. This advice, however, has not to date generated any significant improvements in survival in this complex problem.

Cancer of the ovary

As many patients undergoing hysterectomy are approaching the menopause, it is normal practice to advocate removal of the ovaries during the operation.

Action A diagnosis of ovarian cancer will require consultation and, often, transfer of the patient to a gynaecological oncologist involved in a multidisciplinary clinic (GCC) for future management.

The reporting pathologist must be asked to indicate the type of cancer, the degree of differentiation, the size and any extension of the cancer. The clinician must take blood for tumour marker estimates (CA125). A small intra-ovarian cancer in a single ovary without any extension to the outer surface, and no clinical evidence of extra-ovarian spread reported at the hysterectomy may sound like a very good prospect for all patients; however, although the overall survival figures for stage Ia cancer of the ovary are of the order of 90% or more, there are many reports of lymph-node spread in up to 10% of patients.[5] These data present gynaecological oncologists with a dilemma:

* Should the patient be reassured and no further action taken?
* Should the patient undergo further surgery in order that the true extent of the disease, in particular the lymph node status, can be determined?
* Should tumour marker levels be assessed and future management be based on these levels?
* Should a course of chemotherapy be given and the patient monitored thereafter?

Although there is no perfect answer, the following courses of action should be borne in mind:

1. If the tumour has been reported as a borderline type, then no further action is necessary apart from regular review monitoring.
2. If the tumour is of a mucinous type and (as is usual) the tumour markers are within the normal range, then an expectant policy with intermittent clinical examination is reasonable.
3. If the tumour markers are high around the time of primary surgery (CA125 has a long half-life), and then fall rapidly to normal levels, an expectant policy with frequent monitoring of the tumour markers and clinical examination is realistic.
4. If the cancer is poorly differentiated, or if there is a question about whether it reaches or breaches the outer surface of the ovary, then more information is required. Ultrasound and CT scans have a very limited role in the follow-up of ovarian cancer. The lack of both specificity and sensitivity is disconcerting. The question that must be answered is whether the patient requires further surgery and/or chemotherapy. This is probably best answered by a further intra-abdominal incursion. Clearly, no patient will volunteer to undergo another major procedure involving large scars and prolonged hospitalization and recovery times. The most informative and least invasive procedure is laparoscopic assessment of the abdominal cavity. Using modern safe entry techniques, such as the Hassan technique or the Visiport and Endoview trochars, the abdominal cavity can be entered via small ports so that the cavity can be washed and the nodes can be inspected and sampled. The much-documented risk of port-site implantation appears to be related closely to failure rapidly to treat the ovarian cancer chemotherapeutically once diagnosed, rather than being related to any intrinsic laparoscopic problem. Recently, there has been interest in the possible effects of gas pressure upon metastases in animal models.

Fallopian tube carcinoma
This cancer is rare but can be identified as an incidental finding at hysterectomy and salpingo-oöphorectomy. Survival is related to stage and degree of differentiation of the tumour.

Action   Reference and probable referral to a GCC is recommended. Fallopian tube cancer should be managed in a similar manner to ovarian cancer. Survival for early disease is similar to that for ovarian cancer but at a later stage has a slightly worse prognosis.

Conclusions

When cancer is diagnosed following diagnosis or treatment of a benign condition, expert advice should be sought. Most of these situations can be rectified and the patient given reasonable prospects of cure, even though the treatment may have been suboptimal.

References

1. Mor-Yosef S, Lopes A, Pearson S, Monaghan J M. Loop diathermy cone biopsy. Obstet Gynecol 1990; 73: 884–886

2. FIGO. Staging of gynaecological cancer. Br J Obstet Gynaecol 1992; 96: 889 892

3. Childers J M, Surwit E A. Combined laparoscopic and vaginal surgery for the management of two cases of Stage I endometrial cancer. Gynecol Oncol 1991; 45: 46–51

4. Dinh T, Woodruff J D. Leiomyosarcoma of the uterus. Am J Obstet Gynecol 1982; 144: 817

5. Chen S, Lee L. Incidence of para aortic lymph node metastasis in epithelial carcinoma of the ovary. Gynecol Oncol 1983; 16: 95–100

CHAPTER 19

Vaginal or abdominal hysterectomy?

S. S. Sheth

Introduction

By the time that a woman has attained the age of 55 years, 20% of those in the United Kingdom and 25% in Australia (and 37% by the age of 60 years in the United States) have undergone hysterectomy. Hysterectomy is one of the commonest operations in the United States, where 650,000 hysterectomies are performed yearly; in fact, hysterectomy is the second most frequent major surgical procedure in that country and menorrhagia is the main indication for this.[1]

Studd[2] has drawn attention to the lack of valid data regarding the role of hysterectomy in the treatment of menorrhagia. Unfortunately, vaginal and abdominal hysterectomy are compared in situations where clinical findings clearly indicate that they are not comparable; the results yielded by such comparisons of vaginal and abdominal hysterectomy in different clinical situations are therefore far from impartial.

It is also unfortunate that abdominal hysterectomy — the least-preferred technique for hysterectomy — is being performed in all categories of patients, even those in whom vaginal or laparoscopically assisted vaginal hysterectomy (LAVH) is indicated. As abdominal hysterectomy can be performed more easily, several gynaecologists opt for this route, even in cases where the vaginal approach is the most appropriate.

Abdominal hysterectomy is the best choice in cases where there is associated adherent adnexal pathology or malignancy is suspected and there is a genuine need to visualize the abdominopelvic organs. Although this route gives an unrestricted view of the abdominal structures as a whole, this would be required in only one or two in ten cases; the remaining cases should preferably be operated via the vagina (the occasional one or two with laparoscopic assistance).[3]

Very often, hysterectomy that should have been performed vaginally is carried out abdominally for the sole reason that it is the favoured practice at a particular clinic. The ratio of vaginal to abdominal hysterectomies is 1:3, which should, ideally, be reversed.[4] Regrettably, despite all the advantages offered by the vaginal route, the vast majority of hysterectomies are abdominal, as shown by statistics from multicentre studies.[5] In the series by Brown and Frazer,[1] from Australia, 79% of hysterectomies were performed vaginally; conversely, the Australian Medicare data reveal that as many as 81% of hysterectomies are abdominal. In the author's personal series of 5985 hysterectomies (excluding those indicated for uterine prolapse), 80% were carried out via the vaginal route.

Laparoscopy has had a tremendous influence on vaginal hysterectomy (VH). In the state of Texas, USA, the rate of VH prior to the advent of laparoscopically assisted vaginal hysterectomy (LAVH) in 1991, was 27.7%; with the introduction of LAVH, the incidence of vaginal hysterectomy has almost doubled, to 53.2%.[6] The number of cases of abdominal hysterectomy has been reduced by 29%, with a concomitant increase in the number of cases of VH.[7] These statistics clearly indicate surgeons' acceptance of the supremacy of the vaginal route because of its obvious advantages.

In menorrhagia due to benign conditions requiring hysterectomy, the surgeon chooses the route after analysing the feasibility of the procedure and the difficulties he expects to encounter during surgery. These would broadly comprise the indications and contraindications for conventional vaginal and abdominal hysterectomy. If a laparoscope or laparoscopist is not available what would be the approach — vaginal or abdominal?

After studying hysterectomies performed by generations of gynaecological surgeons, the author has found that certain aspects of this procedure have become crystal clear, as follows:

1. When hysterectomy is possible by either route, the vaginal approach is undoubtedly superior to the abdominal;
2. There are well-defined indications for both vaginal and abdominal hysterectomy;
3. Certain conditions contraindicate VH;
4. There are definite situations in which LAVH is indicated and preferred to a laparotomy;
5. If hysterectomy is possible by all three approaches, in the best interest of the patient the order of preference should be VH, LAVH and abdominal.

Contraindications

It should be borne in mind that vigorous attempts are currently being made, worldwide, to reduce the number of abdominal hysterectomies and replace them (preferably) with VH, or with LAVH as the next choice.[8] In cases where hysterectomy cannot be performed vaginally, laparoscopic assistance should be taken to avoid laparotomy. Therefore the surgeon needs to exercise a choice, keeping in mind the words of Hippocrates: 'Primum, noli nocere' which means 'First, do no harm!' Applying this principle, the choice should be the one that is to the patient's advantage. An experienced gynaecologist will always maintain that some contraindications to VH are relative[9] and never absolute — they vary only with the skill of the surgeon.[10] Such contraindications include the following:

1. Uterus more than 12 weeks' size; however, experienced gynaecologists can use the vaginal approach even in uteri up to 14–16 weeks' size with the help of debulking.[3]
2. Restriction of uterine mobility; however, sometimes, even with slightly restricted uterine mobility, VH can be attempted if there is no associated adnexal pathology.
3. Adherent pathology in contiguous organs such as the tubes and ovaries.
4. Diminished vaginal space.
5. Cervix that is flush with the vagina.

6. Inaccessible cervix.
7. Vesicovaginal fistula repair.
8. Invasive cancer of the cervix.

If these are excluded, the vast majority will have a clear indication for the vaginal route.

Even in the absence of a contraindication for the vaginal route, the author has witnessed hysterectomy by the abdominal route or LAVH being preferred by senior gynaecologists, including teachers in medical colleges. This is then justified on one pretext or the other, such as the following:[4]

1. Absence of uterine prolapse;
2. A large uterus;
3. Presence of a fibroid;
4. Nulliparous patient;
5. Ovaries need to be removed;
6. Adhesions or endometriosis may be present;
7. It is necessary to review the abdominal organs, particularly the appendix;
8. The decision is to be taken only after the patient has been examined under anaesthesia.

Indeed, the impression is often gained that the above situations are used as an excuse to avoid VH — chronic excuses from chronic evaders!

Indications
Dysfunctional uterine bleeding
Dysfunctional uterine bleeding (DUB) is such a common condition that 30–45% of hysterectomies are performed to relieve this condition.[11] From the author's series of 5344 VH, 56.3% were performed in clinically diagnosed cases of DUB or adenomyosis (which are, at times, difficult to differentiate).

In patients with DUB, there is usually no associated adnexal pathology and the uterus is freely mobile and generally not bigger than 10–12 weeks' size; thus, such cases are ideal for VH. It is uncommon in such cases to have a uterus larger than 12–14 weeks' size and it is never beyond 16 weeks unless associated with adenomyosis (which would then call for removal with laparoscopic assistance or by the abdominal route). It is essential to confirm that the endometrium is benign before the decision is made in favour of hysterectomy.

The gynaecologist must use the vaginal route in those patients with DUB who require hysterectomy, and thus sharpen his skills as a vaginal surgeon. It must be emphasized to all students that VH is the procedure of choice in all cases of DUB in the absence of contraindications. Several gynaecologists have now also taken to performing LAVH in cases of DUB or adenomyosis, which is a gross misuse of newer technology. Performing abdominal hysterectomy for DUB amounts to an acknowledgement of the operator's lack of skill and training in performing a highly useful gynaecological operation, as well as in the use of newer technology.

Abdominal hysterectomy would be indicated only in the following circumstances:

1. When vaginal hysterectomy is contraindicated and LAVH is difficult or risky;
2. In cases where oöphorectomy is mandatory and is not otherwise possible;
3. When there is doubt about the benign nature of the endometrium.

Adenomyosis

A definitive diagnosis of adenomyosis can be made only after histopathological examination of the uterus. The clinical diagnosis of DUB is often changed to adenomyosis on histopathological examination (in 65% of cases) (see Chapter 3). The uterus is usually of about 8–12 weeks' size, less commonly 12–14 weeks but never beyond 16 weeks. A uterus of 12 weeks or more will usually display severe adenomyosis, with all-round enlargement (i.e. anteroposterior, transverse and vertical) reducing the uterus-free space.[4]

Adenomyosis is one of the classic indications for vaginal hysterectomy. The decision regarding the route is greatly influenced by absence of adnexal pathology and free mobility of the uterus. At times, a very large uterus may preclude VH. All uteri 12 weeks or less in size should be dealt with per vaginam: it is usually unnecessary to have recourse to laparoscopic assistance or to use the abdominal route in these cases, whereas removal of larger uteri may need to do so (although an experienced vaginal surgeon may be able to debulk uteri of 14–16 weeks or even more without laparoscopic assistance to complete hysterectomy vaginally). The author has carried out 3012 vaginal hysterectomies, and has never used the abdominal route or taken laparoscopic assistance for DUB or adenomyosis, unless there were specific contraindications to VH.

In cases where the vaginal approach is contraindicated because of size or associated conditions, the alternatives appear to be VH with debulking, LAVH, or abdominal hysterectomy — in that order. Total laparoscopic hysterectomy is performed in very few centres globally and hence cannot be the procedure of choice.

Fibroids

As well as large, submucosal fibroids causing menorrhagia, small fibroids may sometimes coexist with other pathology. Menorrhagia in such cases could be due either to DUB or to adenomyosis. The route for hysterectomy in such cases should be determined by uterine size: where there are no other contraindications and the uterus is not larger than 12 weeks, the route should ideally be vaginal; in larger uteri when vaginal debulking is inadequate and/or difficult, laparoscopic assistance or the abdominal route are preferred (Table 19.1).

Hysterectomy for uteri with fibroids should be via the vaginal route (a) if the uterus is 12 weeks or smaller in size; (b) if uterine volume on sonography is 300 cm^3 or less, or (3) in the absence of any contraindication to VH.

It must always be remembered that, when deciding on the route, accessibility to the fibroid is more important than its size; this is particularly valid for large fibroids. A large fibroid at the fundus towards the peritoneal cavity, which leads to a larger uterus than 12–14 weeks, with all-round enlargement, makes descent and access difficult and therefore may lead to difficult debulking or LAVH. However, as previously stated, where conditions are favourable it is possible for the experienced vaginal surgeon to perform VH even in uteri up to 14–16 weeks in size;[3] these uteri are debulked and removed vaginally. It appears that, if the size of an accessible

Table 19.1 Route of choice for hysterectomy compared with size of uterus

Size of uterus in weeks	≤12	13–17	18–24	>24
Route of choice	VH	Tentative VH (experienced vaginal surgeon) LAVH TLH* TAH	LAVH TLH* TAH	TAH

*This technique is employed at only a few centres, and not many can afford it in terms of equipment or operators.

LAVH, laparoscopically-assisted vaginal hysterectomy; TLH, total laparoscopic hysterectomy; TAH, total abdominal hysterectomy; VH, vaginal hysterectomy.

fibroid is 5–7 cm and uterine volume (including that of the fibroid) does not exceed 300–400 cm³, the vaginal approach can be used. It is inadvisable to appear to be struggling to remove a large uterus via the vagina; however, this is a relative phenomenon and is largely determined by the experience of the vaginal surgeon — an important factor.

Factors favouring VH for uterine fibroids are as follows:

1. A freely mobile uterus;
2. A large uterus-free space that allows manoeuvrability;
3. A large fibroid that can be debulked;
4. A surgeon experienced in the debulking procedure;
5. The availability of sonographic details regarding size and location of fibroid and total uterine volume;
6. In some cases, counselling the patient that the vaginal route is tentative and that a switch to LAVH or abdominal hysterectomy may be required;
7. Experience.

Factors favouring abdominal hysterectomy for uterine fibroids are as follows:

1. When VH is contraindicated and LAVH is risky or very difficult;
2. Associated dense adhesions due to endometriosis or pelvic inflammatory disease (PID);
3. Suspicion of malignancy — rapidly growing tumour;
4. Adnexal pathology suspicious of malignancy;
5. Broad-ligament fibroid;
6. Associated extragenital surgery.

More than 50 years ago, Campbell[12] maintained that the size or bulk of the uterus to be removed is not a contraindication to the vaginal route. Until 1990, in uteri larger than 12 weeks, abdominal hysterectomy was the route of choice. Hillis et al.[13]

note that, in women with leiomyomas, where the uterine weight exceeds 500 g there is an increased risk of complications from abdominal hysterectomy. It is not surprising, therefore, that according to Schneider et al.,[14] the incidence of abdominal hysterectomy has fallen precipitously to 12% from 66%, with a concurrent rise in LAVH from 0 to 40%. In the coming years a significant number of uteri will be subjected to morcellation in order to expedite their removal.[15]

Submucous myomatous polyps

Mattingly and Thompson[16] suggest that, in the presence of a prolapsed submucous fibroid, abdominal hysterectomy is contraindicated and it is necessary first to perform a vaginal myomectomy. In these cases, the cervix and vagina dilate and broaden; this places the ureters at increased risk of injury at abdominal hysterectomy. The risk of postoperative peritonitis also increases because of infection of the polyp.

If hysterectomy is the treatment chosen because of associated factors, the prima facie case against VH can change radically in favour of such a procedure if the polypectomy is performed vaginally, with subsequent assessment under anaesthesia (Fig. 19.1).[17] The situation can, however, be dealt with in three stages — first, vaginal myomectomy, followed by hysteroscopic examination and evaluation under anaesthesia, followed by vaginal hysterectomy, which is then easy and successful. In

Figure 19.1 A submucous myomatous polyp: the dotted line shows excision before examination under anaesthesia.

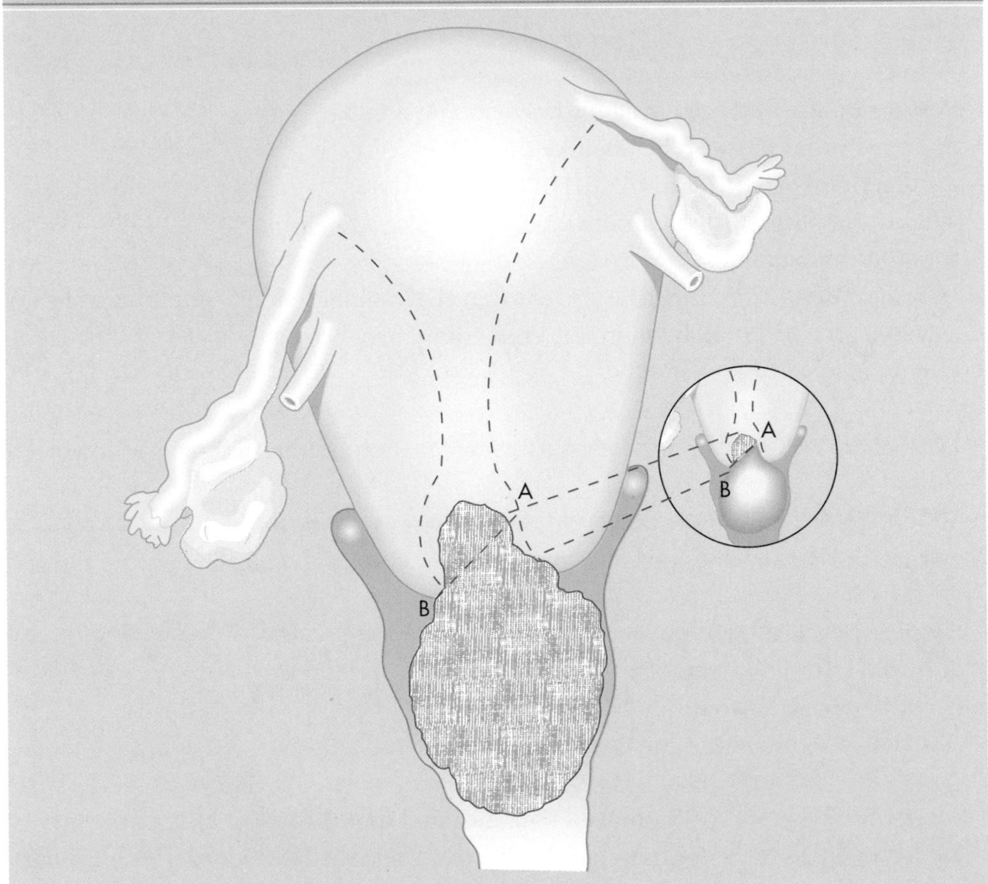

the author's personal series of 32 cases, in not a single case was laparoscopic assistance or abdominal hysterectomy required. The two precautionary measures taken for vaginal surgery were (1) keeping close to the uterocervical border and (2) paying attention to the increased oozing that was a consequence of increased vascularity.

Endometriosis

Endometriosis presents as tiny areas diagnosed at laparoscopy, or as a pelvic mass, or with adhesions that are sufficiently significant to warrant laparoscopic assistance or the abdominal route for hysterectomy. However, it must be remembered that advanced endometriosis is likely to lead to adhesions necessitating extra care and difficult separation by dissection, which may threaten the safety of the bladder and/or bowels and/or ureters and pose a problem even for the experienced operator. Early endometriosis with free mobility of the uterus and adnexa should be managed vaginally. The presence of adhesions and/or restricted mobility of the uterus and/or adnexal swelling calls for laparoscopic assistance or, often, abdominal hysterectomy, and is a strong contraindication to the vaginal approach; the larger the mass and/or the denser the adhesions, the less difficult and the more safe than other alternatives abdominal hysterectomy will prove to be.

Adnexal mass

This condition clearly indicates the need for laparoscopic assistance and/or an abdominal and not a vaginal hysterectomy. An adherent adnexal mass is an absolute contraindication to the vaginal approach. Preoperatively, the surgeon must ensure that the mass is benign through sonography, CT scan or magnetic resonance imaging (MRI) and the assessment of haematological CA125 levels; during the procedure, a frozen-section specimen must be made available for histopathological examination.[18–21] However, nothing can guarantee, preoperatively, the benign nature of the adnexal pathology.

The traditional ('standard textbook') approach of removing a benign teratoma or allied disorder would be a laparotomy. Parkar et al.[22] recommend laparoscopic removal of suitable ovarian cysts. Laparoscopic resection of benign teratomas of the ovary is safe, well tolerated and shortens hospital stay.[23] Teng et al.[24] suggested a combined laparoscopic colpotomy approach and have cautioned that, before undertaking any transvaginal surgery, laparoscopy is necessary. In fact, Reich,[25] after laparoscopic management of an ovarian teratoma, removed the cyst wall by a posterior colpotomy. However, if the cyst needs to be removed finally through a colpotomy incision, then why not debulk and remove the entire ovarian cyst through the vaginal route, which provides plenty of room after uterine extirpation (Fig. 19.2). Why inflict the insult of abdominal incisions? Thus, experienced vaginal surgeons should seriously consider the vaginal route for removing a benign ovarian or adnexal mass/cyst that can be debulked, particularly in multiparous women.[26] One absolute prerequisite for this is the operator's experience of VH with prophylactic bilateral salpingo-oöphorectomy (BSO).

An adnexal mass has been a long-standing contraindication for VH because of problems such as 'fears' of complications and 'lack of expertise' of vaginal surgery. Today, with the availability of a wide range of antibiotics, highly advanced surgical and anaesthetic techniques, and accurate predictions from laboratory and imaging

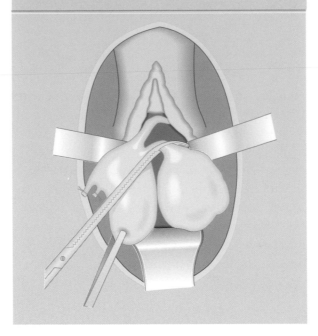

Figure 19.2 A benign, mobile ovarian teratoma clamped for its excision. This was followed by completion of hysterectomy with bilateral adnexectomy.

sciences, the scenario needs to change in favour of VH. An adnexal mass that is freely mobile and benign should no longer be taken as a contraindication for vaginal hysterectomy.[3,26]

The vaginal approach is to be encouraged for the following reasons:

1. It is the least invasive and requires minimal access;
2. The mobile mass can be excised without difficulty per vaginam;[27]
3. After hysterectomy (or near its completion) there is adequate space and the mass descends together with the uterus; the head-high position, relaxants and traction on the uterus make access easier;
4. The risk of spillage is minimal or nil;
5. Isolation aided by lavage and gravity minimizes contamination;
6. The benign nature of the mass can be reasonably ascertained (imaging technique and tumour markers);
7. The approach makes the entire mass available for study;
8. If this approach fails, (a) nothing extra has been excised or incised and (b) there is no harm in switching to laparoscopic assistance or laparotomy;
9. It avoids multiple abdominal cuts;
10. It encourages learning, promotes expertise, and makes the operator a better vaginal surgeon;
11. Science needs to progress, and previous contraindications should no longer be relevant in today's modern world.

Nevertheless, abdominal hysterectomy in the presence of an adnexal mass should be performed in the following circumstances:

1. Mass suspected to be malignant;
2. Histopathological reports on the frozen section indicate possible malignancy;
3. Possibility of trauma to bowel and/or ureter;
4. Uncontrollable bleeding;
5. Large and/or inaccessible mass;
6. Laparoscopy appears very difficult or risky;
7. Laparoscopic method fails;
8. No facility for frozen section and/or inadequate counselling;
9. Laparoscopic equipment and/or laparoscopic surgeon not available;
10. During the early part of the surgeon's learning curve;
11. Possibility of litigation.

Laparotomy is the management choice of many gynaecologists, followed by LAVH, which should be acceptable as an ideal approach by most. The vaginal route without laparoscopic assistance needs strong consideration when the adnexal pathology is benign, the mass is freely mobile and the operator is an experienced vaginal surgeon.

Endometrial cancer

The regular mode of treatment for endometrial cancer is total abdominal hysterectomy (TAH) with BSO and excision of the cuff of vagina with or without radiotherapy, in most patients. Occasionally, there are high-risk patients in whom the surgeon and anaesthetist would hesitate to adopt the abdominal route. Such patients, if examined under anaesthesia, may prove to be operable by the vaginal route — a procedure that would be acceptable to the patient, the anaesthetist and the surgeon.

Quinlan[28] suggests VH with BSO, followed by radiotherapy when required, in such cases. In Ingiulla's series of 573 cases of corpus cancer, 460 were treated by VH:[29] the survival rates were 73.2% in the vaginal group compared with 71.4% in the abdominal group. The high cure rates in endometrial cancer stage I suggest the use of VH in obese patients or those of poor surgical risk, as well as in a few low-risk cases (where the procedure is ideal). The time has come to consider a less radical procedure for endometrial cancer[30] as, in 95–97% of cases, bilateral oöphorectomy or BSO with VH should be possible.[31] If necessary, the surgeon may use laparoscopic assistance for oöphorectomy, which will also help lymphadenectomy; alternatively, laparotomy may be performed.

Carcinoma in situ of cervix

Abdominal or vaginal hysterectomy are both acceptable for cervical intra-epithelial neoplasia (CIN) III, but would normally be performed only in the presence of coexisting gynaecological disease.[32] When the preferred mode of treatment is not conservative, the route should always be vaginal. Besides the well-accepted advantages of VH, cuff removal (which is essential in these conditions) is more easily accomplished vaginally than abdominally, as the latter is accompanied by increased risk of injury to the ureters at the point of entry to the bladder. Unless definitely indicated by coexisting pathology, ovarian removal is not recommended and this leads to the vaginal route being preferred by many. It is necessary for all oncologists to realize that, when they do not perform hysterectomy vaginally, they are not providing their patient with surgery that is the least invasive and minimally accessed, and thus may not be acting in the best interest of their patients.

Postmenopausal bleeding
In patients with persistent or recurrent postmenopausal bleeding without any documentable cause, VH involves very little risk. Ovarian removal, however, becomes necessary in these cases as the ovaries could be harbouring tiny tumours secreting oestrogen.

In a series of 346 cases of postmenopausal bleeding where the endometrium was found to be benign, VH with BSO was performed in 188 cases. In such patients, in the author's opinion, the decision on the route of hysterectomy needs to be taken after due consideration of multiple factors such as endometrial thickness, endometrial histopathology, family history of genital cancer, the surgeon's experience in vaginal surgery and patient counselling. Occasionally, high-placed atrophic and/or retracted ovaries may necessitate laparoscopic assistance for removal at hysterectomy.

Associated conditions and situations
Of the last 1000 consecutive cases of VH, 356 had a history of previous abdominal surgery (Table 19.2), which is more than one in three cases. Previous abdominal surgery could be classified into one of four categories:

1. Operations performed on the uterus,[4] such as caesarean section, hysterotomy and myomectomy; these demand extra care, but do not constitute a contraindication unless they have led to adhesions restricting uterine mobility.
2. Ventrofixation, which is now obsolete, and sling operations for prolapse make vaginal access difficult and are generally a contraindication for VH. Only a very experienced vaginal surgeon will be able to cope in this situation without resorting to laparoscopic assistance or abdominal hysterectomy.
3. Previous surgery on the tubes, broad ligament or ovaries.
4. Previous surgery on abdominal organs other than the bladder and the rectum.

Uncommonly, there are dense adhesions between the uterocervical surface and the bladder with the abdominal wall making the cervix inaccessible by the vaginal route — known as the cervicofundal sign.[33] An endoscopic surgeon may choose laparoscopic assistance to tackle these adhesions but will also have to be very careful while inserting the trocar at the start of the operation.

Previous caesarean section or myomectomy
Currently, 20% or more of deliveries are carried out by caesarean section in most countries.[5] With this trend likely to continue and flourish, it is conceivable that the surgeon of tomorrow will increasingly have to confront the problem of hysterectomy in patients with a previous caesarean section. According to Coulam and Pratt,[34] the chief concern in this group of patients is risk of injury to the bladder and the difficulty of gaining entry through the scarred anterior cul-de-sac. Kovac[35] have discussed the role of LAVH, which is to be preferred to abdominal but not vaginal hysterectomy in these patients.

One of the techniques that the author finds useful in circumventing dense

Table 19.2 Preferred route* for hysterectomy, according to previous history of abdominopelvic surgery

Surgical history	Routine VH	Needs extra care at VH	Tentative VH	LAVH	TAH
ABDOMINAL					
Uterine					
Previous caesarean		1			
Myomectomy		1			
Caesarean + myomectomy		1			
Hysterectomy		1			
Metroplasty		1			
Sling operation			2	1	
Ventrofixation			2	1	2
Tubes and ovaries					
Tubal sterilization	1				
Salpingectomy	1				
Tubal microsurgery	1				
Ovarian cystectomy	1				
Oöphorectomy	1				
Salpingo-oöphorectomy	1				
VAGINAL					
Cervix					
Internal os tightening	1				
Amputation					1
Conization		1			
Anterior colporraphy		1			
Posterior colpoperineorraphy	1				
Colpotomy–tubal sterilization		1			
Fothergill's					1
Shirodkar's (modified Manchester)	1				
Bartholin's abscess	1				
SURGERY ON EXTRAGENITAL ORGANS					
Bladder					
VVF repair					1
Cystotomy					1
Bladder neck repair		1			
Rectum					
RVF repair		1			
Abscess		1			2
Piles	1				
Abdominal contents					
Appendicectomy	1				
Intestinal	1				
Cholecystectomy	1				

*1, first choice; 2, second choice.

Abbreviations as in Table 19.1, plus RVF, rectovaginal fistula; VVF, vesicovaginal fistula.

adhesions is use of the lateral window or the uterocervical broad ligament space,[36] (Fig. 19.3); this allows access to the vesico-uterine fold of peritoneum from the lateral aspect. It can be used to gain access comfortably to the bladder. MRI studies confirm the presence of this space (Fig. 19.4) and Monaghan finds its use of increasing interest in vaginal surgery.[37]

When the clinical findings are not conclusive, especially in the early years of practice, the gynaecologist may take advantage of laparoscopic assistance to perform VH and this would be preferable to abdominal hysterectomy.

Previous vaginal operations
Previous surgery in the vaginal region would include the following:

1. Operation in the region of the vaginal epithelium;
2. Cervical amputation;
3. Fothergill's operation, which includes both 1 and 2 above;
4. Operation through the vaginal epithelium where the peritoneum is entered; this had occurred in 84 of 5344 vaginal hysterectomies in the author's series.

Figure 19.3 Finger points to the entry for uterocervical broad ligament space between the lateral part of the bladder and uterocervical surface and broad ligament laterally.

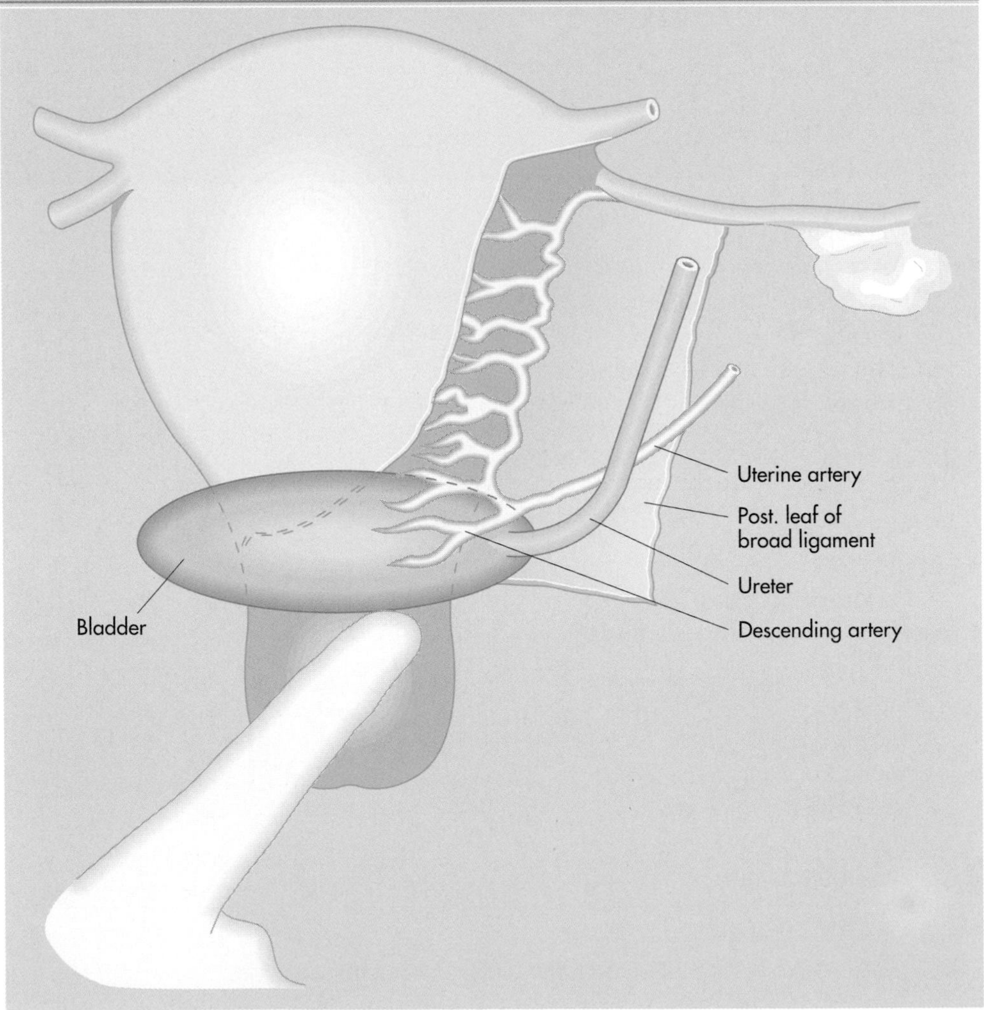

Uterine artery

Post. leaf of broad ligament

Ureter

Descending artery

Bladder

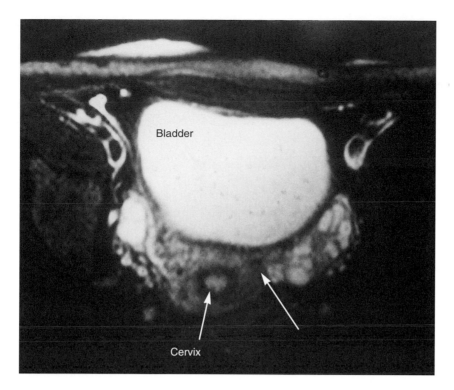

Figure 19.4 A MRI study confirms uterocervical broad ligament space as shown (arrow).

Previous surgery in the vaginal region per se is no contraindication to the vaginal route for hysterectomy. Nevertheless, the surgeon needs to exercise extra caution in these cases. Cervical amputation and Fothergill's operation both considerably distort the anatomy in the genital area and hysterectomy should be performed by the abdominal route.

Nulliparity
Uterine descent is plainly evident in the multiparous woman, but may not be manifest in the nulliparous. Most surgeons, therefore, consider nulliparity to be an indication for abdominal hysterectomy. However, even in the nulliparous woman, generally, there appears to be sufficient uterine descent to facilitate VH, provided that the uterus is freely mobile, not larger than 12 weeks in size and without associated adnexal pathology. Before the advent of LAVH, 90% of hysterectomies in nulliparous women were by the abdominal route.[5]

A series of 368 vaginal hysterectomies in nulliparous women (including 112 virgins), for fibroids, adenomyosis, DUB and severe mental handicap,[38] clearly indicates that nulliparous women, even in the absence of prolapse, have sufficient downward mobility of the uterus and that hysterectomy by the vaginal route is possible in such patients.

If the pelvic findings are favourable, hysterectomy ideally should be by the vaginal route, never by the abdominal route and may occasionally need laparoscopic assistance if the operator is in doubt of success. Diagnostic laparoscopic evaluation will allay any fears and doubts that VH is not appropriate.

High-risk group
Some patients requiring hysterectomy for menorrhagia may have associated clinical

problems — such as interstitial pulmonary fibrosis (which markedly restricts pulmonary function), poor cardiac status, diabetes and/or hypertension — that put these patients at high risk. Two-dimensional sonography of the heart may reveal a poor ejection fraction; the vaginal route, with low spinal or epidural anaesthesia and an expeditious procedure, would be safer in such patients. Those with low haemoglobin should receive haematinics, with adequate control of bleeding with lynoestrenol/norethisterone for 2–3 weeks (or more), and preferably should be subjected to VH.

Tentative VH or trial of vaginal route for hysterectomy

Sometimes it is felt that hysterectomy by the vaginal route is difficult and relatively contraindicated, but that (if and when attempted) it might succeed. A trial of the vaginal route is recommended in such cases, even where the surgeon is experienced.[4] A trial by the vaginal route is undertaken after discussing the patient's condition, the options available and the advantages of each option, with the patient and her family; failure to discuss this can result in the patient losing confidence in the surgeon. Meanwhile, everything is kept in readiness to switch to the abdominal route intra-operatively, if necessary. The situation may be compared to a trial forceps delivery in obstetrics. The option of the vaginal route is attempted in order to reap such benefits as reduced morbidity, shorter hospital stay and faster recovery.

The patients likely to fall into this category are as follows:

1. Those with uterus greater than 12–14 weeks' size;
2. Those with a previous caesarean section and/or myomectomy or with possible adhesions;
3. Nulliparous women;
4. Those with diminished uterus-free pelvic space;
5. Those with doubtful adnexal pathology;
6. Those with an inexperienced operator.

If a thorough preoperative examination and assessment under anaesthesia has been carried out, the necessity for a switch to the abdominal route is unlikely. A sound assessment under anaesthesia is required and the operator should not hesitate to take laparoscopic assistance or the abdominal route, as and when appropriate.

Debulking

Sometimes during the course of VH, all accessible tissue has been cut and no further uterine descent is possible. An important point to remember is that if the fundal top cannot be reached by fingers passed from behind or in front of the uterus, delivery of the fundus is unlikely without debulking.

If uterine enlargement is due to adenomyosis, the bulging uterine wall or adenomatous area can be debulked by morcellating myometrial chunks. Bisection will often give easy access to a fibroid that is close to the endometrium and/or uterine isthmus. In larger uteri, bisection may facilitate debulking by enucleation and/or morcellation. Alternatively, Lash's method[39] can be used for non-myomatous uteri, but is rarely required if morcellation by dechunking is used.

Kovac[40] recommends coring to remove larger uteri by the vaginal route. The author has used the debulking technique in 534 cases without resorting to either Lash's or Kovac's technique, by enucleating the fibroid and/or morcellating myometrial chunks, with or without bisecting the uterus. Suprapubic pressure by the assistant pushes the fibroid into the operative field, particularly in a slim woman. Strategic planning is necessary, based on sonography and uterine findings on the operation table. The author debulks large uteri in a specific order,[41] as shown in Figures 19.5 and 19.6. The essence is to proceed methodically, to enucleate or morcellate systematically, in order to create space and facilitate access.

When debulking a myomatous uterus, access to the fibroid is easier from the posterior aspect. As a rule, the largest and most accessible fibroid must be removed first. Posterior-wall fibroids are more easily accessible than those on the anterior wall and therefore are more easily removed. Once the fundus is accessible, further debulking is unnecessary and hysterectomy can be completed.

Preoperative detailed sonographic assessment regarding the exact location of the fibroid, its size and volume along with the total uterine volume, and thorough examination under anaesthesia (EUA), are great intra-operative assets during debulking. There is no preset limit of uterine weight or volume at which gynaecologists are forbidden to attempt VH; they must all define their own limits keeping in mind their surgical constraints. One gynaecologist may be very reluctant to debulk uteri weighing 200 g, whereas another may comfortably debulk a uterus weighing more than 500 g. It is essential to increase slowly the criteria for operation on an increasingly larger size of uterus to be removed vaginally, rather than

Figure 19.5 Debulking of a uterus of about 14 weeks' size through enucleation of the proximal central fibroid (1) after bisection of the cervix followed by enucleation of the distal fibroids in ascending numerical order (2, 3). (Number 3 is repeated since the fibroid may be on the left and/or right in the uterine wall.)

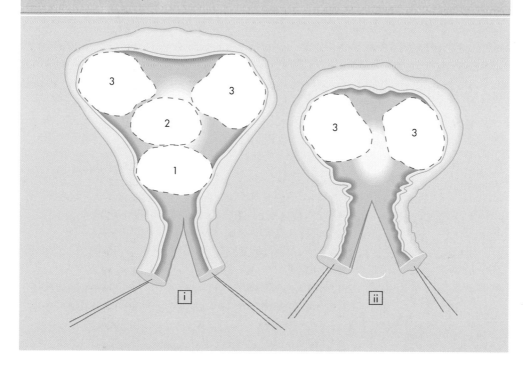

Figure 19.6 Debulking of a uterus of about 18 weeks' size due to fibroids with a uterine volume of 550 cm³. After cervical bisection, the large central proximal fibroids (1, 2) are enucleated first, followed by the lateral wall fibroids in ascending numerical order (3, 4, 5). (If the fibroid is on both sides, the promixal is enucleated first followed by the same number from the other side or whichever is accessible.)

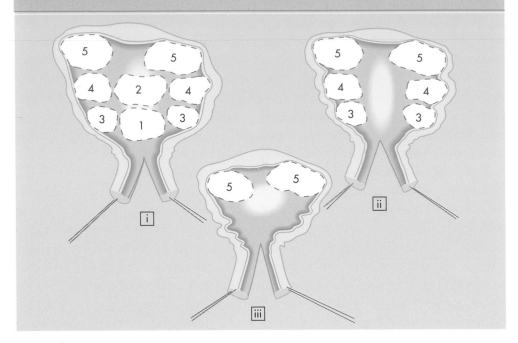

ambitiously attempt too much and suffer a setback. Table 19.3 gives guidance on the basis of uterine volume (cm³).

In selected cases, gonadotrophin-releasing hormone (GnRH) as leuprolide acetate (3.75 mg i.m.) is administered once a month for two doses,[42] to reduce the size of the fibroid; this reduction may be just sufficient to allow VH to be performed.

Examination under anaesthesia

'Give me reliable findings of EUA and I will give you an unambiguous decision on the approach for hysterectomy'. This is a singularly important examination, which

Table 19.3 Uterine volume and vaginal hysterectomy (VH)

Volume (cm³)	Comment
≤ 100	Easy, average gynaecologist should be able to do it
101–200	Interested gynaecologist should be able to do it easily
201–400+	Best performed by gynaecologist with expertise
300–350+	Needs debulking
401–500	Should be scheduled as tentative or trial VH; needs debulking; consider availability of LAVH and/or abdominal hysterectomy

LAVH, laparoscopically-assisted vaginal hysterectomy.

should form an integral part of the management of every patient needing hysterectomy. This will be a great learning experience. Abdominal hysterectomy should not be considered unless there is a contraindication to VH on EUA and LAVH is ruled out.

EUA should include the following:

1. Exclusion of any contraindication to the vaginal route;
2. Assessment of uterine mobility, size and descent;
3. Determination of the descent of the cervix when traction is applied with a vulsellum on both lips (as a rule, there is descent, even in a nullipara, sufficient to permit vaginal hysterectomy);[4]
4. In patients with a history of previous pelvic surgery or doubtful adnexal pathology, further evaluation to assess adhesions or the exact nature of the adnexal pathology, if any, is necessary;
5. Visualization of the cervix on speculum examination;
6. In women with menorrhagia, diagnostic dilatation and curettage provides an excellent opportunity for careful EUA and evaluation of the route for hysterectomy. This must be utilized by experienced and novice gynaecologists alike.

Findings under anaesthesia that favour the vaginal route are as follows:

1. Absence of any contraindication;
2. Mobility of the uterus in all planes;
3. Physiological uterine descent (in the absence of prolapse);
4. Adequate uterus-free pelvic space around the uterus (testing anteroposterior and side-to-side mobility helps to assess the uterus-free pelvic space);
5. Free vaginal mucosa around both the pouches;
6. Normal cervical length of portio vaginalis with deep fornices.

Abdominal hysterectomy is indicated when the clinical findings as well as those under anaesthesia indicate that VH is unsuitable. However, if LAVH can be performed, it should be preferred to abdominal hysterectomy as it resolves the difficulties or contraindications to VH. The flow chart in Figure 19.7 indicates how a decision can be reached, and Table 19.4 indicates the preferred approach or route for hysterectomy for various indications and associated conditions.

Oöphorectomy at hysterectomy

Jones recommends that routine oöphorectomy is performed at VH for all women above the age of 45 years[43] and in all cases where the family or previous history indicates the possibility of future ovarian problems or pathology.

Prophylactic oöphorectomy is clearly indicated at hysterectomy for postmenopausal women, whether the surgery is by the abdominal or the vaginal route.[44] It is a paradox that most gynaecologists consider prophylactic oöphorectomy at abdominal hysterectomy but almost routinely leave the ovaries in place at VH. This is convincingly demonstrated by the statistics: oöphorectomy is performed in only 10% of all VH.[45]

Removal of the ovaries and tubes can be achieved in two-thirds of VH with

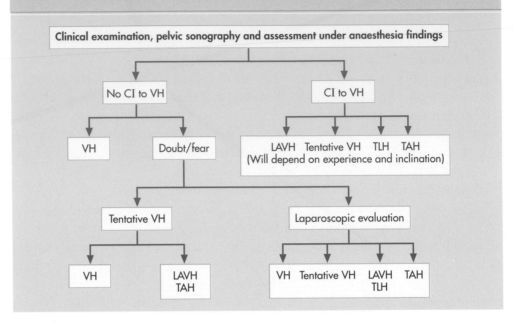

Figure 19.7 A decision-making flow chart for the approach to hysterectomy, based on findings from clinical examination, pelvic sonography and assessment under anaesthesia: CI, contraindication; LAVH, laparoscopically assisted vaginal hysterectomy; VH, vaginal hysterectomy; TAH, total abdominal hysterectomy; TLH, total laparoscopic hysterectomy.

Table 19.4 Choice* of hysterectomy: indications/associated situations

Indication/situation	Route			
	Vaginal	Tentative vaginal	LAVH	Abd
Dysfunctional uterine bleeding	A			
Adenomyosis	A			
Fibroid(s): uterus up to 12 weeks size	A			
Fibroid(s): uterus 13 to 16 weeks size		B1(A**)	A	B2
Fibroid(s): uterus 17 to 22–24 weeks size			A	B1
Fibroid(s): uterus >22–24 weeks size				A
Endometrial hyperplasia	A			
Polyp: cervical/endometrial	A			
Previous abdominopelvic surgery		see Table 19.2		
Nulliparity	A	B1	B2	
Severe mental handicap	A			
Cervical intra-epithelial neoplasia	A			
Endometrial malignancy	B2		B1	A
Benign mobile adnexal pathology		B1	A	B2
Benign adherent adnexal pathology			A	B1

*A, first choice; B1 first alternative; B2 second alternative.

Abd, abdominal; LAVH, laparoscopically-assisted vaginal hysterectomy.

A** for an experienced vaginal surgeon.

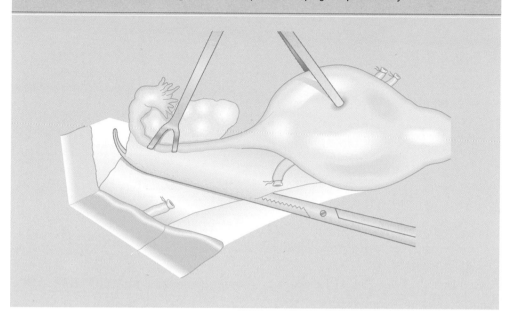

Figure 19.8 The round ligament is cut separately and laterally for the application of an ovarian clamp on the infundibulo-pelvic ligament and to perform salpingo-oöphorectomy.

minimal or no increase in operating time and morbidity.[46] In the author's series of 740 vaginal hysterectomies, BSO was possible in 95% without laparoscopic assistance,[31] which has been extended to successful oöphorectomy in 1186 of 1224 vaginal hysterectomies (96.8%), as shown in Figures 19.8 and 19.9. An experienced vaginal surgeon can safely accomplish oöphorectomy during VH and should adhere to the accepted indication for oöphorectomy irrespective of whether the route is vaginal or abdominal. Transvaginal endoscopic oöphorectomy at VH, which avoids laparoscopic assistance, has been reported in recent literature.[47,48] Hefni and Davies,[48] as well as Davies et al.,[49] have reported successful vaginal oöphorectomy at VH without laparoscopic assistance in 82 cases, and in 39 of 40 cases, respectively, using endoscopic or other techniques. Oöphorectomy is contraindicated in the following cases:

• Where tubovarian adhesions are present;
• Where the ovaries are immobile and atrophic;
• Where the ovaries are placed high up in the pelvis and retracted laterally.

Paying special attention to the following details should help simplify the procedure of oöphorectomy at VH:

• The round ligament should be clamped and cut separately;
• A specially designed clamp should be used;
• Exposure should be improved;
• Speculum and bladder retractors with incorporated fibre-optic light should be used;
• A competent assistant should be available.

It is possible to perform oöphorectomy at VH without laparoscopic assistance.

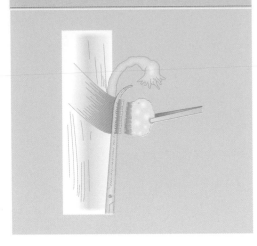

Figure 19.9 The mesoovarium is clamped by an ovarian clamp for excision of the ovary (oöphorectomy).

Some surgeons resort to LAVH, which is in order if the operator is not comfortable about performing oöphorectomy with VH, as opening the abdomen merely for removal of the ovaries should be avoided.

Subtotal hysterectomy

There is a recent trend towards saving the cervix at hysterectomy (subtotal hysterectomy). Subtotal hysterectomy may be abdominal, laparoscopic or vaginal. Gynaecologists in favour of this procedure claim several advantages of retaining the cervix: cervical mucus is believed to promote orgasmal function, although there are no scientific data to support this claim. However, this has induced gynaecologists to perform subtotal hysterectomy laparoscopically and thus to avoid trauma to the uterine artery and the ureters. Ewen and Sutton[50] have reported the first British experience of laparoscopic subtotal hysterectomy.

Subtotal hysterectomy is less easy to perform vaginally than total VH. Under the circumstances, it is not worth recommending this procedure, especially as the advantages of the retained cervix are nebulous.

Subtotal hysterectomies are currently performed and taught by laparoscopic surgeons and this may be interpreted as an admission of lack of skill in endoscopic surgery, or that total hysterectomy is fraught with risk. It is also a way of obscuring the fact that at laparoscopy it is very difficult to remove the uterine cervix and this step adds to the complications — an ingenious way of converting a disadvantage (of having to conserve the cervix) into an apparent advantage![51]

After subtotal hysterectomy, cancer of the cervical stump occurs in 1–3% of cases.[52] This is of great import in the developing world, which harbours 80% of the global estimate of 450,000 new cases of cervical cancer detected every year. An estimated 5% of women in the developing countries have been screened for cancer of the cervix in the last 5 years, compared with 45–50% in the developed world.[53] This is tragic, as leaving behind the cervix in the guise of safe supracervical hysterectomy and basking in the glory of laparoscopic surgery are pretexts that can prove devastating for a woman who subsequently suffers from cervical cancer, and traumatic for her family. It is far better to have a live, healthy woman without a cervix than a dead woman with an ornamental but carcinomatous cervical stump!

Nevertheless, subtotal hysterectomy is indicated in the following circumstances:

1. When the patient's condition demands a rapid hysterectomy. In such situations, retaining the cervix shortens the procedure significantly and saves time, which is of essence in such patients.
2. In the presence of inseparable adhesions that increase the danger of trauma to the sigmoid colon or ureters or are associated with other complications that force the operator to leave behind the cervix, as in cases of severe pelvic endometriosis.
3. When the patient insists on retaining the cervix.

A moot point worthy of consideration by all endoscopic surgeons is whether they routinely perform subtotal hysterectomy at abdominal or vaginal hysterectomy and save the cervix!

Ureteral, bladder and other injuries

The incidence of bladder injury has been assessed as 0.4% at abdominal hysterectomy compared with 1.8% at LAVH;[54] in another study, the incidence of bladder injury was also highest with LAVH.[55] In the author's series of 5344 vaginal hysterectomies, there was one ureteric injury, one rectal injury, one bowel injury and six bladder injuries.

Morbidity and mortality

Morbidity

As a general rule, the incidence of complications following abdominal hysterectomy is 70% higher than that following VH.[56] Postoperative ileus, intestinal obstruction and septic pelvic thrombophlebitis are seen more often with abdominal hysterectomy.

Currently, the trend is to mobilize the patient early and recommend an early discharge from hospital.[57] A short hospital stay has other obvious advantages to the patient in terms of reduced morbidity and complications. In one study involving a short stay, 100% patient satisfaction was recorded.[58] In recent years, a marked swing to minimal hospital stay has been noted, owing to minimally invasive surgery as one of the advantages of laparoscopic surgery.

Anaesthetic complications are more common with abdominal than with vaginal hysterectomy. Similarly, the incidence of blood transfusions is greater with the abdominal[59] than the vaginal route (8.6% in the abdominal vs 2.3% in vaginal hysterectomy) and is best avoided, especially in the current context of the risk of HIV contamination of blood. The risk of leaving behind a sponge is very small with VH but this can easily happen with abdominal hysterectomy. These are real and very relevant advantages of the vaginal over the abdominal route.

Mortality

The mortality rate associated with VH at most centres is less than 0.1%.[60] Although abdominal hysterectomy is the safer procedure, mortality is between 4.1 and 14.6 per 10,000.[61] At King's College Hospital, London, in the last 15 years, there have been no deaths following hysterectomy;[2] similarly, Pratt[62] did not record any deaths after VH. The present author has not had any fatalities after vaginal or abdominal hysterectomy for menorrhagia in the last 16 years; however, he insists on a meticulous preoperative work-up, a competent anaesthesiologist and special precautions for extra care.

Conclusions

Whenever a hysterectomy is to be performed for menorrhagia, whatever its cause, the gynaecologist should endeavour to consider the vaginal route; only when there is a contraindication to this route should the abdominal route be resorted to, as shown in Figure 19.7. There is no doubt that vaginal hysterectomy is the least morbid, least expensive technique, associated with the most rapid postoperative recovery.[63]

In the absence of uterine prolapse, DUB, adenomyosis and fibroids comprise more than 80% of the indications for hysterectomy, and 90% of these hysterectomies can be performed vaginally. In other words, the vast majority of hysterectomies can easily be converted to this least-invasive and minimally accessed route in the best interest of the patients. Debulking and oöphorectomy, if required, should become part and parcel of routine hysterectomy, to facilitate vaginal removal of the uterus.

In the past, prior to the development of LAVH, the master vaginal surgeon Feroze[64] advocated simple abdominal hysterectomy when the uterus is larger than 12 weeks, although this can be tackled by morcellation or splitting. As the frontiers of science advance, operative techniques are becoming increasingly sophisticated, with the use of the laparoscope. However, several gynaecologists continue to practise the techniques that they have acquired from their teachers. Laparoscopy has demonstrated unequivocally the superiority of the vaginal route over the abdominal route by reducing the latter and promoting the former: LAVH is designed to replace abdominal hysterectomy and not VH.[65] A study of VH, TAH and LAVH[66] resulted in higher test scores in favour of VH which conferred a better postoperative quality of life, postoperative outcomes and earlier recovery. Only when VH is contraindicated and LAVH is not possible, should abdominal hysterectomy to be considered (Table 19.4).

The rapid strides taken by surgery have permitted surgeons to improve their skills and to undertake difficult procedures in risky situations. Now, not only is it essential to assess the patient for surgery, but, with advances in surgery, every gynaecologist must also assess himself as a surgeon for a particular type of surgery.

Vaginal surgery has always been the hallmark of the gynaecological surgeon. After all, what is the difference between a gynaecological surgeon who performs an abdominal hysterectomy for DUB in the absence of any contraindication to hysterectomy via the vagina, and a general surgeon who can remove the uterus through the abdomen as competently? In fact vaginal hysterectomy is the least invasive route; after all, it uses the portal designed by God.

References

1. Brown D A, Frazer M I Hysterectomy revisited. Aust N Z J Obstet Gynaeecol 1991; 31: 148–152

2. Studd J W W. Hysterectomy and menorrhagia. Baillieres Clin Obstet Gynaecol 1989; 3: 415–424

3. Sheth S S, Malpani A. Vaginal surgery — what can't we do? In: Downes E, O'Donovan P (eds) Progress in gynecologic surgery. London: Greenwich Medical Media 1999: in press

4. Sheth S S. Vaginal hysterectomy. In: Studd J (ed) Progress in obstetrics and gynaecology. London: Churchill Livingstone, 1993: 317–340

5. Chapron C, Dubuisson J B. Total hysterectomy by laparoscopy: advantage for the patient or only a surgical gimmick? J Gynecol Surg 1996; 12: 75–88

6. Bost B W. Assessing the impact of introducing laparoscopically assisted vaginal hysterectomy into a community based gynecology practice. J Gynecol Surg 1995 11: 171–178

7. Johns D A, Carrera B, Jones J et al. The medical and economic impact of laparoscopically assisted vaginal hysterectomy in a large, metropolitan, not-for-profit hospital. Am J Obstet Gynecol 1995; 172: 1709–1715

8. Dorsey J H, Holitz P M, Griffiths R I et al. Costs and charges associated with 3 alternative techniques of hysterectomy. N Engl Med J 1996; 335: 476–482

9. Moore J G. Vaginal hysterectomy with intra pelvic adhesions: clinical problems. In: Nichols D H (ed) Injuries and complications of gynecologic surgery. Baltimore: Williams and Wilkins, 1988: 102–107

10. Krige C F. Vaginal hysterectomy and genital prolapse repair — a contribution to the vaginal approach to operative gynecology. Johannesburg: Witwatersrand University Press, 1965

11. Goldfarb H A. A review of 35 endometrial ablations using Nd:Yag laser for recurrent menometrorrhagia. Obstet Gynecol 1990; 76: 833–835

12. Campbell Z B. A report on 2798 vaginal hysterectomies. Am J Obstet Gynecol 1946; 52: 598–609

13. Hillis S D, Marchbanks P A, Peterson H B. Uterine size and risk of complications among women undergoing abdominal hysterectomy for leiomyomas. Obstet Gynecol 1996; 87: 539–543

14. Schneider A, Merker A, Martin C et al. Laparoscopically assisted vaginal hysterectomy as an alternative to abdominal hysterectomy in patients with fibroids. Arch Gynecol Obstet 1997; 259: 79–85

15. Pelosi M A III, Pelosi M A. A comprehensive approach to morcellation of the large uterus. Contemp OB/GYN 1997; 106–125

16. Mattingly R F, Thompson J D. Leiomyomata uteri and abdominal hysterectomy for benign disease. In: Mattingly R F, Thompson J D (eds) Te Linde's Operative gynecology, 6th edn. Philadelphia: Lippincott, 1985: 203–255

17. Sheth S S, Shinde L. Vaginal hysterectomy for myomatous polyp. J Gynecol Surg 1993; 9: 101–103

18. Togashi K, Nishimura K, Itoh K et al. Adenomyosis: diagnosis with MR imaging. Radiology 1988; 166: 111

19. Moss A A, Gamsu G, Genant H K et al. Computed tomography of the body with magnetic resonance imaging. In: Scoutt L M et al. (eds) Abdomen and pelvis, 2nd edn. 1992: 1181–1265

20. Scoutt L M, McCarthy S M, Lange R et al. Evaluation of ovarian masses on MRI with ultrasound correlation. (In press)

21. Zarwin M, McCarthy S, Scoutt L M et al. High-field MRI and US evaluation of the pelvis in women with leiomyomas. Magn Reson Imaging 1990; 8: 371

22. Parkar W, Childer J M, Cains M et al. Laparoscopic management of benign cystic teratomas during pregnancy. Am J Obstet Gynecol 1996; 174: 1499–1501

23. Shalev E, Bustan M, Romano S et al. Laparoscopic resection of ovarian benign cystic teratomas: experience with 84 cases. Hum Reprod 1998; 13: 1810–1812

24. Teng F Y, Muzsnai D, Perez R et al. A comparative study of laparoscopy and colpotomy for the removal of ovarian dermoid cysts. Obstet Gynecol 1996; 87: 1009–1013

25. Reich H. Laparoscopic oophorectomy and salpingo-oophorectomy in the treatment of benign tubo-ovarian diseases. Int J Fertil 1987; 32: 233

26. Sheth S S. Adnexal pathology. In: Sheth S S, Studd J. Vaginal hysterectomy. Oxford: Isis Medical Media, 1999: in press

27. Pardi G, Carminati R, Ferrai M M et al. Laparoscopically assisted vaginal removal of ovarian dermoid cysts. Obstet Gynecol 1995; 85: 129–132

28. Quinlan D. Consultant Obstetrician & Gynaecologist, Chelmsford Medical Centre, Durban, South Africa. Personal communication, 1997

29. Ingiulla C. Vaginal hysterectomy for the treatment of carcinoma endometrium. Am J Obstet Gynecol 1968; 100: 541–543

30. Massi G, Savino L, Susini T et al. Vaginal hysterectomy vs abdominal hysterectomy for the treatment of stage I endometrial adenocarcinoma. Am J Obstet Gynecol 1996; 174: 1320–1326

31. Sheth S S. The place of oophorectomy at vaginal hysterectomy. Br J Obstet Gynaecol 1991; 98: 662–666

32. Bigrigg A, Browning J. The treatment of cervical intraepithelial neoplasia. Prog Obstet Gynecol 1993; 10: 359–375

33. Sheth S S, Goyal M V, Shah N. Uterocervical displacement following adhesions after caesarean section. J Gynecol Surg 1997; 13: 143–146

34. Coulam C B, Pratt J H. Vaginal hysterectomy — is previous operation a contraindication? Am J Obstet Gynecol 1973; 116: 252–260

35. Kovac S R. Guidelines to determine the route of hysterectomy. Obstet Gynecol 1995; 85: 18–23

36. Sheth S S. An approach to vesicouterine peritoneum through a new surgical space. J Gynecol Surg 1996; 12: 135–140

37. Monaghan J J. Gynaecological Cancer Center, Queen Elizabeth Hospital, UK. Personal communication, 1992

38. Sheth S S, Malpani A. Vaginal hysterectomy for the management of menstruation in mentally retarded women. Int J Gynecol Obstet 1991; 35: 319–321

39. Lash A F. A method for reducing the size of uterus in vaginal hysterectomy. Am J Obstet Gynecol 1941; 42: 452–459

40. Kovac S R. Intramyometrial coring as an adjunct to vaginal hysterectomy. Obstet Gynecol 1986; 67: 131–136

41. Sheth S S. Uterine fibroids. In: Sheth S S, Studd J. Vaginal hysterectomy. Oxford: Isis Medical Media, 1999: in press

42. Stovall T G, Ling F W, Henry L C et al. A randomised trial evaluating leuprolide acetate before hysterectomy as treatment for leiomyomas. Am J Obstet Gynecol 1991; 164: 1420–1425

43. Sheth S S. The place of oophorectomy at vaginal hysterectomy. Obstet Gynecol Surv 1992; 47: 332–333

44. Sheth S S, Malpani A. Routine prophylactic oophorectomy at the time of vaginal hysterectomy in postmenopausal women. Arch Gynecol Obstet 1992; 251: 87–91

45. Kammerer-Doak D N, Magrina J F, Weaver A et al. Vaginal hysterectomy with and without oophorectomy — the Mayo Clinic experience. J Pelvic Surg 1996; 2: 304–309

46. Ballard L A, Walters M D. Transvaginal mobilization and removal of ovaries and fallopian tubes after vaginal hysterectomy. Obstet Gynecol 1996; 87: 35–39

47. Magos A L, Bournas N, Sinha R et al. Transvaginal endoscopic oophorectomy. Am J Obstet Gynecol 1995; 172: 123–124

48. Hefni A A, Davies A E. Vaginal endoscopic oophorectomy with vaginal hysterectomy: a simple minimal access surgery technique. Br J Obstet Gynaecol 1997; 104: 621–622

49. Davies A, O'Connor H, Magos A L. A prospective study to evaluate oophorectomy at the time of vaginal hysterectomy. Br J Obstet Gynaecol 1996; 103: 915–920

50. Ewen S, Sutton C J G. Initial experience with supracervical laparoscopic hysterectomy and removal of the cervical transformation zone. Br J Obstet Gynaecol 1994; 101: 225–228

51. Sheth S S, Malpani A. Inappropriate use of new technology: impact on women's health. Int J Gynaecol Obstet 1997; 58: 159–165

52. Hannoun-Levi J M, Peiffert D, Hoffstetter S et al. Carcinoma of the cervical stump: retrospective analysis of 77 cases. Radiother Oncol 1997; 43: 147–153

53. WHO Collaborating centre: International Network on control of Gynecological Cancers. Report FIGO. Geneva: WHO, 1998

54. Meikle S F, Nugent E W, Orleans M. Complications and recovery from LAVH compared with abdominal and vaginal hysterectomy. Obstet Gynecol 1997; 89(2): 304–311

55. Ostrzenski A, Ostrzenska K M. Bladder injury during laparoscopic surgery. Obstet Gynecol Surv 1998; 53: 175–180

56. Dicker R C, Scally M J, Greenspan J R et al. Hysterectomy among women of reproductive age — trends in USA 1970–78. JAMA 1982; 248: 323–327

57. Mackenzie I Z. Reducing hospital stay after abdominal hysterectomy. Br J Obstet Gynaecol 1996; 103: 175–178

58. Stovall T G, Ling R L, Braun D F et al. Outpatient vaginal hysterectomy — a pilot study. J Obstet Gynecol 1992; 80: 145–149

59. Mintz P D, Sullivan M F. Pre-operative crossmatch ordering and blood use in effective hysterectomy. Obstet Gynecol 1985; 63: 389

60. Jeffcoate N. Hysterectomy and its aftermath. In: Tindall V R (ed) Jeffcoate's Principles of gynecology. London: Butterworths, 1987: 706–709

61. Bachmann G A. Hysterectomy: a critical review. Reprod Med 1990; 35: 831–862

62. Pratt J H. A personal series of 1000 vaginal hysterectomies. South Med J 1980; 73: 1360

63. Richardson R, Bournas N, Magos A L. Is laparoscopic hysterectomy a waste of time? Obstet Gynecol Surv 1995; 50: 590–591

64. Feroze R M. Vaginal hysterectomy and radical hysterocolpectomy. In: Monaghan J M (ed) Bonnie's Gynecological surgery. London: Baillière Tindall, 1986: 60–86

65. Sutton C. Laparoscopic hysterectomy. Curr Obstet Gynecol 1992; 2: 225–228

66. Van Den Eeden S K, Glasser M, Mathais S D et al. Quality of life, health care utilization and costs among women undergoing hysterectomy in a managed care setting. Am J Obstet Gynecol 1998; 178: 91–110

Which hysterectomy? A detailed comparison of laparoscopic, vaginal and abdominal hysterectomy

R. Garry

Introduction

It is important, but difficult, to assess the role of any new surgical technique. The questions to be answered are as follows:

1. Is the procedure possible?
2. What are the benefits?
3. What are the complications and costs?
4. Does it work?

Not all clinical data in the literature are of equal importance when assessing the worth of a technique: individual case series are of least value; non-randomized controlled trials, cohort and case-controlled studies are of somewhat greater value, and randomized controlled trials (RCTs) are of even more value. Perhaps of most value are meta-analyses of a number of good RCTs. Many scientific and funding bodies are increasingly insisting that evidence is categorized according to quality before it is presented. One method of doing this is to divide data into three grades, namely:

- Class A evidence, which is based on a number of well-conducted RCTs;
- Class B evidence, which is based on good-quality case-controlled and other non-randomized trials;
- Class C evidence, which is based on personal series or on experts' consensus views.

The first planned vaginal hysterectomy was performed by Conrad Langenbeck in 1813 and the first elective abdominal hysterectomies by Charles Clay in Manchester, UK, in 1863, followed by Koeberle in Strasborg a few weeks later.[1] The techniques were progressively refined over the remainder of the 19th century and by the early years of the 20th century had become established as the 'classic' techniques. Since then, these procedures have been tested in the clinical setting many millions of times and have been passed down essentially unaltered to successive generations of gynaecological surgeons.

Problems of choice: abdominal versus vaginal hysterectomy

Almost every gynaecologist is aware of the 'classic' approaches to effective and safe abdominal and vaginal hysterectomies. Almost every gynaecologist also believes he is aware of the correct indications for performing each of these procedures and when each should be performed. For example, the brilliant French gynaecological surgeon Denis Querleu,[2] in a prospective study reported in *Gynaecological Endoscopy* in 1993, stated that he was able to perform a hysterectomy by the vaginal method in 77% of 149 patients requiring a hysterectomy. Similarly, Kovac[3] reported that, in his hands, 548 of 617 (89%) patients requiring hysterectomy could be successfully treated by the vaginal method. In contrast to these individual experiences, a national survey of every hysterectomy performed in Finland[4] indicated that in 1990, 8474 of 9095 (93%) cases involved the abdominal route but that, by 1995, the proportion of vaginal hysterectomies had risen to 11% of the total. Similarly, in the UK, the Vaginal, Abdominal and Laparoscopic Uterine Extirpation (VALUE) study was recently reported by Hall et al.,[5] who found that in 1995, some 74% of 15,379 hysterectomies conducted, in the absence of structural disease, for dysfunctional uterine bleeding were performed by the abdominal route.

This wide variation in proportions of abdominal and vaginal hysterectomies between different units — and, indeed, different surgeons in the same unit — indicates that, after more than 100 years of experience of the world's most commonly performed major surgical operation, the gynaecological profession as a whole has no clear indication of the optimum method of hysterectomy in differing situations. Individual gynaecologists can perform anything between almost nil and close to 100% of their hysterectomies by either classic route: the choice of method of operation depends more upon the experience and biases of the surgeon than on critical evaluation of the operative and outcome data. Alan Johns has memorably summarized the situation: 'The route of hysterectomy is usually determined by the skill, experience, and preferences of the operating gynaecologist. Few other parameters matter.'[6]

The problem about belief in the concept of evidence-based medicine is that convincing evidence should lead to changes in daily practice; this causes most gynaecological surgeons considerable discomfort and inconvenience. It is essential that, to be effective, surgeons should believe that whatever operation they recommend is the best available. It is not helpful to their patients if there are substantial doubts about the superiority of the procedure recommended. Change, however, must be preceded by doubt, and development must follow dissatisfaction with the existing situation. Are the current standard methods of hysterectomy as good as they can be; are the indications for each, sound?

It is accepted that abdominal hysterectomy can be used for every indication and can be considered to be the 'default operation' — i.e. when a procedure cannot be performed by another method it will be done by the abdominal route. Most consider that vaginal hysterectomy should be reserved for specific indications, which will usually include a uterus of fairly normal size. Such-minded gynaecologists consider that fibroids and the need to remove the adnexa are relative contraindications to the vaginal route. Some authors have challenged this widely held view and have recently clearly demonstrated again, what had been known for many years — that both ovaries and large uteri can be safely removed by the vaginal route.[2,3,7–9] Having proved that such operations are possible vaginally, they go on to suggest that the vaginal route is to be preferred in most circumstances; there is, however, a surprising lack of data to support this view. Amazingly, these two approaches to the world's most common major surgical operation have never been subjected to a single formal prospective randomized trial and, until the recent introduction of laparoscopic methods of hysterectomy, had attracted relatively few comparative studies; most studies that have been published were single-centre retrospective studies covering many years. Those published before 1970 generally found vaginal hysterectomy to be associated with more morbidity than abdominal hysterectomy.[10–12] Premenopausal women who underwent vaginal hysterectomy were found to be at particular risk.[13,14]

In 1982, an important and much-quoted study was published by Dicker et al.[15] that examined data from the multicentre, prospective, observational Collaborative Review of Sterilization (CREST) project. As this study is so often quoted, it should be examined, with its conclusions, in some detail. The study collected data from 1851 patients undergoing hysterectomy, of whom 568 (31%) had a vaginal hysterectomy and 1283 (69%) an abdominal hysterectomy. Patients in the latter group were older and had significantly higher percentages of women who were Black or nulliparous or who had previously undergone caesarean section. The indications for surgery in the two groups differed markedly: the primary indications for surgery in the abdominal hysterectomy group were principally fibroids (40%) and pelvic pain/endometriosis in 22%; in contrast, in the vaginal group the main indications were pelvic relaxation (30%), bleeding (27.5%) and cervical dysplasia (20.5%), with only 7% for fibroids. The groups had different demographic features and markedly different pathologies. The headline and much-quoted overall complication rate was 42.8% following abdominal hysterectomy and 24.5% following vaginal hysterectomy. These figures are often taken as 'proving the superiority of the vaginal route'. Closer analysis of the data, however, reveals that most of this observed difference was due to differences in febrile morbidity, with a 32.3% incidence in the abdominal hysterectomy group compared with 15.3% in the vaginal group. This difference was probably completely explained by the differential use of prophylactic antibiotics, for 82% of those having vaginal surgery, but only 32% of those undergoing abdominal surgery were given such prophylaxis. Detailed subgroup analysis stratifying for antibiotic use continued to demonstrate a relative-risk benefit in favour of vaginal hysterectomy, but this evidence is much less compelling than is often claimed.

Harris and Daniell[16] have produced a review of 65 large series of complications associated with either abdominal and/or vaginal hysterectomy that have been published since the CREST study. This complex analysis gave some general conclusions, including the following:

1. A higher incidence of bleeding complications occurs after vaginal than abdominal hysterectomy;
2. The overall blood transfusion rate has fallen but the rate is still higher after abdominal hysterectomy;
3. Abdominal hysterectomy probably still has a higher rate of unexplained infection than vaginal; however, the rate of urinary tract infections is now similar in both groups, with a lower incidence than noted in the CREST study;
4. There appears to be a greater risk of bladder injury after vaginal hysterectomy and Harris and Daniell warn that, as more difficult vaginal procedures are performed, the risk of inadvertent bladder injury will rise;
5. Ureteric injuries appear to be more common after abdominal hysterectomy.

There is not a single class A evidence trial comparing abdominal and vaginal hysterectomy: most studies contain poor-quality class C personal series data, and even the class B prospective comparative studies compare mostly surgical methods for different indications in different population groups and the conclusions are, therefore, usually invalid. This lack of relevant data allows all gynaecological surgeons to continue to perform the type of conventional hysterectomy that they prefer, when they choose to, without the inconvenience of having to test their approach against validated evidence.[17]

Laparoscopically-assisted hysterectomy

Into this field dominated by tradition, personal preferences and biases, Harry Reich's seminal paper about the first hysterectomy performed entirely with laparoscopic techniques burst in 1989.[18] The potential benefits and risks of this approach have been much discussed in recent years.[19] What chance is there of assessing the role of this new group of procedures if the relative roles of abdominal and vaginal hysterectomy have not been determined over the course of more than 100 years? Paradoxically, however, the introduction of this new approach to hysterectomy has stimulated a much greater interest in proper scientific evaluation of all forms of hysterectomy: the first class A randomized trials to address any aspect of hysterectomy have all been directed at laparoscopically assisted vaginal hysterectomy (LAVH).

Laparoscopically-assisted vaginal hysterectomy versus abdominal hysterectomy

There have been at least six RCTs comparing laparoscopic (LAVH) and abdominal hysterectomy (TAH). Those by Nezhat et al.,[20] Phipps et al.[21] and Raju and Auld were short studies of a total of 112 patients, which each concluded that laparoscopic procedures took significantly longer to perform and yet were associated with significantly less postoperative pain, shorter hospital stays and quicker return to work and normal activities. Raju and Auld[22] also reported a significant reduction in postoperative fever in the LAVH group. Olsson et al.[23] reported a larger series of 143 patients in greater detail, and Langebrekke et al.[24] reported a series of 100 cases. These studies again indicated that LAVH took significantly longer to perform than conventional TAH, but was associated with much shorter postoperative stay and convalescent time. The amount of blood lost, as assessed by measurement of the erythrocyte volume fraction, was significantly less after LAVH, as was the number of patients requiring blood transfusion. The overall complication rates appeared similar in both groups in all studies but there was a single vesicovaginal fistula in the laparoscopic arm of Olsson's study and two ureteric injuries in the laparoscopic arm of the Langenbrekke[24] study. The most recent RCT was reported by Marana et al.;[25] interestingly, this study concentrated specifically on a group of patients most would consider unsuitable for vaginal hysterectomy and in whom the mean uterine weight was in excess of 300 g. Despite such adverse factors, this study showed for the first time, with class A evidence, that LAVH could be performed in the same operative time as TAH (mean 91 min in each group). They also confirmed that blood loss was less and postoperative pain (as assessed by analogue pain scores) was significantly less on postoperative days 1, 2 and 3 in the LAVH group.

LAVH versus vaginal hysterectomy

There have also been two small RCTs comparing vaginal hysterectomy (VH) with LAVH. The first, by Summit et al.,[26] unusually reported the comparison of these two approaches in an outpatient setting; it included 56 patients who had adequate uterine mobility and a good-shaped pelvis. Again, the operating time in the LAVH group was significantly longer than in the conventional hysterectomy, but other measures suggested little difference between the two approaches, apart from the fact that operative blood loss after conventional VH was significantly greater. A single patient developed a vesicovaginal fistula in the vaginal hysterectomy arm, but there were no statistically significant differences in the complication rates between the two procedures. The second RCT of 45 patients was reported by Richardson et al.:[27] the operating time was, again, much longer with the LAVH approach, and other measures of recovery and morbidity were similar in the two groups.

Complications

These RCTs give useful information about some aspects of the comparative performance of the three methods of performing a hysterectomy; however, perhaps the most important statistics are missing from these studies. Marginal benefits in the size of scars and in postoperative pain and recovery times will be irrelevant if it can be shown that there are significant differences in major complications between the techniques. According to the review by Harris and Daniell,[16] the accepted incidence of intra- and postoperative haemorrhage with conventional hysterectomies is about 2–4% and the need for blood transfusion about 2–12%; the incidence of bowel damage is lower, at about 0.1–0.8% and of ureteric damage about 0.1–0.2%. The largest of the RCTs quoted above had 70+ patients in each arm. To detect a reduction/increase in incidence of 50% of all major complications with a total incidence of (say) 9%, with $\alpha = 0.1$ and $\beta = 0.1$, would require at least 540 patients in each arm. None of the studies quoted here is at all powered to detect such changes and therefore can provide no meaningful guidance about relative complication risks. There can be no confidence in conclusions relating to the incidence of complications based on studies of this size.

If a summation of small-number class A type evidence is of little value in determining the relative complication rates, then it is likely that the summation of poorer-quality data will simply increase the number of patients in the study but not improve the quality of the conclusions derived. Meikle et al.[28] did perform such a study based on a MEDLINE search in which 33 papers listing comparative complication rates of various types of hysterectomy were analysed; data on 3112 LAVH, 1618 TAH and 690 VH were collected. The only significant differences between LAVH and TAH were a higher rate of bladder damage in the LAVH group (1.8% vs nil) and a higher rate of haemorrhage in the TAH group (2.65% vs 1.4%). The incidence of ureteric damage in the LAVH group was 0.3% and again nil in the TAH group, but this was not statistically significant. There was no significant difference in bowel, bladder and ureteric injuries between the LAVH and VH groups. This type of study clearly indicates the shortcomings of simply summating the results of a large number of small, highly selective class B and C trials.

Several much larger studies have been performed in an attempt to obtain a clearer picture of the relative complication rates. The most comprehensive is a series reported by Harkki-Siren et al.:[29] a national register for all laparoscopic hysterectomies performed in Finland over a 2-year period was obtained and details of some 1165 operations were collected, which represents an astonishing 96% of all the procedures performed in that country. Of 51 major complications that occurred (an overall rate of 3.5%), there were 14 vascular complications (1.2%), 17 bladder lesions (1.5%) and 15 ureteric lesions (1.3%); there were also five electrosurgical burns of the bowel (0.4%). These rates of ureteric lesions appeared high and were subsequently subjected to a more detailed investigation.[30] In this study, 142 urinary tract injuries that occurred after all forms of hysterectomy over a 6-year period between 1990 and 1995 were reviewed. The overall rate of ureteric damage was 1.0/1000 cases, but there was a considerable discrepancy in rates associated with each form of hysterectomy: the incidence after LAVH was 13.9/1000, that after TAH 0.4/1000 and that after VH only 0.2/1000. This represents an astonishing 35-fold higher rate of ureteric injury after LAVH than after TAH. If this figure is representative of the world experience, then there will be no future for LAVH. More detailed inspection of the data reveals that the remarkable statistic in this series is not the rate of ureteric injuries after LAVH but the amazingly low rate of damage reported after TAH: only 18 damaged ureters were found in 43,149 abdominal hysterectomies. This rate of 0.4/1000 compares with the CREST figure of 2/1000,[15] and a range of 1–5/1000 in the subsequent review by Harris and Daniell,[16] and represents a 5–10 times lower incidence of ureteric damage than is usually quoted.

This worrying discrepancy encouraged the author to look for other studies that investigated the incidence of ureteric damage. Even more worrying was the single-unit series reported by Tamussino et al.,[30] in which he described three ureteric injuries out of only 70 cases of LAVH (which represents a rate of 43/1000; there were no cases of ureteric damage in 641 other operative laparoscopies performed by the same group). In another study, looking specifically at urinary tract injuries after LAVH, Saidi et al.[31] reported one case of ureteric injury in 489 LAVH procedures, which is a rate of 2/1000. Deprest et al.[32] found 19 ureteric injuries from a total of 4502 LAVH cases reviewed (4.2/1000). The Scottish audit of laparoscopic surgery[33] noted a rate of ureteric damage of 8/1000 from 458 cases. Many of these data were collected retrospectively; in contrast, in the large UK prospective VALUE study, in 15,379 procedures performed for dysfunctional uterine bleeding (1198 of which were performed laparoscopically),[5] there was no significant difference in the incidence of any form of visceral damage, including ureteric lesions. The total number of hysterectomies included in the study was 34,969, which represents about 50% of all hysterectomies performed in England and Wales during the study period. The most important figure — and perhaps an important clue to making sense of all the previous data — is buried in the wealth of data contained in this study:[34] of 192 surgeons undertaking some form of LAVH, the vast majority reported performing under ten procedures during the year of the study; only 33 performed ten or more procedures/year and only two surgeons reported doing more than 50 procedures/year, which is equivalent to only one LAVH each week. Not surprisingly, those who performed less than ten procedures/year were significantly more likely to note complications (such as haemorrhage, visceral damage and return to theatre) than those who performed the operation more frequently.

Performing a new and unfamiliar surgical operation is not the same as giving a new drug. Nevertheless, both new therapies require evaluation and RCTs would appear to be the most critical way to determine the effectiveness of both new types of therapy. The Cochrane method of assessing the worth of clinical trials gives clear guidance about evaluating the structure and value of their format. For surgical procedures, a well-planned trial alone is not sufficient: technical proficiency and competence in the new techniques must be reached before it can be meaningfully compared with the standard procedure, which, almost inevitably, will be performed in an efficient and well-proven manner. Most of the studies reviewed in this chapter were performed during the 'world learning curve for laparoscopic hysterectomy'. For example five of the six class A studies of LAVH versus TAH and both the class A studies of LAVH versus VH indicated that the LAVH procedures took much longer to perform than the conventional equivalent. These studies were all performed early in the 'world experience' of LAVH and, in most cases, early in the participating surgeons' experience of the new procedure. Certainly, in no case was the surgeon as experienced in the new technique as in the conventional technique that was being compared. In contrast, the class A study presented first in 1997 by the Italian group[25] appears to demonstrate greater laparoscopic skills. This, the latest of these studies to be published, is the first to target specifically those patients with significant pathology such as fibroids, moderate and severe endometriosis and adnexal disease. In this study, operating times were identical in each group and significant other benefits of the laparoscopic approach were demonstrated. The VALUE study clearly indicated the importance of experience in influencing outcome.[34] It is essential to compare personal experience with established norms when establishing a new surgical procedure.

Personal experience

The author's experience reflects most of the difficulties and problems reflected in the studies above. In 1985, he performed 99 hysterectomies, of which 27 were vaginal and the remaining 73% were abdominal. These figures mirrored the national figures precisely and the author continued with this pattern until performing his first laparoscopic hysterectomy in 1991. In 1997 he performed 127 hysterectomies, of which 27 (21%) were by the abdominal method, four (3%) by the vaginal method and 96 (76%) by various laparoscopic techniques. The early experience was full of technical difficulties and problems; a number of different approaches and a number of differing technologies were attempted: for example, the diathermy equipment, which had been found quite satisfactory for open surgery, was clearly inadequate for laparoscopic bipolar diathermy work and needed to be replaced (which, of course, took many months to achieve). There were innumerable such problems associated with minor equipment and procedure, which will be familiar to those who have attempted this type of surgery. Even when it was thought that most of the technical difficulties had been overcome, a number of serious clinical problems were still encountered.

Initially, the author found laparoscopic hysterectomy much more difficult to perform than anticipated: in his first series of 100 reasonably standard LAVH procedures, there was a depressing 20% serious complication rate, which included 13 cases of vault haematoma, three of cystotomy, two of ureteric injury, one epigastric artery injury and one pulmonary embolism. Of course, results are appreciated only in retrospect. These figures match some of the worst results reported above and were certainly much worse than the author had expected — in fact he seriously contemplated giving up the procedure at this stage. Nevertheless, impressed by the excellence of the postoperative recoveries in the 80% of patients who did not develop complications, he continued to perform laparoscopic hysterectomies, but only after undertaking an in-depth look at the procedure and the possible causes of the problems encountered. The main difficulty, of course, was excessive bleeding from the vaginal vault during transection of this and the associated uterine and vaginal vessels. That the author was not the only UK gynaecologist encountering these difficulties was subsequently revealed in the VALUE study, for this showed that the rate of haemorrhage associated with LAVH was significantly higher than that after VH, which was in turn higher than after TAH.[5] This difficulty led to a combination of unexpectedly heavy bleeding with the frequent need for blood transfusion and the development of vault and peritoneal haematomata and/or the excessive use of diathermy, with the consequent risk of diathermy or clip damage to the ureter.

Döderlein's method

The author reviewed the literature to look for guidance as to ways of overcoming this group of problems,[35] during which he encountered a fairly obscure paper by Saye et al.,[36] describing a laparoscopic version of Döderlein's method of hysterectomy. The principles of this approach are, first, that the laparoscopic component of the dissection should stop above the level of the uterine artery, which is subsequently secured from below; this ensures that the ureter in the canal is not threatened during this stage of the operation. Second, only the anterior cul-de-sac is opened from below and the uterus is inverted through this incision. This permits the lateral vaginal angles and the posterior vaginal walls to be divided, after first being secured by clamps, which substantially reduces the amount of vault bleeding. Third, during the vaginal dissection the bladder is mobilized and placed behind a vaginal retractor, thus removing the ureter from the operative field and enabling the uterine vessels to be secured under direct vision. The combined result of these steps is that the uterus can be removed without threatening the deep ureter and vaginal vault bleeding can be kept to a minimum. The author's initial experience with this approach has already been reported,[37] and his experience of 300 consecutive cases is in press. Many of these patients had significant pelvic pathology. The results are encouraging and much less depressing than some of the studies outlined above. They are shown in Table 20.1 with the CREST 'gold standard' figures and the author's earliest LAVH figures for comparison.

The combination of increasing experience, better equipment, and much greater attention to the technical details of the procedure have allowed a transformation in results from the unacceptable to levels significantly better than the accepted standard levels. The laparoscopic Döderlein technique allows a variety of patients — with all the conditions referred to a general gynaecologist, and with a higher proportion of advanced endometriosis than usual — to obtain all the benefits of the laparoscopic approach without unacceptable level of risk of complications. These figures are now better than most of the series reported above.

There are, of course, many other surgical strategies that can achieve good vault haemostasis with minimal risk of ureteric damage, including subtotal approaches, use of illuminated ureteric stents and the use of vaginal delineators. The purpose of this section was not to claim that the Döderlein approach is the optimum method

Table 20.1 Percentage of complications following the Döderlein approach to hysterectomy compared with those following LAVH, abdominal and vaginal hysterectomy

Complication	Percentage of complications according to method of hysterectomy			
	Döderlein	LAVH	Abdominal	Vaginal
Unexplained fever	0.7	n.a.	16.8	7.2
Urinary infections	3.0	n.a.	7.0	3.4
Blood transfusions	1.7	27	15.4	8.3
Bladder injury	1.0	3	1.6	0.3
Ureteric injury	0	2	0.2	0
Bowel trauma	0.3	0	0.3	0.6

LAVH, laparoscopically-assisted vaginal hysterectomy; n.a., not available.

of LAVH but to illustrate that it requires careful thought and attention to surgical details to achieve satisfactory results. It is self-evident that surgical operations should not be performed in a suboptimal manner. It is equally evident that studies of such suboptimal procedures, performed during the learning curve of experience, should not be compared with the most highly developed and worked-out reference procedures. In the author's opinion, most of the studies that have gone before are therefore of limited value; what is now required is large-scale well-designed prospective RCTs comparing the established techniques.

Building on classic methods

Early in this chapter, the author wondered whether the 'classic' methods of hysterectomy described and refined in the early parts of this century were so well developed that no further improvement was possible. One of the works of an English master of this 'golden age' of gynaecological surgeons — Victor Bonney — is entitled *The Technical Minutiae of Extended Myomectomy and Ovarian Cystectomy*.[38] In this monograph, this surgical giant of his times makes several observations of great relevance today. The first is the amazing attention to the surgical detail that he exhibited: he takes 282 pages and 242 original drawings (made by himself) to describe two operations that, in their time, were revolutionary but now seem mundane and obvious. He advocates the adoption of the conservative operation of ovarian cystectomy in the following manner:

> *Ovarian cystectomy is easy and safe but it requires of the surgeon that he should forgo a procedure which achieves a striking result in a startlingly short time for one which, though it takes longer, has a far greater appeal to the connoisseur. There is a pleasure, a pride, and a satisfaction in these conservative operations which cannot be appreciated save by those who have performed them.*

In this book, Bonney also answers the author's earlier question in the following manner — which appears even more appropriate at the end of the century than it did earlier:

> *This century has witnessed immense progress in all branches of surgery, not least in those whose concern is in reparation. Each generation would fain believe its self the*

acme; each succeeding generation disproves the belief, and so the advances go on, and the amazement of today becomes the commonplace of tomorrow. We surgeons form one small group of a great host whose marching cry is 'something better,' and therein lies our certainty of the future; for even while we sit talking here, somewhere or other in the world minds are at work plotting discoveries to astonish the coming years.

Relief of symptoms

So far it has been demonstrated that the new laparoscopic methods of hysterectomy:

1. Can be done;
2. Can result in faster and less painful recovery from surgery with acceptably low complication rates;
3. Can result in serious complications that can be reduced to an acceptable minimum by paying careful attention to the minutiae of technique.

It has not, however, been demonstrated whether the new or, indeed, the conventional forms of hysterectomy work. *It must be considered whether the aim of performing a hysterectomy is to remove the uterus or to cure the patient of her symptoms.* It has been assumed in every one of the studies quoted above that the successful removal of the uterus is inevitably associated with relief of all the patient's symptoms. It has also been assumed that each method of hysterectomy is equally effective in producing this relief. In part, this must, of course, be true: if the only symptom is excessive uterine bleeding, then every form of hysterectomy must work every time. If pain, dyspareunia, and general ill health are also components of the patient's symptom complex it is, however, by no means certain that hysterectomy will always work and there is almost no evidence to indicate if each form of hysterectomy is equally effective in improving such symptoms: in an Australian study of women who had undergone hysterectomy, some 82% reported feeling better, 10% noted no change and 8% felt worse;[39] in a quality assurance exercise by the Australian College of Obstetricians and Gynaecologists, all patients surveyed after LAVH reported that they had been helped by the operation, but only 84% of women with abdominal pain and 68% of those with painful intercourse reported an improvement in these symptoms.[40]

In the opinion (as yet unproven) of the author, all forms of hysterectomy will not be equal in terms of the patient's perception of long-term outcome. In a small study shortly to be published from the author's unit, looking at the laparoscopic removal of large fibroid uteri, significant previously unsuspected additional pelvic pathology was found in 25% of cases, including three (15%) cases of coexisting severe endometriosis. Leaving such lesions untreated must increase the risk of the presenting symptoms persisting after the uterus has been removed. In the author's opinion, it is unacceptable to perform a major operation such as hysterectomy without taking care to ensure that all the pathology contributing to the patient's symptoms has also been removed. The widespread adoption of the relatively 'blind' vaginal hysterectomy, in which much of the pelvis cannot be inspected, may result in substantial numbers of such significant pathology being missed, with a consequent reduction in the effectiveness of the operation. There is absolutely no evidence to support or refute this suggestion at present, but the effectiveness of each type of hysterectomy in relieving patient symptoms must form a major component of future studies.

Conclusions

What do all these personal, single-site, multicentre, case-controlled and randomized clinical studies tell us about the optimal method of hysterectomy to use as we approach the millennium? It is clear that both vaginal and laparoscopic techniques, when performed well, can replace (with benefit) the abdominal method in most circumstances. As these approaches are less painful and are associated with a more rapid recovery and lower complication rate, they appear to be the preferred methods. Patients' symptoms, as well as their physical findings, should influence the choice between these two methods. Vaginal hysterectomy is usually completed more rapidly than LAVH and is therefore likely to be the more cost-effective method when bleeding alone is the presenting symptom. When other symptoms — particularly pain — are present it is probable that the ability to visualize the pelvis may improve the long-term outcome measures; in these circumstances, in the author's opinion the laparoscopic approach may be best.

References

1. Sutton C. Hysterectomy: a historical perspective. Baillieres Clin Obstet Gynaecol 1997; 11: 1–22
2. Querleu D, Casson M, Parmenter D, Debodinance P. The impact of laparoscopic surgery on vaginal hysterectomy. Gynaecol Endosc 1993; 2: 89–91
3. Kovac S R. Guidelines to determine the route of hysterectomy. Obstet Gynecol 1995; 85: 18–23
4. Harkki-Siren P, Sjoberg J, Tiitinen A. Urinary tract injuries after hysterectomy. Obstet Gynecol 1998; 92: 113–118
5. Hall V, Overton C, Hargreaves J, Maresh M J A. Hysterectomy in the treatment of dysfunctional uterine bleeding. Br J Obst Gynaecol 1998; 105(Suppl 17): 60 (abstr.)
6. Johns D A, Carrera B, Jones J et al. The medical and economic impact of laparoscopically assisted vaginal hysterectomy in a large, metropolitan, not-for-profit hospital. Am J Obstet Gynecol 1995; 172: 1709–1715
7. Sheth S S. The place of oöphorectomy at vaginal hysterectomy. Br J Obstet Gynaecol 1991; 98: 662–666
8. Davies A, O'Connor H, Magos A L. A prospective study to evaluate oöphorectomy at the time of vaginal hysterectomy. Br J Obstet Gynaecol 1996; 103: 915–920
9. Magos A, Bournas N, Sinha R et al. Vaginal hysterectomy for the large uterus. Br J Obstet Gynaecol 1996; 103: 246–251
10. Amrikia H, Evans T N. Ten year review of hysterectomies: Trends, indications and risks. Am J Obstet Gynecol 1979; 134: 431–437
11. White S C, Wartel J, Wade M E. Comparison of abdominal and vaginal hysterectomies. A review of 600 operations. Obstet Gynecol 1971; 37: 530–537
12. Leventhal M L, Lazarus M C. Total abdominal and vaginal hysterectomy: a comparison. Am J Obstet Gynecol 1951; 61: 289–293
13. Pratt J H, Galloway J R. Vaginal hysterectomy in patients less than 36 or more than 60 years of age. Am J Obstet Gynecol 1965; 93: 812–821
14. Taylor E S, Hansen R R. Morbidity following vaginal hysterectomy and colpoplasty. Obstet Gynecol 1961; 17: 346–350

15. Dicker R C, Greenspan J R, Strauss L T et al. Complications of abdominal and vaginal hysterectomy among women of reproductive age in the United States. Am J Obstet Gynecol 1982; 144: 841–848

16. Harris W J, Daniell J F. Early complications of laparoscopic hysterectomy. Obstet Gynecol Surv 1996; 51: 559–567

17. Davies A, Magos A. Vaginal hysterectomy: attitudes and practice. Br J Obstet Gynaecol 1998; 105(Suppl 17): 60 (abstr.)

18. Reich H, Decaprio J, McGlynn F. Laparoscopic hysterectomy. J Gynecol Surg 1989; 5: 213–216

19. Garry R. How safe is the laparoscopic approach to hysterectomy? Gynaecol Endosc 1995; 4: 77–79

20. Nezhat F, Nezhat C, Gordon S, Wilkins E. Laparoscopic versus abdominal hysterectomy. J Reprod Med 1992; 37: 247–250

21. Phipps J H, John M, Nayak S. Comparison of laparoscopically assisted vaginal hysterectomy and bilateral salpingo-oöphorectomy with conventional abdominal hysterectomy and bilateral salpingo-oöphorectomy. Br J Obstet Gynaecol 1993; 100: 698–700

22. Raju K S, Auld B J. A randomised prospective study of laparoscopic vaginal hysterectomy versus abdominal hysterectomy each with bilateral salpingo-oöphorectomy. Br J Obstet Gynaecol 1994; 101: 1068–1071

23. Olsson J H, Ellstrom M, Hahlin M. A randomised prospective trial comparing laparoscopic and abdominal hysterectomy. Br J Obstet Gynaecol 1996; 103: 345–350

24. Langebrekke A, Eraker R, Nesheim B I et al. Abdominal hysterectomy should not be considered as a primary method for uterine removal. A prospective randomised study of 100 patients referred to hysterectomy. Acta Obstet Gynecol Scand 1996; 75: 404–407

25. Marana R, Busacca M, Garcia N et al. LAVH versus AH. J Am Assoc Gynecol Laparosc 1997; 4 (S): S5

26. Summit R L, Stovall T G, Lipscomb M H, Ling F H. Randomised comparison of laparoscopy-assisted vaginal hysterectomy with standard vaginal hysterectomy in an outpatient setting. Obstet Gynecol 1992; 80: 895–901

27. Richardson R E, Bournas N, Magos A L. Is laparoscopic hysterectomy a waste of time? Lancet 1995; 345: 36–41

28. Meikle S F, Nugent E, Orleans M. Complications and recovery from laparoscopy-assisted vaginal hysterectomy compared with abdominal and vaginal hysterectomy — reply. Obstet Gynecol 1997; 89: 1050–1051

29. Harkki-Siren P, Sjoberg J, Makinen J et al. Finnish national register of laparoscopic hysterectomies: a review and complications of 1165 operations. Am J Obstet Gynecol 1997; 176: 118–122

30. Tamussino K F, Lang P F, Breinl E. Ureteral complications with operative gynecologic laparoscopy. Am J Obstet Gynecol 1998; 178: 967–970

31. Saidi M H, Sadler R K, Vancaillie T G et al. Diagnosis and management of serious urinary complications after major operative laparoscopy. Obstet Gynecol 1996; 87: 272–276

32. Deprest J A, Munro M G, Koninckx P R. Review on laparoscopic hysterectomy. Zentralbl Gynakol 1995; 117: 641–651

33. Lumsden M A, Hawthorn R, Davis J et al. A prospective audit of operative laparoscopic surgery, particularly hysterectomy and operations for ectopic pregnancy. Br J Obstet Gynaecol 1998; 105 (Suppl 17): 60 (abstr.)

34. Hall V, Overton J, Hargreaves J, Maresh M J A. Laparoscopic hysterectomy: Do we do enough? Is there a learning curve? How much training do we need? Br J Obstet Gynaecol 1998; 105 (S17): 109

35. Gary R. Various approaches to laparoscopic hysterectomy. Curr Opin Obstet Gynaecol 1994; 6: 215–222

36. Saye W B, Espy G B, Bishop M R et al. Laparoscopic Döderlein hysterectomy: a rational alternative to traditional abdominal hysterectomy. Surg Laparosc Endosc 1993; 3: 88–94

37. Garry R, Hercz P. Initial experience with laparoscopic-assisted Döderlein hysterectomy. Br J Obstet Gynaecol 1995; 102: 307–310

38. Bonney V. The technical minutiae of extended myomectomy and ovarian cystectomy. London: Cassel, 1946

39. Ryan M M, Dennerstein L, Pepperell R. Psychological aspects of hysterectomy: a prospective study. Br J Psychiatry 1989; 154: 516–522

40. Petrucco O, Maher P, Molloy D, Ryan M M. The laparoscopically assisted hysterectomy (LAH) project. R Coll Obstet Gynaecol Bull 1996; 10: 22–23

CHAPTER 21

Vaginal hysterectomy or TCRE?

C. J. G. Sutton

Early development of vaginal hysterectomy

Although there are reports of vaginal hysterectomy being performed by Themison of Athens 50 years before the birth of Christ,[1] the first elective hysterectomies performed vaginally date from 1800. Baudelocque in Paris introduced the technique of artificially prolapsing and then (in favourable cases) cutting away the uterus and appendages. He performed 23 such procedures during the first 16 years of the 19th century but gave Lauvariol the credit for having performed the first operation in France.

Most of these procedures were performed on puerperal uteri and were undertaken on an emergency basis, but the first planned procedure was by Friedrich Osiander of Gottingen in 1801, during which he amputated the vaginal portion of a carcinomatous uterus.[2] Rather than rush into print in the way of his modern counterpart, he wisely did not report the procedure until he had operated on his ninth patient! In 1810, Wrisberg wrote advocating vaginal hysterectomy for cancer, in a prize essay read before the Vienna Royal Academy of Medicine; two years later, Dr. G. B. Paletta of Milan performed the operation. It was, however, almost accidental, because he intended to amputate a malignant cervix and, to his surprise, found that he had extirpated the entire uterus by the vaginal approach. The patient soon died of peritonitis.[3] This early case illustrates one of the problems of vaginal hysterectomy in that it is almost a blind procedure compared with a laparoscopic hysterectomy and thus is very much more difficult to teach apprentice surgeons.

The first planned vaginal hysterectomy for cancer

Wrisberg's paper, and the report of Paletta's case, encouraged the first deliberate planned vaginal hysterectomy for carcinoma. This was undertaken by Conrad Langenbeck (Fig. 21.1), the Surgeon-General of the Hanoverian army, who performed the operation in 1813 but did not report it until 1817.[4] Langenbeck, having little precedent to follow, dissected the uterus out of its peritoneal investment, taking great care not to enter the peritoneal cavity. Unfortunately, he encountered torrential haemorrhage from one of the uterine pedicles and called upon his assistant, an elderly army surgeon crippled with gout, to come to his aid. Unfortunately, the gentleman concerned could not rise from his chair, so Langenbeck had no alternative but to pass a ligature round the bleeding pedicle, tie it by grasping one end between his teeth and then throw a single-handed tie with

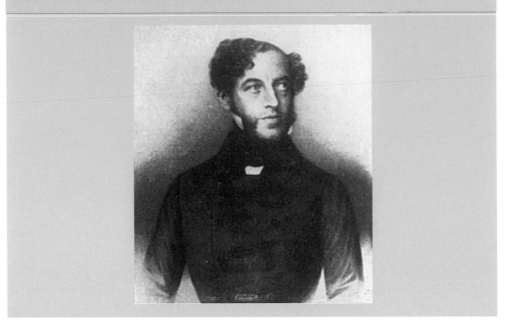

Figure 21.1 Conrad Langenbeck, Surgeon-General to the Hanoverian army, who performed the first vaginal hysterectomy for endometrial cancer in 1813.

his right hand. At the end of the procedure he could not detect an opening into the peritoneal cavity and the patient made an uneventful recovery.

A series of unfortunate events occurred, following this brilliant display of surgical virtuosity: not only did the specimen get lost, but the assistant died of gout the following week. The patient herself was unable to corroborate the story because she suffered from dementia and none of Langenbeck's colleagues believed that he had actually performed the operation; he was, therefore, subjected to jibes, ridicules and vilification for the rest of his professional career. He was finally vindicated some 26 years later, when the woman died of senility and a necropsy clearly showed that the uterus had, indeed, been removed by vaginal surgery.

Comparative development of abdominal and vaginal hysterectomy

The first abdominal hysterectomy was performed by Charles Clay of Manchester in 1843; the patient died almost immediately afterwards. Clay did not, in fact, have a patient who survived the procedure until he performed a procedure 20 years later — a few days before Koeberle of Strasburg performed the first successful abdominal hysterectomy in continental Europe. It can be seen, therefore, that vaginal hysterectomy was performed much earlier than abdominal hysterectomy and it was not until 1883 that Thomas Keith from Scotland realized that the massive mortality of abdominal hysterectomy, as high as 73% in the hands of Spencer Wells, was largely due to the archaic and dangerous practice of leaving the cervical stump to discharge pus through a long ligature. Keith cauterized the stump and returned it to the abdomen, and thus brought the mortality down to a much more respectable 8%.

The latter years of the 19th century witnessed further developments and the technique for abdominal hysterectomy was refined and standardized by Freund. Czerny, following Langenbeck's original description, did the same for vaginal hysterectomy.[5]

With the introduction of specially modified instrumentation, anaesthesia and antisepsis, the mortality rate for vaginal hysterectomy dropped precipitously and by 1886 was approximately 15%. By 1890 it had reached 10% and by 1910 it was as low as 2.5%. Abdominal hysterectomy lagged far behind and was formally condemned by the Academy of Medicine of Paris in 1872. In spite of this, 8 years later, T G Thomas reported on 365 collected cases, which revealed a horrific mortality of 70%.

Modern hysterectomy

Over the past 60 years, the introduction of antibiotics, intravenous therapy, anti-coagulation and blood transfusion have further reduced the mortality for both vaginal and abdominal hysterectomy to about 0.1%; however (given the very rocky start of abdominal hysterectomy), it is surprising that it has outstripped vaginal hysterectomy to the extent that, in the United States, approximately 25% of hysterectomies are performed vaginally,[6] (Figs. 21.2 and 21.3) compared with only 11.9% in England,[7] despite the fact that a large series has shown a lower rate of morbidity for vaginal hysterectomy (24.5%) than for abdominal hysterectomy (42.8%).[8] Nevertheless, although there is undoubtedly a lower morbidity and faster recovery from vaginal hysterectomy, this study[8] is seriously flawed and provides an eloquent testimony to the efficacy of prophylactic antibiotics, since those who underwent vaginal hysterectomy had the benefit of these drugs, whereas those who underwent abdominal hysterectomy did not.

The history of endometrial ablation

Menorrhagia is probably the commonest indication for hysterectomy and, once organic causes have been excluded, there remains a group of patients with abnormal bleeding without an organic cause; this group, labelled as those with 'dysfunctional

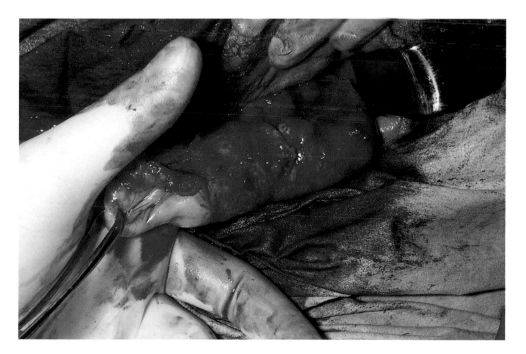

Figure 21.2 Schauta's vaginal hysterectomy, being performed by Daniell Dargent from Lyon, for the treatment of Stage I cervical carcinoma.

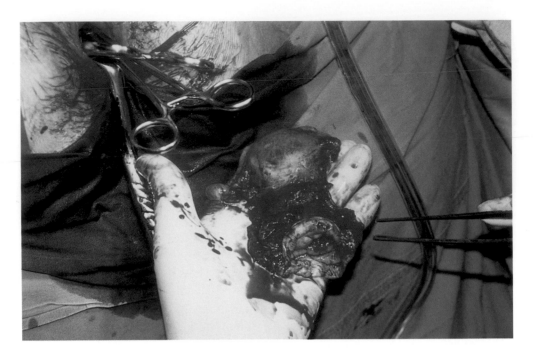

Figure 21.3 Schauta's radical vaginal hysterectomy for early cervical carcinoma. This is now usually proceeded by laparoscopic pelvic lymphoderectomy. Note the large amount of parametrium removed.

uterine bleeding' (DUB), accounts for 35% of all hysterectomies.[7,9] This is a diagnosis of exclusion and other chapters in this book describe in detail how that diagnosis is arrived at.

The fact that so many uteruses are removed that appear to be completely normal and yet the operation has been done for a very good indication — namely, excessive menstrual loss that is either socially unacceptable or leading to ill health — inspired one of the most profound original thoughts in the history of gynaecology. Credit for that must go to Professor Milton Goldrath of Detroit, who reasoned that, if one could destroy the endometrium selectively, then there should be no reason to remove the uterus itself. Already an accomplished hysteroscopist, he administered danazol to thin the endometrium in order to get a clearer view with less bleeding and then inserted a neodymium:yttrium aluminium garnet (Nd:YAG) laser fibre through the operating channel of the hysteroscope and ablated the endometrium by dragging the fibre from the fundus towards the internal os until the entire endometrium had been destroyed. This technique depends on the deep penetration of laser energy at this wavelength (1064 nm) and also relies for its safety on the fact that the myometrium is relatively thick and it is unlikely that the Nd:YAG laser energy could damage internal organs unless perforation has occurred (this should be recognized instantly and, if perforation occurs, the laser energy should be switched off immediately). Initially, he was concerned that the thermal effect could be transmitted to the internal organs and possibly damage the bowel; however, by a simple experiment (in which he held the uterus in his hand while the laser fibre was activated but the uterus did not become warm) he reasoned that, in the situation in vivo it would become even less warm since the circulation would dissipate the heat. His next step was to verify this with the use of thermocoupling devices attached to the uterus; once he found that his hypothesis was correct, he progressed to using the technique on patients and published some very impressive results in 1981.[10]

Endometrial laser ablation (ELA)

Further contributory evidence of the efficacy and safety of ELA came from other centres in the United States[11,12] and from the United Kingdom.[13] The main disadvantage of the Nd:YAG laser for endometrial ablation is the very high cost of the laser itself and the laser fibre. The latter used to be cleaved back and used repeatedly, but since the company have stamped 'Single Use Only' on the packaging, health authorities in these litigious days have limited the use of the fibre to one patient for fear of spreading bizarre new viruses and other infections. Unfortunately, it is possible to titrate the result of the procedure with the wattage employed and Davies[14] has shown that the results obtained with a 50 W laser are considerably inferior to those obtained with one of 80–100 W. Unfortunately, the price of these lasers rises proportionally to the wattage, and £80,000–£100,000 represents a considerable capital investment when much cheaper electrosurgical generators are available in all hospitals. This is probably why this technique is now employed in relatively few centres and is also the reason for its commendable safety record, because it is used only in centres of excellence in this type of surgery.

Transcervical resection of the endometrium (TCRE)

It has often perplexed the author that gynaecological surgeons are so slow to learn from colleagues in other surgical disciplines. Some 20 years ago, general surgeons looked with disdain at gynaecologists' early attempts at operative laparoscopy: the relatively simple operation of laparoscopic cholecystectomy took a long time to arrive on the surgical scene and, even then, was first performed by a gynaecologist in Lyons, France. Now, the laparoscope has revolutionized many general surgical operations — and, to listen to general surgeons talking, one could be forgiven for thinking that they had invented the technique! Gynaecologists were equally slow to learn from their urological colleagues, because it now seems blindingly obvious that the technique of transurethral resection of the prostate could easily be applied to resection of the endometrium with an operating hysteroscope. Credit for the first electrosurgical loop resection must go to Alan DeCherney who was then Professor at Yale University in the United States and who reported a series of patients who were too ill to undergo hysterectomy and were successfully treated by electrosurgical endometrial resection.[15] In fact, Robert Neuwirth from New York had used a similar technique several years previously for the removal of submucous fibroids.[16] Endometrial resection was popularized in Europe by Jacques Hamou, who became aware of the problem of intravenous infusion of irrigating fluid when large vessels were opened up by the resectoscope loop: he invented an automated perfusion pump to control the intra-uterine pressure and fluid flow in order to minimize this problem. He also introduced the technique to British gynaecologists at a memorable meeting organized by Adam Magos under the aegis of Sir Alec Turnbull (who was Regius Professor of Obstetrics and Gynaecology at the University of Oxford in 1987). Magos went on to publish his first series, the results of his initial experience in 1989.[17] This also highlighted the problems of excessive absorption of glycine (which occurred in a few patients) and the need to monitor carefully input and output and to stop the procedure in the event of a deficit of more than 1.5 litres.

One of the problems with endometrial resection is that it has tended to look too simple when performed by an expert: many people, having seen a video of the procedure, have thought that it was only a matter of getting the instrument manufacturers to attend an operating list and to perform endometrial resections without any formal training. This resulted in a series of very unfortunate accidents and even a few fatalities from perforation of major vessels or peritonitis and septicaemia following unrecognized bowel perforation. The British Society for Gynaecological Endoscopy established protocols for the teaching of this new technique and training courses were provided in several centres throughout the country. Gynaecologists are now aware of the need to learn this technique initially on simulators and models of a uterus made from advanced plastic materials that are very similar to endometrium when electroresected. Following this, surgeons are expected to have close supervision during their first practical cases and, even then, should probably perform the procedure on uteri that have been removed at abdominal or vaginal hysterectomy in an in vitro situation. As most accidents occur during the learning curve (which probably includes the first 25–50 cases), trainee surgeons should be closely supervised during this initial phase of learning. Subsequently, the chance of an accident occurring is relatively remote, as long as the strict rules laid down for this technique are adhered to: when the Royal College of Obstetricians and Gynaecologists asked Michael Maresh to undertake a prospective audit in all hospitals in the United Kingdom performing endometrial ablation techniques, it was concluded that the procedure is essentially very safe compared with hysterectomy.[18]

Women who should be advised to undergo vaginal hysterectomy
Women with prolapse
If the patient is complaining of symptoms of prolapse, with a feeling of a lump coming down in her vagina that gradually worsens as the day proceeds, then, clearly, a vaginal hysterectomy and repair operation would be the procedure of choice. It is sometimes difficult to assess the degree of prolapse in the outpatient setting; putting a single-tooth tenaculum on the cervix and pulling down can be uncomfortable and distressing, and can often result in bleeding. Nevertheless, some information can be achieved by merely getting the patient to push down as if in labour; however, the fear of passing flatus or leaking urine often prevents patients from doing this and many actually contract their pelvic floor muscles — which has the completely opposite effect. Nevertheless, the amount of access can be assessed and the angle of the sub-pubic arch estimated in order to assess the suitability for vaginal hysterectomy; if there are symptoms of prolapse, then, clearly, this would be a better option, as the patient is likely to need a prolapse repair procedure during the forthcoming few years.

Women with a family history of ovarian cancer
It is becoming increasingly obvious that some families exhibit a strong tendency to breast or ovarian cancer and, when investigated, members of the family can be shown to have the BRCA 1 or 2 gene. At present it is known that there are at least five genes that predispose to breast cancer in families. BRCA 1 has been identified on chromosome 17 and has a strong link between breast and ovarian cancer; families with this gene will often have a history of several female members dying of an ovarian cancer — although the further back one goes, the more unreliable the information becomes and, often, the cause of death is attributed to terminal

malignancy, secondary carcinomatosis or even liver cancer. It is known that the lifetime risks of someone carrying BRCA 1 is around 85% for breast cancer and possibly around 60% for ovarian cancer.[19] Obviously, such families are always going to be worried about this high risk and, as ovarian screening has not conclusively been able to show that it can detect early disease, then such patients are usually advised to have the ovaries removed at the time of hysterectomy. Most ovaries are accessible at the time of vaginal hysterectomy but, clearly, this does depend on the skill of the surgeon.[20] There remains a group of patients who have significant adhesions or endometriosis sticking the ovaries to the pelvic side-wall; obviously, there would be considerable technical difficulty in removing these ovaries, although this can be facilitated by performing a laparoscopic oöphorectomy as part of a laparoscopically assisted vaginal hysterectomy.

At the time of endometrial resection the ovaries are not involved in the operation. For this reason, many surgeons would recommend that an ovarian ultrasound scan is performed prior to endometrial resection and that, if there is any doubt about the ovaries, they should be examined laparoscopically and biopsied — and that, probably, consent also should be given for laparoscopic oöphorectomy or even laparotomy if their appearance gives rise to suspicion of carcinoma.

Women seeking complete amenorrhoea

The operation of endometrial resection or ablation is designed to restore a woman's heavy menstrual loss to normality — or at least to a level that is personally and socially acceptable. It is fortuitous that, in some women, amenorrhoea does result and the patient is usually happy with this. The rate of amenorrhoea, which is around 35% in most series, gradually rises with age and is, therefore, to some extent age dependent rather than dependent on the technique or operator. Some modern women, who are involved in an intensely competitive and demanding business schedule or in some other occupation, such as top-flight athletics, may wish to be rid of their menses altogether and, if this is their particular concern, then probably a vaginal hysterectomy would be a more satisfactory operation. It is for this reason that some of the randomized control trials comparing hysterectomy with ablation have shown greater satisfaction following hysterectomy,[21-23] although the same studies show that hysteroscopic surgery is associated with a shorter operating time, fewer complications, reduced analgesic requirements and faster return to normal activities and work; however, the lesser degree of satisfaction is based on an interview at 1 year, when (presumably) the upheaval, pain and distress caused by hysterectomy have long been forgotten, whereas menstrual bleeding and pain are still present in a certain proportion of the patients who have had endometrial ablation.

Patients with significant dysmenorrhoea

The currently perceived wisdom among endoscopic surgeons is to perform endometrial ablation techniques only on women with significant menorrhagia due to either dysfunctional bleeding or submucous fibroids but, generally, to reserve the technique for those patients who do not have a significant degree of dysmenorrhoea or pelvic pain. For those patients that do, hysterectomy is usually advised and, depending on the cause of the pain, then either abdominal or vaginal hysterectomy is usually employed. If the pain is due to endometriosis, then almost certainly abdominal hysterectomy is the treatment of choice because all endometriotic deposits and adhesions can be removed at the same time and a bilateral salpingo-oöphorectomy performed (often with difficulty in advanced cases) to avoid any recurrence of the disease.[24]

Nevertheless, many patients with primary dysmenorrhoea and those with endometriosis in the uterosacral ligaments can achieve significant relief from dysmenorrhoea by laparoscopic uterine nerve ablation, which can be performed at the same time as the endometrial resection.[25,26] This is a relatively simple procedure that takes only a few minutes to perform and patients undergoing endometrial resection concomitantly can still be treated as day cases. A few years ago, the author and Simon Ewen published a paper looking at a small series of patients who had menorrhagia and dysmenorrhoea and who were successfully treated by a combination of endometrial resection and laparoscopic laser uterine nerve ablation using the carbon dioxide laser.[27]

The main problem is to distinguish those patients who have adenomyosis as the reason for their pelvic pain and dysmenorrhoea rather than endometriosis externa. These patients quite often have had a negative laparoscopy, and continue to have pelvic pain and dysmenorrhoea and sometimes also dyspareunia; this is a very real trap for the unwary because it is easy to be lulled into a false sense of security by the failure to see any cause of pelvic pain at the time of laparoscopy. The experienced or fastidious laparoscopist, however, would probably note a dusky red or blotchy appearance to the uterus, which often — when compressed with a stainless steel probe — will retain the indentation of the probe, indicating considerable oedema of the myometrium; characteristic appearances can also be noticed on hysteroscopic examination. The 'give-away' clue is to examine these patients at the time of menstruation: they feel marked discomfort if the uterus is palpated bi-manually and compressed between the examining hands; this differs markedly from the pain elicited during cervical excitation when the cervix is rocked forward, which is usually due to deposits of endometriosis in the uterosacral ligaments; it also has to be differentiated from the pain caused by the nodular deposits of deeply infiltrating endometriosis in the rectovaginal septum. Adenomyosis is often a diagnosis made only retrospectively when the histologist slices through the uterus with a microtome and finds the classic pathognomonic features of endometrial glands and stroma within the myometrium. Nevertheless, it is important to try to arrive at this diagnosis by clinical acumen, taking a careful history and following this up with a very thorough pelvic examination; often, the diagnosis can be confirmed by changes in the junctional zone on magnetic resonance imaging that are highly suggestive of adenomyosis.[28] It is vital to exclude adenomyosis because this group of patients do extremely badly following endometrial resection: the operation will often relieve them of the very heavy bleeding of which they initially complained, but it will be replaced by extremely unpleasant menstrual pain. These patients are often extremely upset because, essentially, the socially unacceptable condition of very heavy menstrual loss has merely been replaced by agonizing pelvic pain that requires extremely strong painkillers to effect any relief. Sometimes this is due to an adhesion at the level of the internal os, or higher up in the uterine cavity, stopping the egress of menstrual blood — and this can, quite often, be overcome merely by breaking down the adhesion by inserting an operating hysteroscope and using the rollerball electrode to eradicate any residual endometrium. In the majority of cases, however, it is due to adenomyosis and this unpleasant consequence of the procedure can be avoided by a careful evaluation of the patient before deciding on the method of treatment. The author's undoubted opinion is that, if adenomyosis is suspected, then vaginal hysterectomy is the treatment of choice.

Women who should be advised to undergo endometrial ablation
Women presenting with menorrhagia who have completed their families
In the absence of prolapse and any good reason to remove the ovaries, and an absence of symptoms suggestive of endometriosis or adenomyosis, women should be encouraged to opt for the simplest possible procedure — and that is undoubtedly endometrial ablation using either the Nd-YAG laser[13] loop resection[29,30] or ablation by the electrosurgical rollerball.[31,32] If the equipment is available, consideration should be given to the newer techniques of endometrial ablation using the Vestablate Thermal Ablation Device (Valleylab, Boulder, Co, USA)[33], the endothermal hot water balloon (Cavaterm, UK) or the newer microwave techniques[34] (described more fully in Chapter 26) and photodynamic therapy (Chapter 17).

Endometrial ablation should always be offered as the first surgical option for the treatment of menorrhagia because it can be performed as a simple day-case procedure; the patient is in hospital for only a few hours and any postoperative cramps and discomfort can be virtually abolished by giving a paracervical block with 5 ml 0.5% bupivacaine injected at 7 o'clock and 5 o'clock into the cervix, aiming at the insertion of the uterosacral ligament, at the end of the procedure. Although some surgeons advise patients to be off work for 1–2 weeks, the author advises patients to return to full activity as soon as the effects of the anaesthetic have worn off. They are told that they must expect a watery pink discharge that can last anything from 10 days to 6 weeks and they are also warned that they might have a couple of heavy periods during the healing phase — because it does take 6 months before full intra-uterine scarring takes place and it is pointless to see patients before that time in order to assess the true result of surgery. Any woman who is complaining of excessive bleeding or an offensive discharge about 1 week to 10 days following surgery should consult her family doctor and be given a prescription for antibiotics, in view of the rare occurrence of endometritis; however, this can usually be prevented by giving prophylactic antibiotics intravenously at the time of the initial surgery.

Most women with an endometrial cavity of 12 cm or less, undergoing endometrial ablation performed by an experienced operator, can be expected to avoid a hysterectomy. The author's figures, at the Royal Surrey County Hospital, Guildford, suggest that 75% of women at the end of 5 years are still satisfied with the result of this simple day-case procedure; if the operation is performed by a single, experienced operator, then that figure rises to 83%.[30] Employing a life-table analysis of their results, O'Connor and Magos[29] have shown that over 90% of patients avoid a hysterectomy and 80% any further gynaecological surgical intervention over a 5-year period. Objective assessment of menstrual loss has also confirmed the therapeutic efficacy of these techniques.[35,36] The further advantage over hysterectomy is that endometrial ablation can be performed without general anaesthesia[37] and that, despite the small failure rate associated with the technique, the treatment cost of endometrial ablation is considerably less than that for hysterectomy.[38,39] Although it is clear that endometrial ablation is a popular and accepted alternative to hysterectomy, it has not been associated with a decline in hysterectomy rates — which was prophesied when these techniques were introduced. This may be due to the fact that there is now a considerably lower threshold in offering such surgery, with its low morbidity and discomfort that is little more than that associated with a dilatation and curettage and it is possible that such techniques are being used as an alternative to medical treatment.[40]

In view of the satisfactory long-term results alluded to above, it is likely that endometrial resection has secured a permanent place in our armamentarium for the treatment of dysfunctional uterine bleeding and that most modern women find it more user-friendly, cosmetic and less defeminizing than the alternative of vaginal hysterectomy, even though that remains one of the most acceptable minimal-access surgical techniques.

References

1. Lameras K. Galen and Hippocrates. Athens: Papyrus, 1975

2. Ricci J V. Genealogy of gynecology. Philadelphia: Blakiston, 1950: 350

3. O'Dowd M J, Philipp E E. The history of obstetrics and gynaecology. Carnforth: Parthenon Press, 1994: 409

4. Matthieu A. History of hysterectomy. West J Surg Obstet Gynecol 1934; 42: 1–24

5. Ricci J V. One hundred years of gynaecology. Philadelphia: Blakiston, 1945

6. Sutton C J G. Advances in hysterectomy techniques. In: Studd J, Edwards L (eds) Hysterectomy and HRT. London: RCOG Press, 1997: 43–50

7. Vessey M P, Villard-Mackintosh L, Macpherson K et al. Epidemiology of hysterectomy: findings of a large cohort study. Br J Obstet Gynaecol 1992; 99: 402–407

8. Dicker R C, Greenspan J R, Strauss L T et al. Complications of abdominal and vaginal hysterectomy among women of reproductive age in the United States. Collaborative review of sterilisation. Am J Obstet Gynecol 1982; 144: 841–848

9. Lee N C, Dicker R C, Rubin G L, Ory H W. Confirmation of the pre-operative diagnosis for hysterectomy. Am J Obstet Gynecol 1984; 74: 327–335

10. Goldrath M H, Fuller T, Segal S. Laser photovaporisation of the endometrium for treatment of menorrhagia. Am J Obstet Gynecol 1981; 140: 14–19

11. Lomano J N. Photocoagulation of the endometrium with the Nd:YAG laser for the treatment of menorrhagia. J Reprod Med 1986; 31: 148–150

12. Loffer F D. Hysteroscopic endometrial ablation with the Nd:YAG laser using a non-touch technique. Obstet Gynecol 1987; 69: 679–682

13. Garry R, Shelley-Jones D, Mooney P, Phillips G. Six hundred endometrial laser ablations. Obstet Gynecol 1995; 85: 24–29

14. Davies J A. Hysteroscopic endometrial ablation with the neodymium:YAG laser. Br J Obstet Gynaecol 1989; 96: 928–932

15. De Cherney A H, Polan M L. Hysteroscopic management of intrauterine lesions and intractible uterine bleeding. Obstet Gynecol 1983; 61: 392–397

16. Neuwirth R S. A new technique for and additional experience with hysteroscopic resection of submucous fibroids. Am J Obstet Gynecol 1978; 131: 91–94

17. Magos A L, Baumann R, Turnbull A C. Trans-cervical resection of the endometrium in women with menorrhagia. Br Med J 1989; 298: 1209–1212

18. Royal College of Obstetricians and Gynaecologists Audit Unit. Bull 4 (April) London: RCOG Press, 1994

19. Evans G. Consultant Clinical Geneticist, Regional Genetic Service, St. Mary's Hospital, Manchester. Personal communication, 1997

20. Sheth S S. The place of oophorectomy at vaginal hysterectomy. Br J Obstet Gynaecol 1991; 98: 662–666

21. Dwyer N, Hutton J, Styrett G M. Randomised control trials comparing endometrial resection with abdominal hysterectomy for the surgical treatment of menorrhagia. Br J Obstet Gynaecol 1993; 100: 237–243

22. Pinion S B, Parkin E E, Abramovich D R et al. Randomised trial of hysterectomy, endometrial laser ablation and trans-cervical endometrial resection for dysfunctional uterine bleeding. Br Med J 1994; 309: 979–983

23. Alexander D A, Naji A A, Pinion S H et al. Randomised trial comparing hysterectomy with endometrial ablation for dysfunctional uterine bleeding: psychiatric and psycho-social aspects. Br Med J 1996; 312: 280–284

24. Henderson A F, Studd J W W. The role of definitive surgery and hormone replacement therapy in the treatment of endometriosis. In: Thomas E, Rock J (eds) Modern approaches to endometriosis. Lancaster: Kluwer Academic, 1991: 275–290

25. Sutton C J G. Laser uterine nerve ablation. In: Donnez J (ed) Laser operative laparoscopy and hysteroscopy. Belgium: Nauwelaerts, 1989: 43–52

26. Sutton C J G. Laparoscopic treatment of dysmenorrhoea. In: Sutton C J G, Diamond M (eds) Endoscopic surgery for gynaecologists. Chapter 25. 2nd edn. London: Saunders, 1998: 249–260

27. Ewen P, Sutton C J G. A combined approach for painful heavy periods. Laparoscopic uterine nerve ablation and TCRE. Gynaecol Endosc 1994; 3(3): 167–168

28. Brosens J J, de Souza N M, Baker F G et al. Endovaginal ultrasonography in the diagnosis of adenomyosis uteri: identifying the predictive characteristics. Br J Obstet Gynaecol 1995; 102: 471–474

29. O'Connor H, Magos A L. Endometrial resection for menorrhagia: evaluation of the results at 5 years. N Engl J Med 1996; 335: 151–156

30. Pooley A, Sutton C J G. Five year follow-up of endometrial resection. J Am Assoc Gynecol Laparosc 1998; 00: 000–000

31. Vancaillie T G. Electro-coagulation of the endometrium with the ball and resectoscope. Obstet Gynecol 1989; 74: 425–427

32. Townsend D E, Richart R M, Paskowitz R A, Woolfork R E. 'Rollerball' coagulation of the endometrium. Obstet Gynecol 1990; 76: 310–313

33. Dequesne K, Gallinat A, Garza-Leal J H et al. Thermo-regulated radio frequency endometrial ablation. Int J Fertil 1997; 42(5): 311–318

34. Sharn N C, Feldberg I B, Hodgson D A et al. Microwave endometrial ablation. In: Sutton C J G, Diamond M (eds) Endoscopic surgery for gynaecologists. Chapter 63. 2nd edn. London: Saunders, 1998: 630–640

35. Cooper M J W, Magos A, Baumann R, Rees M C P. The effect of endometrial resection on menstrual blood loss. Gynaecol Endosc 1992; 1: 195–198

36. McLure N, Mamers B M, Healy D L et al. A quantitative assessment of endometrial electro-cautery in the management of menorrhagia and a comparative report of argon laser endometrial ablation. Gynaecol Endosc 1992; 1: 199–202

37. Lockwood G N, Magos A, Bowman R, Turnbull A C. Extensive intrauterine surgery without general anaesthesia. Gynaecol Endosc 1992; 1: 15–21

38. Sculpher M J, Bryan S, Dwyer N et al. An economic evaluation of transcervical endometrial resection versus abdominal hysterectomy for treatment of menorrhagia. Br J Obstet Gynaecol 1993; 100: 244–252

39. Molloy D, Taylor P T. Gynaecological surgery after endometrial ablation. Aust Med J 1994; 161: 604–606

40. Coulter A. Trends in gynaecological surgery [letter]. Lancet 1994; 344: 1367

CHAPTER 22

Should ovaries be removed at hysterectomy?

D. H. Oram and J. Johns

Introduction

It has been suggested that the clinical practice of gonad removal is influenced by an underlying attitude that 'an ovary is not good enough to be saved, whereas a testis is not bad enough to be removed'. Although these two situations are not analogous in surgical or, indeed, other terms, one can easily identify with the philosophy. Nevertheless, the only real reason to consider the removal of apparently healthy ovaries at the time of hysterectomy for benign disease is as prophylaxis against the subsequent development of epithelial ovarian cancer. Reoperation for benign pathology in conserved ovaries is necessary in 1–5% of cases[1] and, perhaps, should not be dismissed with the alacrity suggested in the previous sentence; however, it is not really a major determinant in clinical decision-making. If ovaries are obviously diseased (e.g. involved in endometriosis), then the issue is entirely different and is not really part of the underlying theme of this chapter.

Whatever the rights and wrongs of prophylactic oöphorectomy, there is no doubt that an increasing number are being performed. Thirty years ago, bilateral salpingo-oöphorectomy (BSO) accompanied total abdominal hysterectomy (TAH) in 26% of cases; the most recent data indicate that this figure has now risen to 48%. With increasing confidence in long-term hormone replacement therapy (HRT), as well as wider usage of laparoscopic surgery, the age limits at which gynaecologists are prepared to consider prophylactic oöphorectomy are being progressively reduced, and the numbers of such procedures are unquestionably set to rise even further. Support is lent to this prediction by a survey of UK gynaecologists conducted in 1988, in which Jacobs and Oram[2] reported that only 2.4% of Fellows and Members of the Royal College of Obstetricians and Gynaecologists (RCOG) routinely removed ovaries at the time of hysterectomy in women under the age of 45 years. This figure rose to 20% only in women aged between 45 and 49 years, and clinical practice really changed only when postmenopausal status had been attained, at which stage 85% of respondents were prepared to perform oöphorectomy. It was significant that this study identified that the more senior the clinician (as measured by years since passing the MRCOG examination), the less likely he or she was to remove ovaries prophylactically. Nearly ten years on, it is not unreasonable to assume that, as this subset of gynaecologists pass into retirement, a less-conservative practice will ensue. However, more recent data are limited and the only evidence to endorse the suggestion of more-aggressive practice comes from a small survey of Alaskan gynaecologists published in 1996 by Conklin et al.[3] in this study they found that 40% of their members would perform oöphorectomy in women with normal ovaries and 81% for patients between the ages of 45 and 49 years. In the United Kingdom, however, in spite of any possible changes in overall practice, attitudes among currently practising clinicians still vary between ultra conservative and positively cavalier.

This range of opinion and practice reflects the paucity of data, in particular the absence of long-term prospective studies assessing the value of prophylactic oöphorectomy in the prevention of ovarian cancer. As a result, this issue, which forms part of a gynaecologist's weekly decision-making, is devoid of guidelines and continues to be managed in a completely arbitrary fashion. Implicit in the decision-making process is the patient herself: while not wishing to diminish the importance of her contribution, it is naïve to think that her wishes are paramount, because her decision is often based on the advice she is given and (most importantly) on the way in which it is presented to her (see below). So what is the correct advice?

Prophylactic oöphorectomy: the case for

Ovarian cancer: the problem

Epithelial ovarian cancer is the commonest type of gynaecological cancer in the United Kingdom, and the largest cause of mortality from gynaecological malignancy. The vast majority of cases (95–97%) are sporadic events. Familial or hereditary ovarian cancer appears to account for a small proportion of cases and should be considered as a separate issue (see below). The advent of platinum-based chemotherapy in the late 1970s and 1980s, and of paclitaxel (Taxol) in the 1990s, has had an effect on medium-term survival figures, but long-term cures remain elusive. The benefits of screening and early diagnosis are as yet unproven and this subject is still very much within the realms of research. For as long as this is the case, the concept of prevention is of relevance.

Medical prevention

Medical prevention with the oral contraceptive pill is of enormous importance. Pill usage appears to afford a sustained reduction in the risk of the subsequent development of ovarian cancer. Ovulation inhibition with the pill is associated with a 40% reduction in risk compared with that in women who have never used it;[4] with prolonged usage (> 10 years) the risk reduction might be as high as 80%.[5] The evidence for the protective effect of the pill is sufficiently strong that many groups are recommending it for prophylaxis in women with strong family histories and confirmed mutations,[6] although no studies have been conducted that demonstrate that the pill is protective in this group.

Widespread long-term pill usage in women in their forties, however, might not be considered to be appropriate, and it is in this group that the issue of surgical prevention of ovarian cancer is particularly relevant.

Surgical prevention

Prophylactic oöphorectomy works: it is an effective method of preventing ovarian cancer. It has been estimated that approximately 12% of ovarian cancers are already prevented by the current practice of BSO at the time of hysterectomy.[7] Several studies have examined the frequency of the 'missed opportunity'. Sightler et al.[8] examined all cases of ovarian cancer in their institution over a 14-year period: they

Table 22.1 Reported incidence of previous surgery in women subsequently developing ovarian cancer

Author	Year	Surgery* Abdominal hysterectomy	Pelvic operation
Speert[12]	1949	9/260 (3.5)	52/260 (20)
Golub[13]	1953	16/210 (7.6)	n.a.
Counsellor[14]	1955	67/1500 (4.5)**	n.a.
Fagan[15]	1956	2/172 (1.2)	8/172 (4.7)
Bloom[16]	1962	14/141 (9.9)	n.a.
Terz[17]	1967	27/624 (4.3)	50/624 (8.0)
Gibbs[18]	1971	21/236 (8.9)	38/236 (16.1)
Kofler[19]	1972	45/556 (8.1)	66/556 (11.9)
Grundsell[20]	1981	N/A	21/352 (6.0)
Jacobs and Oram[21]	1986	28/407 (6.9)	37/407 (9.1)
Total		229/4106 (5.6)	272/2607 (10.4)

* Percentages in parentheses.

** Number of abdominal and vaginal hysterectomies not specified.

n.a., not assessed.

From ref. 11 with permission.

found that 12.6% had previously undergone hysterectomy with conservation of one or both ovaries and 7.9% had undergone hysterectomy after the age of 40 years. They calculated that 60 cases of ovarian cancer could have been prevented if prophylactic oöphorectomy had been practised routinely in women over the age of 40 years. Several other studies support this theory[9,10] (see Table 22.1).[11–21] The consensus from these reports is that a further 10–15% of ovarian cancers could be prevented if a more aggressive approach to prophylactic oöphorectomy was adopted; in UK terms, this represents 500–800 cases/year.

Reoperation for benign disease and ovarian longevity There are two other arguments that can be used to support the practice of prophylactic oöphorectomy. First, as mentioned, reoperation for benign disease is a requirement in approximately 1–5% of cases. Secondly, there is some evidence to suggest that ovarian function and longevity is compromised after hysterectomy. Interestingly, this is only partially borne out by recent work by Stillwell et al.,[22] who examined ovarian function following radical hysterectomy and suggested that ovarian compromise might be related to the woman's age at the time of hysterectomy. The study showed that whereas 58% of women over 40 years of age had gonadotrophins in the menopausal range within 2 years of hysterectomy, only 3% of women who were less than 40 years old had compromised ovarian function within this timescale. Four years after surgery, the difference between the two groups was maintained (73% vs 13%).

Prophylactic oöphorectomy: the case against

Long-term HRT

It is axiomatic that, if the ovaries are removed from a premenopausal woman, then HRT is indicated on a long-term basis. The risk-benefit analysis of prophylactic oöphorectomy and long-term HRT versus ovarian conservation has been reported by Speroff et al.[23] They demonstrated that in order for an improvement in life expectancy to be achieved, long term compliance with HRT was essential. Viewed another way, if a woman is not prepared to take HRT on a long-term basis, she would be better served if her ovaries were left in situ (Fig. 22.1). The variables involved in such risk–benefit calculations centre around the balance between the decrease in mortality from ovarian cancer and the increased mortality associated with osteoporosis and cardiovascular disease in the absence of oestrogen. For the balance in terms of improved life expectancy to change in favour of prophylactic surgery, long-term compliance with HRT is required in 70–80% of any given population. Such long-term use of HRT and the subsequent increased risk of breast cancer has been a cause for concern for those considering premenopausal oöphorectomy. Recent data suggest that the incidence of breast cancer being diagnosed is slightly increased in women that have used HRT, this risk increasing with increasing duration of use. This effect stops when HRT is withdrawn, and no significant excess in risk was seen 5 years after cessation.[24] It should be noted, however, that these studies were performed upon postmenopausal women and that, although the incidence of breast cancer was increased, there was no increase in mortality and therefore when considering survival and life expectancy it should not be a factor (unlike osteoporosis).

Psychological sequelae

The psychological sequelae associated with gonad removal are difficult to quantify but are of undoubted relevance and obvious to all in clinical practice. Data on this

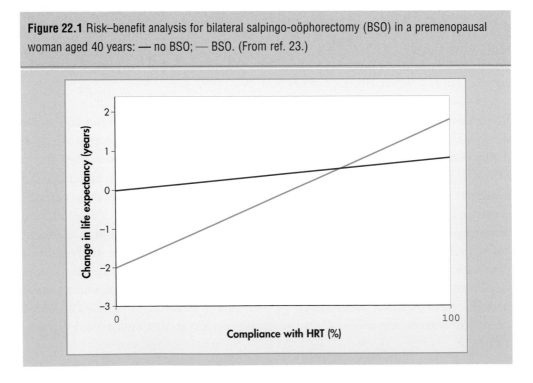

Figure 22.1 Risk–benefit analysis for bilateral salpingo-oöphorectomy (BSO) in a premenopausal woman aged 40 years: — no BSO; — BSO. (From ref. 23.)

subject are extremely limited; nevertheless, they are easily (and all too frequently) underestimated.

The number of oöphorectomies required

Although, as already stated, the diligent practice of prophylactic oöphorectomy at the time of hysterectomy might prevent 15% of ovarian cancers, the counter argument is that ovarian cancer is, in fact, a relatively rare disease and a very large number of oöphorectomies would have to be performed in order to prevent a single case. Because of the lack of long-term follow-up in the studies that have addressed the frequency with which ovarian cancer occurs in conserved ovaries, the exact ratio of prophylactic oöphorectomies to ovarian cancer is unknown (Table 22.2).[25–31]

Table 22.2 Incidence of ovarian cancer in ovaries retained at surgery for benign gynaecological disorders

Author	Year	Length of follow-up	Cases of ovarian cancer	Total no. of patients
Grogan[25]	1957	1.2 years average	0	391
Whitelaw[26]	1959	Min 1, max 28 years	0	1215
Randall[27]	1963	20 years average	2	915
Randall[28]	1962	15 years average	4	345*
De Neef[29]	1966	Min 3 weeks, max 21 years	0	207
McKenzie[30]	1968	n.a.	0	252
Ranney[31]	1977	7.5 years average	4	1265
Total			10 (0.2%)	4590

* Unilateral oöphorectomy for benign tumour of contralateral ovary.

n.a., not assessed.

From ref. 11 with permission.

Failure of prevention

It is a well-known fact that (albeit, extremely rarely), in certain genetically disposed high-risk individuals oöphorectomy fails to prevent intraperitoneal carcinomatosis. This was initially reported by Tobacman et al.,[32] who described the results of prophylactic oöphorectomy in 28 female members of 16 families at high risk of ovarian cancer: three of these women subsequently developed disseminated intra-abdominal malignancy of uncertain origin, which was histologically indistinguishable from ovarian cancer. This report questioned the ability of prophylactic oöphorectomy to reduce the risk of ovarian cancer to zero, and in high-risk women with a genetic susceptibility any tissue derived from the coelomic epithelium may potentially undergo malignant transformation. Further reports[33–36] also illustrated the possible development of intraperitoneal carcinomatosis between 1 and 27 years after oöphorectomy, either because of an individual's genetic propensity or, in a small number of cases, because microscopic malignancy was present but unidentified at the time of oöphorectomy,[37] or because a small amount of ovarian tissue was inadvertently left behind at the time of surgery. Salazar et al.[38] reported the findings of a comparison of the histological features of the ovaries of women at increased risk of ovarian cancer with women whose ovaries were removed for reasons unrelated to cancer risk: they suggested that certain histological characteristics were associated with the 'high-risk' ovaries (in two cases, microscopic or near-microscopic malignant neoplasms were found). The need for thorough examination of the abdominal cavity and even formal staging in these high-risk women becomes apparent. It is important to stress that these cases, although well known, are, in fact, extremely rare even within the family history group and should not detract from the value of prophylactic oöphorectomy in such individuals. Of course, these findings should have no influence on decision-making in the general population.

What is correct clinical practice?

Against this background of conflicting argument it is readily apparent that individual assessment and counselling is the only rational practice. Any woman's decision-making, as mentioned above, is influenced not only by her fears of the development of ovarian cancer or the apprehension of losing her ovaries but also by the way in which the facts are presented to her. This has been regularly demonstrated by one of the authors (DHO), by placing undue emphasis on one or other argument to successive groups of medical students and then asking for a vote on what constitutes correct clinical practice. The results can vary between abhorrence at the mere contemplation of gonad removal to the view that castration is a woman's right and should not be denied!

In calculating an individual's risk and determining appropriate practice, factors such as age, parity, pill usage, ovulation stimulation and a past history of breast cancer are all relevant. Perhaps the overriding factor in the mix, however, is the presence of a positive family history of ovarian cancer.

The influence of family history

After the age of 40, any woman's lifetime risk of developing ovarian cancer is 1.6%. With one first-degree relative with the disease, this lifetime risk increases to approximately 5%. If a woman has two first-degree relatives with ovarian cancer there is a 66% risk that an autosomal dominant predisposing gene is in the family; there is therefore a 33% chance that the woman has inherited the gene. The penetrance of the gene, however, is incomplete — around 40% — and so the risk to the woman of developing the disease is about 15%. These figures need to be viewed in the context of any woman's lifetime risk of developing breast cancer being approximately 8% (and the fact that there is no rush for prophylactic mastectomies!). Any family history is an influence, as far as opportunistic prophylactic oöphorectomy is concerned. Primary prophylaxis (i.e. prophylactic oöphorectomy as a primary surgical procedure) is not justifiable with one family member with the disease; it is justifiable with two histologically proven family members and it is justifiable following genetic testing and the proven inheritance of BRCA1 and BRCA2 mutations. In both groups, such advice is given only after very detailed personal risk assessment and counselling, and only on completion of child bearing.[39] Kerlikowske et al.[6] suggest that, among women with one relative with ovarian cancer, the lifetime probability of ovarian cancer is not sufficiently great to recommend oöphorectomy as a primary surgical procedure but would be an influential factor of some significance should that patient require hysterectomy. They also suggest that, in women with hereditary ovarian cancer syndromes with pedigrees suggesting an autosomal dominant mode of inheritance, the lifetime risk of ovarian cancer is high enough to justify oöphorectomy. Despite this, some groups still prefer to advocate more intense surveillance.[6,39]

The removal of ovaries as a primary surgical procedure is, therefore, justifiable only in a very small cohort of women, following careful counselling and individual risk assessment based on a verified history and possible genetic testing to demonstrate BRCA1 or BRCA2 mutations. For women who are at increased (but not very high) risk of ovarian cancer, in whom primary prophylaxis is not justifiable, the opportunity for prevention afforded by incidental pelvic surgery including hysterectomy should, of course, be taken.

Influence of other factors

Age

The single biggest risk factor for ovarian cancer is age: there is a progressive increase in incidence into the sixth decade, with a small decline thereafter.[40] This knowledge is not, however, of great value in decision-making in Western countries, as it must be assumed that all women will reach the high-risk age group. It is of more use in women from families with hereditary ovarian cancer syndromes, who tend to be 7–14 years younger at diagnosis than the general population.[41] With regard to age as an influencing factor for oöphorectomy at the time of hysterectomy, in a premenopausal woman obviously the decision-making is more straightforward the older she is. Perhaps it would not be too controversial to recommend oöphorectomy at the time of hysterectomy for all women over the age of 45 years.

Ovulation interruption

One of the leading theories in the aetiology of ovarian cancer is the 'incessant ovulation' theory.[42,43] The protective effect of the pill has already been mentioned. The association between number of pregnancies and decreased risk of ovarian cancer is well established. Risk decreases with increasing parity among parous women and each additional pregnancy appears to be associated with a percentage risk reduction. Lactation, in the same way, confers protection.[44]

Ovulation stimulation

There has been much debate on the issue of the use of fertility drugs and the risk of ovarian cancer. In keeping with the theory that repeated ovulations disrupt the surface epithelium of the ovary, increasing the risk of malignant transformation, the use of drugs that result in multiple ovulations in one cycle could potentially increase the risk of ovarian cancer. (The same has been postulated for the use of gonadotrophins.) Whittemore et al.,[44] in their analysis of 12 US case–control studies, found an increased risk of ovarian cancer in women who had used fertility drugs [odds ratio (OR) 2.8] relative to women with no history of infertility, whereas women with infertility who had not used these drugs showed no increase in risk (OR 0.91). This risk was greatest in women who had taken clomiphene for more than ten cycles without achieving a pregnancy. It was later stressed by Whittemore[45] that the data did not allow for the separation of treatment effects from abnormalities of ovulation, which may themselves increase a woman's risk of ovarian cancer. Whittemore also commented that the lifetime risk of ovarian cancer in women who have used fertility drugs would be about 4–5%, less than that of breast cancer. Rossing et al.,[46] in a study of 3837 women who had been evaluated for infertility, also found a positive association between the use of clomiphene and ovarian cancer, particularly borderline tumours. This finding was especially valid if treatment had persisted for more than 12 months. To date, however, there are still insufficient data to prove a causal link.

Past history of breast cancer

A past history of premenopausal breast cancer increases an individual's propensity to develop ovarian cancer.[47] If such an individual were to undergo hysterectomy, this would provide a basis for recommending removal of the ovaries at the time of surgery. This has to be tempered by the knowledge that HRT, in these circumstances, carries its own problems. The decision-making is inevitably influenced by discussion, not only with the patient herself but also with her breast-cancer surgeon. Increasingly, HRT is used in such patients and a compromise may be a combination of oestrogen, progesterone and tamoxifen given concurrently, although it must be said that the data in support of such therapeutic manoeuvring are non-existent.

Racial and cultural considerations

When considering an individual's risk of ovarian cancer, it is important to take into account certain racial and cultural factors. Ovarian cancer is a disease of industrialized societies and there are marked geographical incidence rates: the highest incidences are seen in Scandinavia, with the highest rate seen in Sweden; Scandinavia is followed by Germany, the United Kingdom and the United States; the lowest rates are seen in Asia and Africa.[48] Immigration studies have shown, however, that this racial difference is not sustained when Asians and Africans migrate to Western countries.[49] The incidence is higher for professional groups than for the unskilled.[50] Certain ethnic groups are at particular risk of ovarian cancer, which is the most common gynaecological cancer to be diagnosed amongst Israeli Jewish women, with familial aggregation occurring within this population.[51]

Conclusions and recommended practice

Past advocacy of an individualized approach to this controversial subject has been greeted not so much by an appreciation of balance and fairness as by accusations of fence sitting. Lest this chapter be branded similarly indecisive, the authors suggest a schema for clinical practice. They do so in the knowledge that, in the absence of firm scientific data in many areas, their recommendations are open to criticism for not being 'evidence based' (you can't win!).

Oöphorectomy as a primary surgical procedure

In the past, this procedure has been advocated in women with a strong family history of disease (prescribing the oral contraceptive pill is advisable). Primary prophylaxis on completion of child bearing in women with two family members with the disease or genetically proven mutations is justifiable, following careful individual risk assessment and counselling. The reports of primary peritoneal carcinomatosis, although of concern, are rare even in these very high-risk women, and should not detract from the value of oöphorectomy nor deter the clinician from recommending prophylactic surgery. When prophylactic oöphorectomy is performed in this group, there should be careful surgical staging together with thorough histological examination of the ovaries.

Oöphorectomy at the time of pelvic surgery

Opportunistic secondary oöphorectomy should be offered to all women undergoing hysterectomy who are over the age of 40 years, and should be positively recommended to all women over the age of 45 years. Such a recommendation is strengthened if there is any family history of ovarian cancer, or if there is a past history of ovarian stimulation. Greater consideration should be given to the possibility of oöphorectomy at the time of vaginal hysterectomy. The feasibility and safety of this procedure has been demonstrated by Sheth and Malpani.[52] Laparoscopic assistance for this procedure might be chosen by some.

Finally, general surgical colleagues, when operating in the pelvis of postmenopausal women, might be encouraged to consider the possibility of opportunistic bilateral oöphorectomy (Table 22.3).

Table 22.3 Recommended practice for prophylactic oöphorectomy

Prophylactic oöphorectomy	Suitable patients
Primary	• Defined very-high-risk groups*
Secondary	• Offer to all >40 years • Recommend to all >45 years** • Consider at vaginal hysterectomy • Involve surgical colleagues

* Two or more proven first-degree relatives with disease.

** Particularly those with one relative with disease or a past history of ovulation stimulation.

References

1. Randall C L, Hall D W, Armenia C S. Pathology in the preserved ovary after unilateral oophorectomy. Am J Obstet Gynecol 1962; 84: 1233

2. Jacobs I, Oram D. Prevention of ovarian cancer: a survey of the practice of prophylactic oophorectomy by fellows and members of the Royal College of Obstetricians and Gynaecologists. Br J Obstet Gynaecol 1989; 96(5): 510–515

3. Conklin B H, McGuire P A, Weiler P L, Webb D I. A survey of the practice of prophylactic oophorectomy by gynecologists in the state of Alaska. Alaska Med 1996; 38(2): 71–74

4. The Cancer and Steroid Hormone Study of the Centers for Disease Control and the National Institute of Child Health and Human Development. The reduction in risk of ovarian cancer associated with oral contraceptive use. N Engl J Med 1987; 316(11): 650–655

5. Vessey M, Metcalf A, Well C et al. Ovarian neoplasms, functional ovarian cysts and oral contraceptives. Br Med J 1987; 294: 1518–1520

6. Kerlikowske K, Brown J S, Grady D G. Should women with familial ovarian cancer undergo prophylactic oophorectomy? Obstet Gynecol 1992; 80(4): 700–707

7. Howe H L. Age specific hysterectomy and oophorectomy prevalence rates and the risks for cancer of the reproductive system. Am J Public Health 1984; 74(6): 560–563

8. Sightler S E, Boike G M, Estape R E, Averette H E. Ovarian cancer in women with prior hysterectomy: a 14-year experience at the University of Miami. Obstet Gynecol 1991; 78(4): 681–684

9. Jacobs I, Oram D. Prophylactic oophorectomy. Br J Hosp Med 1987; 38(5): 440–449

10. Kontoravdis A, Kaligirou D, Antoniou G et al. Prophylactic oophorectomy in ovarian cancer prevention. Int J Gynaecol Obstet 1996; 54(3): 257–262

11. Jacobs I J, Oram D H. Oöphorectomy and prevention of ovarian cancer. In: Chamberlain G (ed) Contemporary obstetrics and gynaecology. London: Butterworths, 1988: 397–408

12. Speert H. Prophylaxis of ovarian cancer. Ann Surg 1949; 129: 468

13. Golub L J. The diagnosis of ovarian cancer. Am J Obstet Gynecol 1953; 66: 169–177

14. Counsellor V S, Hunt W, Haigler F H. Carcinoma of the ovary following hysterectomy. Am J Obstet Gynecol 1955; 69: 538–542

15. Fagan G E, Allen E D, Klawans A H. Ovarian neoplasms and repeat pelvic surgery. Obstet Gynecol 1956; 2: 418–421

16. Bloom M L. Certain observations based on a study of 141 cases of primary adenocarcinoma of the ovaries. South Afr Med J 1950–1959; 36: 714

17. Terz J J, Barber H R K, Brunschwiz A. Incidence of carcinoma in the retained ovary. Am J Surg 1967; 113: 511

18. Gibbs E K. Suggested prophylaxis for ovarian cancer. Am J Obstet Gynecol 1971; 111: 756–765

19. Kofler E. The incidence of previous hysterectomies and/or unilateral oophorectomies in women with malignant ovarian tumours. Geburtshilfe und Frauenheilkunde 1972; 32: 873–881

20. Grundsell H, Ekman G, Gullberg B et al. Some aspects of prophylactic oophorectomy and ovarian carcinoma. Ann Chir Gynaecol 1981; 70: 36–42

21. Jacobs I J, Oram D H. Prophylactic oophorectomy. Br J Hosp Med 1987; 38: 440–444

22. Stillwell S, Houdmont M, Paterson M E L. Ovarian function after radical hysterectomy for carcinoma of the cervix. Int J Gynecol Cancer 1997; 7: 49–56

23. Speroff T, Dawson N V, Speroff L, Haber R J. A risk-benefit analysis of elective bilateral oophorectomy: effect of changes in compliance with estrogen therapy an outcome. Am J Obstet Gynecol 1991; 164: 165–174

24. Collaborative Group on Hormonal Factors in Breast Cancer. Breast Cancer and Hormone Replacement Therapy: collaborative reanalysis of data from 51 epidemiological studies of 52705 women with breast cancer and 105411 women without breast cancer. Lancet 1997; 350: 1047–1059

25. Grogan R H. Reappraisal of residual ovaries. Am J Obstet Gynecol 1967; 97: 124–129

26. Whitelaw R G. Pathology and the conserved ovary. J Obstet Gynaecol Br Empire 1959; 66: 413–416

27. Randall C L. Ovarian conservation. In: Progress in Gynecology. Volume 4. New York: Grune and Stratton, 1963: 457

28. Randall C L, Hall D W, Armenia C S. Pathology in the preserved ovary after unilateral oophorectomy. Am J Obstet Gynecol 1962; 84: 1233

29. De Neef J C, Hollenbeck Z J R. The fate of ovaries preserved at the time of hysterectomy. Am J Obstet Gynecol 1966; 96: 1088–1097

30. McKenzie L L. Discussion of the frequency of oophorectomy at the time of hysterectomy. Am J Obstet Gynecol 1968; 100: 626–634

31. Ranney B, Abu-Ghazaleh S. The future function and fortune of ovarian tissue which is retained in vivo during hysterectomy. Am J Obstet Gynecol 1977; 128: 626–634

32. Tobacman J K, Tucker M A, Kase R et al. Intra-abdominal carcinomatosis after prophylactic oophorectomy in ovarian cancer prone families. Lancet 1982; ii: 795

33. Weber A M, Hewett W J, Gajewski W H, Curry S L. Serous carcinoma of the peritoneum after oophorectomy. Obstet Gynecol 1992; 80(3 Pt 2): 558–560

34. Piver M S, Tishi M F, Tsukada Y, Naraz G. Primary peritoneal carcinomatosis with prophylactic oophorectomy in women with a family history of ovarian cancer. Cancer 1993; 71(8): 2751–2755

35. Kemp G M, Hsiu J G, Andrews M C. Papillary peritoneal carcinomatosis after prophylactic oophorectomy. Gynecol Oncol 1992; 47(3): 395–397

36. Struewing J P, Watson P, Easton D F et al. Prophylactic oophorectomy in inherited breast/ovarian cancer families. Natl Cancer Inst Monogr 17. Bethesda: NCI, 1995: 33–35

37. Chen K T K, Schooley J L, Flam M S. Peritoneal carcinomatosis after prophylactic oophorectomy in familial ovarian cancer syndrome. Obstet Gynecol 1985; 66(3): 935–945

38. Salazar H, Godwin A K, Daly M B et al. Microscopic benign and malignant neoplasms and a cancer-prone phenotype in prophylactic oophorectomies. J Natl Cancer Inst 1996; 88(24): 1810–1820

39. Burke W, Daly M, Garber J et al. Recommendations for follow-up care of individuals with an inherited predisposition to cancer. II: BRCA1 and BRCA2. JAMA 1997; 277(12): 997

40. Yancik R, Ries LG, Yates J W. An analysis of surveillance, epidemiology, and end results program data. Am J Obstet Gynecol 1986; 154: 639–647

41. Lynch H T, Watson P, Bewtra C et al. Hereditary ovarian cancer: heterogeneity in age at diagnosis. Cancer 1991; 67: 1460–1466

42. Fathalla M F. Incessant ovulation — a factor in ovarian neoplasia? Lancet 1971; ii: 163

43. La Vecchia C, Franceschi S, Gallus G et al. Incessant ovulation and ovarian cancer: a critical approach. Int J Epidemiol 1983; 12: 161–164

44. Whittemore A S, Harris R, Itnyre J. Characteristics relating to ovarian cancer risk: collaborative analysis of 12 U.S. case–control studies. II. Invasive epithelial ovarian cancers in white women. Collaborative Ovarian Cancer Group. Am J Epidemiol 1992; 136(10): 1184–1203

45. Whittemore A S. Characteristics relating to ovarian cancer risk: implications for prevention and detection. Gynecol Oncol 1994; 55(3 Pt 2): S15–19

46. Rossing M A, Daling S R, Weiss N S et al. Ovarian tumours in a cohort of infertile women. N Engl J Med 1994; 331(12): 771–774

47. Prior P, Waterhouse J A H. Multiple primary cancers of the breast and ovary. Br J Cancer 1981; 44: 628–636

48. International Agency for Research on Cancer. Cancer incidence in five continents, Vol 3. IARC Scientific Publication No. 15. Lyon: IARC, 1976

49. Weiss N S, Homonchuck T, Young J L Jr. Incidence of the histologic types of ovarian cancer: the US Third National Cancer Survey 1969–1971. Gynecol Oncol 1977; 5: 161–167

50. Beral V, Fraser P, Chilvers C. Does pregnancy protect against ovarian cancer? Lancet 1978; 1: 1083–1087

51. Menczer J, Ben-Baruch G. Familial ovarian cancer in Israeli Jewish women. Obstet Gynecol 1991; 77(2): 276–277

52. Sheth S, Malpani A. Routine prophylactic oophorectomy at the time of vaginal hysterectomy in postmenopausal women. Arch Gynecol Obstet 1992; 251(2): 87–91

CHAPTER 23

Management of high-risk women

R. P. Soonawala and K. R. Damania

Introduction

Today, many treatment options are available for the management of menorrhagia. Treatment measures are often individualized, depending on the condition causing menorrhagia and the patient's characteristics and needs.

In the management of menorrhagia, two categories of high-risk women need to be addressed — namely, those at risk of a systemic disorder leading to menorrhagia and those at risk from conventional treatment modalities for menorrhagia.

Risk of systemic disorder leading to menorrhagia

A small proportion of the total cases of menorrhagia are caused by these conditions. They usually present as puberty menorrhagia, although presentation throughout the reproductive years is possible. Table 23.1 lists these disorders.

The risk to patients with systemic disorders can stem from a delay in exact diagnosis (incomplete history or investigation) and/or from inappropriate treatment or choice of a treatment modality that would put the patient with a systemic disorder at risk.

Among adolescents and (rarely) even adults[1] without a prior history of bleeding problems, menorrhagia can present as a symptom of von Willebrand's disease,[2] prothrombin deficiency, idiopathic thrombocytopenic purpura or platelet disorder.[3] Women with a history of high-risk factors, adolescents with menorrhagia, women with anovulatory dysfunctional uterine bleeding (DUB) who do not respond to medical or surgical therapy and women with ovulatory DUB without an anatomical uterine lesion should be screened for coagulopathy.[4] Acquired von Willebrand's disease is an unusual manifestation of hypothyroidism and is reversible with

Table 23.1 Systemic disorders leading to menorrhagia

- Coagulation disorders
- Thyroid disorders
- Leukaemia
- Tuberculosis
- Systemic lupus erythematosus
- Liver and renal dysfunction

thyroxine therapy.[5,6] Women unresponsive to 1-desamino-8-D-arginine vasopressin (DDAVP) in von Willebrand's disease often require blood products. The majority, around 90%, respond to oral contraceptive therapy, but a hysterectomy may be needed in non-responders.[7]

Surgery, in the form of therapeutic curettage or hysterectomy, can be performed in patients with congenital blood dyscrasias after adequate stabilization of the coagulation profile. For factor X deficiency, levels between 10 and 20% obtained from fresh-frozen plasma or factor IX are sufficient for haemostasis in the postoperative period.[8] In addition, in cases of severe systemic lupus erythematosus and thrombocytopenic purpura not responding to high doses of steroids, splenectomy may be considered.[9]

Severe hypothyroidism often results in menorrhagia. However, mild or early hypothyroidism can also result in abnormal bleeding patterns. Wilansky and Creisman[10] reported that 20% of menorrhagic women having early hypothyroidism, as evaluated by a thyrotrophin-releasing hormone (TRH) test, responded to L-thyroxine therapy: symptoms disappeared within 3–6 months and did not reappear after 1–3 years follow-up. The concentration of thyroid-stimulating hormone should, thus, be assessed in women not responding to medical therapy; subjecting such individuals to surgery without proper diagnosis would risk problems with anaesthesia. Aspirin, an 'over-the-counter' drug and a commonly taken analgesic, may explain and be a cause of occasional menorrhagia, especially in hypothyroid individuals: a study has indicated that thrombus-induced platelet serotonin release, following aspirin ingestion, is subnormal in hypothyroid patients. Hypothyroid women should be advised to avoid aspirin, as it may cause a sudden episode of menorrhagia.[11]

Genital tuberculosis often presents with infertility and amenorrhoea; however, in early tuberculous endometritis, menorrhagia may be the presenting complaint.[12] Liver dysfunction as a cause of menorrhagia is common in cases of primary biliary cirrhosis compared with cases of chronic active hepatitis or alcoholic liver disease; this could be a consequence of high concentrations of oestrogens in patients with primary biliary cirrhosis.[13] Patients with chronic renal disease often have menorrhagia: in one study of patients with chronic renal disease, 58% had menorrhagia.[14]

Management of these patients with a systemic illness entails the management of the disorder itself. Menorrhagia in most such cases resolves with the treatment of the causative disease, as in coagulopathies, hypothyroidism and tuberculosis. However, in those who do not respond, as often occurs early in the treatment of systemic illnesses, additional/alternative methods with medical drugs are used. These drugs are so selected that they should not be contraindicated in the presence of the primary systemic disease, such as oral contraceptive pills in biliary cirrhosis or prostaglandin synthetase inhibitors in renal disease. Surgical options may have to be resorted to only when there is failure to respond to the treatment of the underlying condition or additional medical treatment. The choice of procedure often takes into consideration the degree of stabilization of the condition, and utilizes techniques of minimal invasion, accompanied by intensive monitoring during anaesthesia and the postoperative period to minimize risk.[15]

It is important to take a proper history, as failure to suspect a systemic disorder can put the patient at risk. Iatrogenic causes of menorrhagia, such as hypothalamic depressants, digitalis, phenytoin, anticoagulants, sex steroids or a lost intra-uterine device, can also put the patient at risk, as such causes can be missed and incorrect treatment therefore given.[16]

Risk from conventional treatment of menorrhagia

Treatment modalities (medical or surgical) chosen for the management of menorrhagia can also pose a risk to certain patients. The choice of management not only should consider its effectiveness but also should take into consideration (a) the risk of existing disease leading to a contraindication, intolerance or side effects (especially when treatment is prolonged) and (b) the high cost of treatment (where cheaper but effective treatment is available). Choosing a suitable option for management of menorrhagia aims at giving maximum benefit while minimizing risk.

Risks of medical options

Studies have shown that the symptom of menorrhagia often returns when medical therapy has ceased;[17] hence, long-term therapy may be necessary. It is therefore important to consider the side effects and contraindications of specific drugs to minimize risk. As the duration of therapy is often prolonged, this leads to the increased risk of adverse effects; hence careful consideration of pharmacodynamics (with regard to absorption, metabolism and excretion) and of drug interactions is necessary before drug selection.

Combined oral contraceptive pills and progesterone   These are the most frequently prescribed drugs for the treatment of menorrhagia. Although they are effective in cases of essential menorrhagia, caution needs to be exercised in prescribing them to older women (especially those who smoke), in view of their cardiovascular risk. As well as being contraindicated in patients at risk of thrombo-embolic disorders, liver dysfunction, recent jaundice, rotor syndrome and Dubin–Johnson syndrome, common side effects such as weight gain, abdominal discomfort, breast enlargement, chloasma and occasional spotting (breakthrough bleeding) limit their long-term use.

Centchroman   Centchroman, a non-steroidal oral contraceptive, has none of these side effects. Its potent anti-oestrogenic activity on the endometrium can be used to benefit patients with menorrhagia in a dosage schedule of one tablet twice a week. Although not useful in acute bleeding episodes owing to its delayed action, it is effective in the long term without side effects or contraindications as with hormonal contraceptives.[18]

Non-steroidal anti-inflammatory drugs   These are well-tested, effective and often well-tolerated agents; however, they are contraindicated in patients with glaucoma or with a history of gastrointestinal ulcerations. Common side effects reported are headache and gastrointestinal disturbance causing dyspepsia, nausea, vomiting or diarrhoea. However, since these drugs are prescribed to be taken only during the time of menstruation (that is, usually for not more than 5 days each cycle), adverse effects associated with long-term use, such as haemolytic anaemia, jaundice or leucopenia, are not seen.

Antifibrinolytics   Tranexamic acid and epsilon-aminocaproic acid (EACA) have been used in menorrhagia. Common side effects of tranexamic acid are nausea and diarrhoea, however, the possibility of arterial thrombosis is of more concern.[19] An ester prodrug of tranexamic acid (Kabi 2161) increases the bioavailability of tranexamic acid, leading to decreased frequency of administration and less-frequent gastrointestinal side effects.[20] EACA, too, is associated with side effects of nausea, dizziness, diarrhoea, headaches and abdominal discomfort; renal disease is a contraindication to its use. An increased risk of thrombo-embolic disease and a case of cerebral sinus thrombosis have been reported with its prolonged use for treatment of menorrhagia.[21]

Danazol   In an effort to reduce common side effects and the risk of hormonal pseudomenopausal symptoms such as weight gain, migraine, headache, hot flushes and emotional lability, but at the same time to maintain efficacy at low cost, danazol in daily doses of 200 mg has been shown to be effective for menorrhagia. Long-term use (more than 6 months) of danazol needs to be monitored by serum liver enzyme studies. Drug interaction with warfarin anticoagulant therapy (potentiating the effect of warfarin), which is a paradoxical effect, has been reported.[22,23] Furthermore, a case report of benign intracranial hypertension (BIH) in a woman receiving danazol therapy for menorrhagia, leading to headache and visual symptoms, emphasizes the need for more careful assessment in order to avoid visual failure due to advanced BIH.[24]

Gonadotrophin-releasing hormone (GnRH) analogues   Although GnRH analogues are highly effective, the high cost of therapy and long-term risk of hypo-oestrogenic effects (including osteoporosis) have limited their use. Combining them with cyclical HRT can control the risk of demineralization without impairing their efficacy.[25]

Radiotherapy   Radiotherapy is not a primary mode of therapy, as the procedure leaves a damaged organ that is liable to develop haematometra, pyometra and even cancers (cancer of the cervix or endometrium, or leukaemias), especially with X-ray irradiation[26,27] or brachytherapy (internal radiation).[28] These risks far outweigh any advantages. However, very rarely, when radiotherapy is decided upon (especially in a patient who is resistant to drug treatment and is at very high risk for surgical options, even those that are minimally invasive), teletherapy (external irradiation) is preferred.

Coagulants   Styptic agents such as flavonoids (Diosmin),[29] rutin, vitamin K, vitamin C, vitamin A[30] and vitamin E[31] have been tried. Injections of haemocoagulase (Botropase, Reptilase) isolated from the venom of Brazilian snakes of the *Bothrops* species have also been use for their astringent properties for emergency haemostasis in menorrhagia. As they are coagulants, there is the risk that they may cause thrombotic episodes in patients liable to these, but they are often used as stopgap regimens in high-risk patients where other medical treatments are contraindicated, owing to systemic illness, or have failed. The patient is normally awaiting surgery and often under investigation for surgical fitness. Coagulants can also be used as adjuvants to other medical regimens for improved effectiveness. It is important to add here that the literature lacks proper studies and that their results are often uncertain.

Risks of surgical options
In spite of the risk of major morbidity and even mortality, surgical options are often preferred by patients and gynaecologist alike, owing to their 'one-off' benefit and better satisfaction over time.

Women undergoing surgery for menorrhagia can risk problems from the anaesthesia or the surgery.

Anaesthesia   Risk conditions for anaesthesia include the following:

- Restricted pulmonary function (intestinal pulmonary fibrosis, bronchiectasis)
- Impaired cardiac status
- Unstable hypertension
- Severe diabetes
- Morbid obesity.

Ways of reducing anaesthetic risk include thorough preoperative assessment, the use of intra-operative monitoring tools, and safer anaesthetic agents associated with intensive postoperative care facilities. In high-risk situations, the choice of anaesthesia (whether regional or general) should be made with regard to safety, rather than according to personal (surgeon or patient) preferences. An anaesthetist in such situations often prefers low regional anaesthesia for pelvic surgery and also prefers the gynaecologist to take the vaginal route, thus avoiding general anaesthesia and the use of muscle relaxants.[32]

Surgical risk Traditionally, dilatation and curettage (D&C) and hysterectomy (either vaginal or abdominal) are the surgical procedures selected for menorrhagia. The surgical operation of hysterectomy has an increased risk in the presence of certain associated conditions, as listed in Table 23.2; and in these cases it is logical to take steps to minimize risk or choose alternative methods.

Table 23.2 Conditions in which hysterectomy is associated with increased risk

Frozen pelvis
- Pelvic inflammatory disease (PID) including genital tuberculosis
- Severe endometriosis
- Previous multiple laparotomies

Leiomyoma
- Multiple and large fibroids
- Cervical fibroids
- Broad-ligament fibroid

Minimizing risk from surgery   Risk from surgical procedures can be reduced in the following ways:

1. Preoperative assessment. In high-risk cases, additional investigations are necessary. These include:

   • Haematology (blood dyscrasias)
   • Ultrasound (size and location of fibroids/pathology, hydronephrotic change)
   • Intravenous pyelography (delineation of ureter)
   • CT/MRI (identify anatomical distortion due to coexisting pathology). These aids help to build a 'virtual reality' picture of gynaecological anatomy and disease pathology in the surgeon's mind so that he is better prepared for the surgical difficulties he may encounter and have no surprises on the operating table.

2. Reducing intraoperative/postoperative risk. Appropriate measures include the following:

   • An examination under anaesthesia to decide route of hysterectomy, assessment of pathology (pelvic inflammatory disease, fibroid) and type of incision.
   • Control of blood loss and achievement of a clearer field of surgery by the use of mechanical devices (Bonney's Myomectomy Clamp, rubber catheter around uterine isthmus) or chemical 'tourniquets' (adrenaline, vasopressin). In cases of continuous bleeding after D&C for acute bleeding, the author has, on occasion, controlled the bleeding by inserting a 50 ml 16 Fr Foley catheter via the cervix, then inflated it and left it in the uterus for 2–4 hours; this was subsequently removed in the recovery room, with success.
   • Use of retroperitoneal approaches for dissection and identification of anatomical structures such as the ureter, bladder and pelvic vascular structures.
   • Acknowledgement by the surgeon of his limitations, with the ability to ask for help as and when necessary.
   • Preoperative use of antibiotics, especially in those at risk of postoperative infection.
   • Intensive postoperative patient monitoring, especially where problems are anticipated or in those who have had intra-operative difficulties.

Alternative surgical techniques Alternative methods, such as hysteroscopic polypectomy or myomectomy and hysteroscopic endometrial resection/ablation, developed for patients at risk and in whom the hysterectomy was undesirable, dangerous or impossible,[33,34] have themselves become standard acceptable modalities of surgical treatment for menorrhagia. The main advantages stem from the possibility of performing these procedures under local anaesthesia using a paracervical block, with or without intravenous sedation, and the fact that, with a transvaginal approach, the problems of a difficult peritoneal approach do not arise.

Furthermore, performing the hysterectomy with laparoscopic assistance, as in minimal invasive or operative endoscopy, has become associated with patient satisfaction and reduced hospital costs; nevertheless, these techniques have brought newer risks of prolonged pneumo-insufflation, fluid overload and bowel burns. Technology, fortunately, has kept abreast: newer equipment for these techniques aims at reducing these risks. Today, non-hysteroscopic thermal coagulation,[35] endometrial cryo-ablation,[36] gasless laparoscopic myomectomy,[37] and radiographic uterine artery embolization[38] are newer techniques suitable in risk situations. These may become standard methods in the future and are discussed in separate chapters in this volume.

Conclusions

In conclusion, it is important to remember that high-risk patients often present with a history of systemic disorder or have an undiagnosed blood dyscrasia. They have already consulted one or more gynaecologists, but medical therapies may have failed or produced adverse effects, whereas surgical options have been associated with complications and are undesirable. Managing such patients is difficult and often a dilemma; treatment mostly has to be tailor-made. The physician should approach the problem with a fresh and open mind, willing to alter dosage or regimen if either, after one or two trial cycles, do not produce results. The patient too, should be made to understand her particular situation and be encouraged to participate in all decisions.

The goal of any high-risk manager is to minimize risk and maintain client satisfaction. This goal, in the treatment of menorrhagia, can be achieved by diligently searching for and identifying the exact cause of the menorrhagia. For the subsequent line of treatment, due consideration should be given to drug contraindications or side effects. Physicians should also understand their surgical capabilities and make surgical decisions with regard to their work environment and terms of practice.

References

1. Weiss R M. Case presentation: a patient with von Willebrand's disease with menorrhagia. Am J Obstet Gynecol 1996; 175: 763–765

2. Ahuja R, Kriplani A, Choudhary VP, Takkar D. Von Willebrand's disease: a rare cause of puberty menorrhagia. Aust N Z J Obstet Gynaecol 1995; 35: 337–338

3. Southeimer S J. Menorrhagia and abnormal vaginal bleeding. In: Benrubi G I (ed) Obstetric and gynecologic emergencies. Philadelphia: Lippincott, 1994: 251–262

4. Brenner P F. Differential diagnosis of abnormal uterine bleeding. Am J Obstet Gynecol 1996; 175: 766–769

5. Attivissimo L A, Lichtman S M, Klein I. Acquired von Willebrand's syndrome causing a hemorrhagic diathesis in a patient with hypothyroidism. Thyroid 1995; 5: 399–401

6. Bruggers C S, McElligot K, Rallison M L. Acquired von Willebrand's disease in twins with autoimmune hypothyroidism: response to desmopressin and L-thyroxin therapy. J Pediatr 1994; 125: 911–913

7. Foster P A. The reproductive health of women with von Willebrand's disease unresponsive to D.D.A.V.P.: results of an international survey. Thromb Haemost 1995; 74: 784–790

8. Knight R D, Barr C F, Alving B M. Replacement therapy for congenital factor X deficiency. Transfusion 1985; 25: 78–80

9. Himan W P, Dineen P. The role of splenectomy in the treatment of thrombocytopenic purpura due to systemic lupus erythematosus. Am Surg 1978; 187: 52–56

10. Wilansky D L, Creisman B. Early hypothyroidism in patients with menorrhagia. Am J Obstet Gynecol 1989; 160: 673–677

11. Zeigler Z R, Hasiba U, Lewis J H et al. Hemostatic defects in response to aspirin challenge in hypothyroidism. Am J Hematol 1986; 23: 391–399

12. Bhaskar Rao K. Pelvic inflammatory disease. In: Ratnam S S, Bhaskar Rao K, Arulkumar S (eds) Obstetrics and gynecology for postgraduates, vol.2. Madras: Longman, 1994: 385–393

13. Stellon A J, William R. Increased incidence of menstrual abnormalities and hysterectomy preceding primary biliary cirrhosis. Br Med J 1986; 293: 297–298

14. Cochrane R, Regan L. Undetected gynaecological disorders in women with renal disease. Hum Reprod 1997; 12: 667–670

15. Berry D L, DeLeon F D. Endometrial abortion for severe menorrhagia in patient with hereditary hemorrhagic telangiectasis. A case report. J Reprod Med 1996; 41: 183–185

16. Brenner P F. Differential diagnosis of abnormal uterine bleeding. Am J Obstet Gynecol 1996; 175: 766–769

17. Shaw R W. Assessment of medical treatments of menorrhagia. Br J Obstet Gynaecol 1994; 101(suppl 11): 15–18

18. Levi J M. Personal communication, Chief Medical Officer, Family Welfare Programme, Nowrosjee Wadia Maternity Hospital, Mumbai, 1998

19. Agnelli G, Gresele P, DeCurto M et al. Tranexamic acid and intrauterine contraceptive devices and fetal cerebral arterial thrombosis. Br J Obstet Gynaecol 1982; 89: 681–682

20. Edlund M, Anderson K, Rybo G et al. Reduction of menstrual loss in women suffering from idiopathic menorrhagia with a novel antifibrinolytic drug (Kabi 2161). Br J Obstet Gynaecol 1995; 102: 913–917

21. Achivon A, Gornish M, Melamed F. Cerebral sinus thrombosis as a potential hazard of antifibrinolytic treatment in menorrhagia. Stroke 1990; 21: 817–819

22. Small M, Peterkin M, Lowe G D et al. Danazol and oral anticoagulants. Scott Med J 1982: 27: 331–332

23. Meeks M L, Mahaffey K W, Katz M D. Danazol increases the anticoagulant effect of warfarin. Ann Pharmacother 1997; 26: 641–642

24. Pear J, Sandercock P A. Benign intracranial hypertension associated with danazol. Scott Med J 1990; 35: 49

25. Thomas E J. Add-back therapy for long term use in dysfunctional uterine bleeding and uterine fibroids. Br J Obstet Gynaecol 1996: 103 (Suppl 14): 18–21

26. Smith P G, Doll R. Late effects of X-irradiation in patients treated for metropathia haemorrhagica. Br J Radiol 1976; 49: 224–232

27. Darby S C, Reeves G, Key T et al. Mortality in a cohort of women given x-ray therapy for metropathia haemorrhagica. Int J Cancer 1994; 56: 763–801

28. Thomas W D, Harris H H, Enden J A. Post irradiation malignant neoplasm of the uterine fundus. Am J Obstet Gynecol 1969; 104: 209–219

29. Darmaillacq R, Sentenac J. A non-hormonal therapeutic agent in menorrhagia. Clinical trial of Daflon. Bord Med 1972; 5: 71–76

30. Lithigon D M, Politzer W H. Vitamin A in the treatment of menorrhagia. S Afr Med J 1979; 51: 191–193

31. Dasgupta P R, Dutta S, Banerjee P, Majumdar S. Vitamin E (alpha tocopherol) in the management of menorrhagia associated with the use of intrauterine contraceptive devices (IUCD). Int J Fertil 1983; 83: 55–56

32. Sheth S S. Vaginal hysterectomy. In: Studd J (ed) Progress in obstetrics and gynaecology, Vol. 10. Edinburgh: Churchill Livingstone, 1993: 317–340

33. DeCherney A H, Polan M L. Hysteroscopic management of intrauterine lesions and intractable uterine bleeding. Obstet Gynecol 1983; 61: 392–397

34. Lockwood M, Magos A L, Baumann R, Turnbull A C. Endometrial resection when hysterectomy is undesirable, dangerous or impossible. Br J Obstet Gynaecol 1990; 97: 656–658

35. Prior M V, Phipps J H, Roberts T et al. Treatment of menorrhagia by radiofrequency heating. Int J Hyperthermia 1991; 7: 213–220

36. Pittroff R, Majid S, Murray A. Transcervical endometrial cryoablation for menorrhagia. Int J Gynaecol Obstet 1994; 47: 135–140

37. Chang F H, Soong Y K, Cheng P J et al. Laparoscopic myomectomy for large symptomatic leiomyoma using airlift gasless laparoscopy: a preliminary report. Hum Reprod 1996; 11: 1427–1432

38. Ravina J H, Herbretan D, Ciraru-Vigneron N et al. Arterial embolization to treat uterine myomata. Lancet 1995; 346: 671–672

The abnormal uterine bleeding clinic: a role in advising family doctors on the management of menorrhagia

P. M. Coats

Introduction

Women who suffer from abnormal uterine bleeding commonly appeal for medical help: 12% or more of new referrals to a general gynaecology outpatient clinic are made because of abnormal uterine bleeding[1] and one-half of all the hysterectomies recorded in the United Kingdom are performed because of menorrhagia.[2]

A patient is seen for the first time by her family doctor and treatment is given to her on the basis of the best clinical judgement that can be made. It is because of this that, in 1993, 822,000 prescriptions were written by medical practitioners for 345,225 women for this complaint.[3] If the patient's symptoms cannot be corrected easily, then sooner or later a precise diagnosis has to be made.

Women who complain of abnormal uterine bleeding are often concerned that their unusual menstrual loss is due to a serious disorder. Chaotic, heavy or frequent periods are commonly the presenting symptoms. After menstruation has ceased, bleeding may appear unexpectedly and many women are worried that they might have cancer. A comprehensive and sympathetic assessment is imperative.

The patient's history and examination are important guides to diagnosis. Investigations by the family doctor should include at least a full blood count, thyroid function testing and, if indicated, a clotting screen. Conditional treatment may be started in primary care.

If the patient's symptoms do not improve, then the family doctor will request a hospital consultation.

The diagnostic service

The outpatient consultation that follows often results in the patient being admitted to hospital for additional investigations. A critical examination of the uterine cavity is necessary to demonstrate the presence (or otherwise) of intra-uterine pathology. A hysteroscopy with sampling of the endometrium is the procedure of choice and is often carried out under general anaesthesia. Most patients are treated as day cases,[4] but Goldrath has proposed that this investigation should be performed on an outpatient basis.[5]

This approach can be developed to assess the patient comprehensively at 'one outpatient visit' and to give her and her family doctor immediate advice. An ideal way to achieve this is to set up a clinic dedicated to investigating the complaint of abnormal uterine bleeding. By creating a team of skilled nurses, doctors, reception staff and secretaries, it is possible to provide the patient with a diagnosis at one visit.[6] If properly structured, a 'one visit clinic' is effective and spares resources.[7]

This chapter describes one such clinic that has been run successfully for more than 6 years at the Royal Surrey County Hospital, Guildford, where it serves a population of 240,000.

Clinic amenities

A 'one stop' diagnostic clinic for abnormal uterine bleeding should ideally be placed at a convenient location within the hospital. It should have a pleasant waiting area and be supported by appropriate patient services. Reception staff need to appreciate the clinic's purpose and support the 'total care' philosophy for the patient's 'one' diagnostic episode.

Small details matter to the patient. Lack of adequate municipal arrangements, such as poor car parking or public transport, can lead to unnecessary anxiety being created in the patient before she is ever seen for consultation. A relaxed and composed patient is much easier to assess and examine by hysteroscope.

Patient selection

It may be difficult to establish the severity of a patient's symptoms on presentation. Whether the patient is suitable for assessment as an outpatient can be gathered from the substance of a good referral letter.

The complaint of abnormal uterine bleeding is frequently difficult to evaluate, as the amount of blood lost by a patient is subjective and it is generally assessed by the patient herself. Her history may not always be accompanied by unequivocal laboratory evidence of anaemia. Various appraisal procedures have been used in an attempt to measure the severity of the symptom: pictorial blood loss assessment charts are one example of this.[8] The author has found that a daily numerical estimation of menstrual loss measured by the patient recorded on a scale of 0–5 has practical value: it encourages the patient to document her bleeding as it evolves (Fig. 24.1), while allowing practised professionals to judge the subjective importance of the complaint.

Figure 24.1 A simple global estimation of menstrual loss recorded on a scale of 0–5 and kept as a daily record by the patient.

Month	1	2	3	4	5	6	7	8	9	10	11	12	13	14	15	16	17	18	19	20	21	22	23	24	25	26	27	28	29	30	31
January														0	5	3	3	2	1								0	0			
February												0	3	3	2	2	1	0						0							
March								1	1	3	3	1	0										0	0	0						
April						0	1	1	3	3	1									0	0										
May																															
June																															
July																															
August																															
September																															
October																															
November																															
December																															

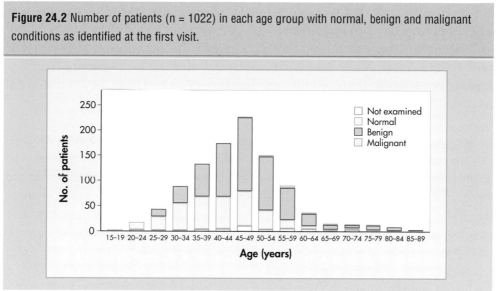

Figure 24.2 Number of patients (n = 1022) in each age group with normal, benign and malignant conditions as identified at the first visit.

There are, of course variations in blood loss within an individual patient[9] and between patient groups.[10–12] A good guide (and strong justification) for investigating the symptom is simply to heed the patient when she senses that her normal menstrual flow is altered: the complaint at that time deserves attention.

It is unnecessary to subject women under the age of 30 years to hysteroscopy; the amount of pathology found is likely to be small. In the author's series of more than 900 outpatient hysteroscopies, less than 7% of the pathology occurred in women under 30 years of age. Between the ages of 30 and 40 years, 22% of all pathology was seen (Fig. 24.2). This is in contrast to the suggestion from epidemiological data,[4] that cervical dilatation and uterine curettage are not justified under the age of 40 years.

Figure 24.3 Scheme of operation of an abnormal uterine bleeding clinic.

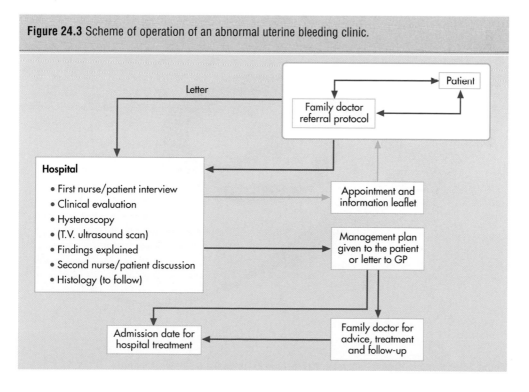

Excessive and prolonged menstrual loss leads women to be anxious[13] and to seek an explanation for their complaint. They are frequently relieved when a logical reason can be given and a sound diagnosis made. If this is then shared with the family doctor, much of the anxiety created by the symptom is eased and a cognitive approach to care can then be followed. The flow chart in Figure 24.3 outlines the elements of a 'one visit clinic'.

Basic equipment

Precise examination of the uterine cavity and pelvis requires special equipment, as listed below. A case can be made for either hysteroscopy or ultrasound[14] but, in reality, each is complementary to the other and, taken together, they will improve the global information available for the clinical decision-making process. The equipment required is as follows:

1. Gynaecological examination chair
2. Cusco's speculum
3. Flexible hysteroscope (Fig. 24.4)
4. Light source of at least 300 watts
5. Hysteroflator
6. Endometrial sampler
7. Sterilization equipment
8. Transvaginal ultrasound.

Staff requirements

The most experienced nursing and medical staff available are needed to run an abnormal uterine bleeding clinic. A skilful nurse is of immeasurable value, particularly if she has a mature understanding of general gynaecology. She is in the best position to talk to the patient initially and to discuss the complaint. An early

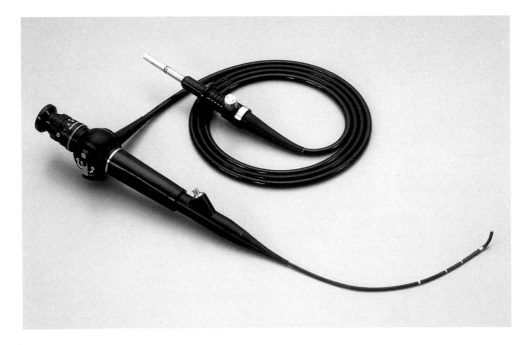

Figure 24.4 Olympus Hystero-Fiberscope HYF Type XP (external diameter 3.1 mm).

empathy with the patient's problem is one of the keys to the success of the outpatient examination.[15]

The nurse specialist verifies the history of the patient's complaint and gathers information on her general medical condition. She carefully notes the patient's menstrual pattern with reference to the cycle length. If there is evidence of endocrine disease, this is recorded. Past obstetric and fertility history are noted on a proforma. Special attention should be paid to how the complaint affects the patient's life: an analogue score is helpful to ascertain this.

The nurse bonds with the patient while establishing the history of the complaint. She can then explain to the patient the basic nature of the examination and describe the procedures of hysteroscopy, transvaginal ultrasound and endometrial sampling (Fig. 24.5).

The doctor can rapidly become conversant with the patient's history, related by the specialist nurse, while the patient is preparing to be examined. During the hysteroscopic procedure, the nurse behaves as the patient's advocate and friend; she can lend support or distraction, as the situation may require, while the patient is examined. A diagnosis is reached by the hysteroscopist and discussed with the patient in front of the nurse. Advice on treatment is then given.

Finally, because of her experience, the nurse is in a position to explain the nature and implications of any pathology found by the doctor. The patient's understanding is reinforced and she leaves the clinic confident in her grasp of the problem. Similar nursing roles are advocated in many other areas of clinical practice.[16–18]

The nursing staff has an important additional role in maintaining equipment and ensuring that it operates reliably.

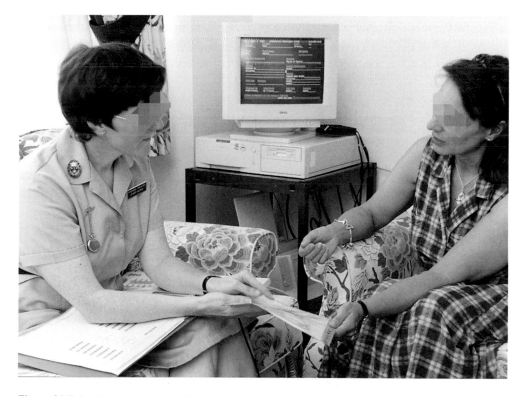

Figure 24.5 A relaxed nurse specialist/patient interview.

Procedure of outpatient flexible hysteroscopy

An unobstructed view of the perineum is easily obtained by using an electronically operated gynaecological examination chair. The cervix is visualized using a bivalve speculum, which permits manipulation of the direction of the cervix in the vaginal vault. A single-toothed vulsellum forceps can then be secured to the ectocervix at a point close to the external os; gentle traction may be applied, if necessary. Mucus is cleared from the cervix and a flexible hysteroscope 3.6 mm in diameter is passed into the canal (Fig. 24.4).

Carbon dioxide is the distension medium and is supplied from a hysteroflator that accurately dispenses a small volume of gas at a low flow rate under limited pressure. The gas flow is set at 38–40 ml/min with a maximum distension pressure of no more than 40 mmHg. The investigation can be completed in less than 2 minutes, using no more than 100 ml carbon dioxide. By adhering to these pressures and flow rate, it is possible to avoid carbon dioxide entering the peritoneal cavity and causing diaphragmatic irritation and shoulder pain. A pan-endoscopic view of the uterine cavity is obtained and with dextrous manipulation of the flexible scope, all areas of the cavity can be explored (Figs. 24.6–24.8). Withdrawal of the instrument must be preceded by the release of the intra-uterine gas pressure. The walls of the collapsed uterine cavity are then opposed and this facilitates Pipelle sampling of the endometrium; histology is requested.

An audit of patients' responses to flexible outpatient hysteroscopy without analgesia was favourable: 80–90% experienced no noticeable pain.

Communications

Although a comprehensive history and examination may provide a preliminary diagnosis it must be noted that the relationship between subjective assessment of menstrual blood loss and the objective appraisal is poor.[9]

The developments in modern hysteroscopy[19] and, to some extent, the slower development of the flexible hysteroscope, has allowed a critical view of the uterine cavity to be obtained; pathology is commonly discovered[7] and remedial non-radical

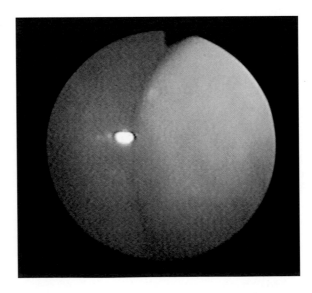

Figure 24.6 A benign endometrial polyp.

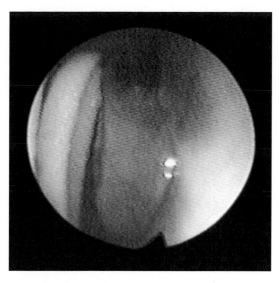

Figure 24.7 A polyp and intra-uterine device.

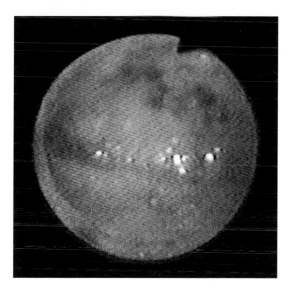

Figure 24.8 An atrophic uterine cavity.

treatment can be planned. Family doctors seek guidance on the best evidence available to plan their patients' future care rationally. They appreciate a precise diagnosis, with swift provision of advice both to themselves and to their patients.

Sensitive and perceptive handling of the patient by all the clinical staff is a fundamental component of care in a 'one visit clinic'. Every effort should be made to provide an appointment within 7–10 days from the date of referral. The patient's concerns are at their greatest when there is a fear of malignant disease. Patients often attend the clinic alone.

Whereas, in 30% of referrals the patient claims to be postmenopausal, the majority of patients simply find their menstrual loss to be of concern to them. Endometrial malignancy is the primary concern of the majority of perimenopausal and menopausal women and their family doctors; the majority can be reassured following outpatient hysteroscopy and evaluation.

Anovulatory cycles are common at the extremes of the fertile years and rational

Table 24.1 Feelings (shown as a percentage) expressed by women who have undergone outpatient flexible hysteroscopy

Feeling	Intensity			
	Very/quite	A little	Not at all	N/R
Embarrassed	21	38	35	6
Fearful	7	38	48	7
In pain	11	42	42	5
Comfortable	72	6	14	8
Undignified	21	39	32	8
Relaxed	62	18	13	7
Anxious	15	49	31	5

N/R, not recorded.

treatment, correcting the fault in the luteal phase, is valuable. Anovulatory bleeding requires further assessment and the exclusion of systemic disease or local pelvic pathology before prudent management can be advised.

Findings

Outpatient flexible hysteroscopy is an especially acceptable investigation for the patient (Table 24.1) when it is carried out by competent staff; it may be argued to be the 'gold standard' of intra-uterine visualization. The results of the clinical examination and the flexible hysteroscopic findings are shared immediately with the patient, the nurse specialist and any other involved person who may be present, such as a chosen family member. This is helped by video-endoscopy (Table 24.2).

More than one-third of the hysteroscopic findings in an abnormal uterine bleeding clinic are normal (Table 24.2); this is of immediate relief to the patient. In those cases where there is an abnormality, the pathology may be visualized by the patient, enhancing her understanding of the problem. This helps particularly in explaining to the patient why treatment is required. In less than 3% of unselected cases, an experienced hysteroscopist cannot perform flexible hysteroscopy on an outpatient basis (Table 24.3).

Advice to the patient and family doctor

Although a final decision on treatment may be delayed until the histopathological results are available, medical or surgical advice can be given and a substantive management plan set out before the patient leaves the abnormal uterine bleeding clinic.

Conservative care may be discussed and limited surgical intervention considered, such as transcervical resection of intra-uterine polyps or fibroids. If more definitive surgery is planned, then this can be further talked over between the patient, her family doctor and her family.

A holistic approach, such as that proposed, sends an important message in terms of the future direction of patient care. It also achieves an objective of cost

Table 24.2 Primary hysteroscopic diagnosis in 916 consecutive patients referred for abnormal uterine bleeding

Diagnosis	No. of patients
Normal uterine cavity	316
Irregular uterine cavity	6
Endometrium	
Adhesions	9
Atrophic	72
Haemorrhagic	4
Inflammation	14
Progesterone effect	4
Hyperplastic	25
Malignant endometrium	12
Uterine anomalies	9
Fibroids	
Intra-uterine	136
Intramural	68
Polyps	
Cervical	57
Intra-uterine	111
?Adenomyosis	19
Unclassified	2
Not examined	
Bleeding	7
Cervical ectopy	1
Cervical polyps	4
Cervical stenosis	4
Vaginitis	2
Hysterectomy	1
Others	22
Haematometria	2
Vaginitis	9

containment that is greatly extolled by health economists. Above all, the patient retains a sense of ownership of her care — something greatly appreciated by many women today.

Key points

The main advantages of the system outlined above are as follows:

1. It is a dedicated clinic for abnormal uterine bleeding;
2. It is staffed by experienced professionals;

Table 24.3 Reasons given why 53/916 (5.8%) clinic attenders did not undergo hysteroscopy

Reason	No. of patients
Cervical stenosis	9
Intramural fibroids	3
Bleeding	8
Vaginitis	5
Hysterectomy	2
Cervical polyps	4
No reason given	22
Technical failure acknowledged	25 (2.7%)

3. No anaesthetic is needed for examination of the uterine cavity with a flexible hysteroscope;
4. All patients are spared general anaesthesia;
5. One-third of patients have a normal uterine cavity;
6. Many patients have intra-uterine pathology that can be treated with moderate surgical intervention only.

References

1. Barlow J, Coulter A, Brooks P. Patterns of referral. Oxford: Health Services Research Unit, 1992.
2. Coulter A, Klassen A, McPherson K. How many hysterectomies should purchasers buy? Eur J Public Health 1995
3. Coulter A, Kelland J, Long A et al. The management of menorrhagia. Effect Health Care Bull 1995; 9: 1–10
4. Coulter A, Klassen A, MacKenzie I, McPherson K. Diagnostic dilatation and curettage: is it used appropriately? Br Med J 1993; 306: 236–239
5. Goldrath M H, Sherman A I. Office hysteroscopy and suction curettage: can we eliminate the hospital diagnostic dilatation and curettage? Am J Obstet Gynecol 1985; 152(2): 220–229
6. Baskett T F, O'Connor H, Magos A L. A comprehensive one-stop menstrual problem clinic for the diagnosis and management of abnormal uterine bleeding. Br J Obstet Gynaecol 1996; 103(1): 76–77
7. Coats P M, Haines P, Kent A S H. Flexible hysteroscopy: an outpatient evaluation in abnormal uterine bleeding. Gynaecol Endosc 1997; 6: 229–235
8. Higham J M, O'Brien P M, Shaw R W. Assessment of menstrual blood loss using a pictorial chart. Br J Obstet Gynaecol 1990; 97(8): 734–739
9. Hallberg L, Nilsson L. Determination of menstrual blood loss. Scand J Lab Invest 1964; 16: 224–228
10. Barer A P, Fowler W M. The blood loss during normal menstruation. Am J Obstet Gynecol 1936; 31: 979–986
11. Hallberg L, Hogdahl A, Nilsson L, Rybo G. Menstrual blood loss — a population study. Acta Obstet Gynecol Scand 1966 45: 320–351
12. Cole S L, Billewicz W Z, Thomas A M. Sources of variation in menstrual blood loss. J Obstet Gynaecol Br Commonw 1971; 78: 933–939

13. Sherry S, Notman M T, Nadelson C C et al. Anxiety, depression, and menstrual symptoms among freshman medical students. J Clin Psychiatry 1988; 49(12): 490–493

14. Al-Azzawi F. Hysteroscopy or ultrasound? Curr Opin Obstet Gynecol 1996; 8(4): 246–249

15. Quinn P. Developing a direct access outpatient hysteroscopy service. Nurs Stand 1996; 10(33): 40–42

16. Albarran J W, Whittle C. An analysis of professional, specialist and advanced nursing practice in critical care. Nurse Educ Today 1997; 17(1): 72–79

17. Poole K. The evolving role of the clinical nurse specialist within the comprehensive breast cancer centre. J Clin Nurs 1996; 5(6): 341–349

18. Jary J, Franklin L. The role of the specialist nurse in breast cancer. Prof Nurse 1996; 11(10): 664–665

19. Kowdley K V, Silverstein F E. Future developments in endoscopic imaging. Baillieres Clin Gastroenterol 1995; 9(1): 173–183

CHAPTER 25

Choice of treatment for menorrhagia

G. Khastgir and J. Studd

Introduction

Menorrhagia is rarely life threatening but can result in considerable inconvenience, embarrassment and ill health. Lives may need to be adjusted around a menstrual calendar, with social and work commitments being cancelled during the bleeding days. Excessive menstrual flow is often painful and many suffer from chronic pelvic pain, premenstrual syndrome (PMS) and menstrual migraine. In some women, iron-deficiency anaemia may ensue if the diet fails to compensate for the excessive menstrual loss. Prolonged suffering from such physical incapacities and social limitations is likely to make these women depressed and to affect their sexual function. Thus, the main purpose of any treatment is to relieve the symptoms and, in consequence, to improve the overall quality of life.[1]

There is considerable debate about whether and how the problem should be treated. This is reflected by wide national and international variation in the referral for treatment and surgical rates for menorrhagia.[2] There are two main limitations in selecting the most appropriate treatment: first, many women with menorrhagia have no apparent organic pathology, and this often leads to a choice of non-specific and less-radical treatments;[3] the other practical problem is of an objective measurement of menstrual loss that is not feasible in routine clinical practice. Clinicians rely on women's inaccurate perception of the heaviness of loss[4] and any adverse effect on their quality of life as the main guidelines to decide the need for treatment. Hence, efficacy of any treatment is ultimately judged by subjective views on its benefits and limitations.

Menorrhagia is most commonly treated by drugs that may be temporarily effective in some women. However, in the long term, such treatments are often of little benefit, owing to their inability to cure the problem and also because of their side effects, which lead to discontinuation.[5–7] Thus, hysterectomy is often accepted or demanded for permanent relief.[5,8,9] With the concern over hysterectomy in the absence of gross pelvic pathology, considerable interest has developed in alternative treatments. This has led to the widespread introduction of hysteroscopic endometrial ablation, which has also lowered the threshold for surgical treatment. However, menstrual problems recur after about one-quarter of endometrial ablations and the surgical workload has actually increased, with more hysterectomies being performed.[10] With the introduction of hormone-releasing intra-uterine systems, there is a real prospect of avoiding hysterectomy in achieving a long-term cure for menorrhagia.

Table 25.1 Comparison of factors influencing the choice of drug therapy for menorrhagia

Factor	Drug therapy					
	Prostaglandin inhibitors	Antifibrinolytics	Progestogens	OCP	Danazol	GnRH analogue
Reduction in menstrual loss (%)	20–40	45–55	10–30 (ovulatory) 50 (anovulatory)	50	60–80	90
Additional use	• Dysmenorrhoea • Menstrual migraine	• Dysmenorrhoea	• Irregular cycle	• Dysmenorrhoea • Irregular cycle	• Dysmenorrhoea	• Dysmenorrhoea • Menstrual migraine • Severe PMS
Side effects	Nausea, vomiting, gastric irritation, diarrhoea, rashes, headache, dizziness, bronchospasm	Nausea, vomiting, diarrhoea, tinnitus, dizziness, colour vision disturbances, abdominal cramp, skin rashes	Nausea, bloating, oedema, weight gain, headache, leg cramp, acne, skin rashes, depression, adverse lipid change	Nausea, headache, migraine, weight gain, breast tenderness, hypertension, thrombotic episodes, cholestatic jaundice, mood changes	Headache, weight gain, acne, rashes, hirsutism, flushes, voice change, muscle cramp, breast atrophy, tiredness, vertigo, skin rashes, adverse lipid changes	Flushes, sweats, headache, lethargy, vaginal dryness, loss of libido, irritability, loss of bone mineral density
Relative cost (6-month course)	£5	£50	£30	£5–10	£60	£350

GnRH, gonadotrophin-releasing hormone; OCP, oral contraceptive pill; PMS, premenstrual syndrome.

In this chapter the effectiveness, benefits, limitations and costs of four main types of treatment for menorrhagia are analysed. The choice of treatment for a patient depends on individual preferences and circumstances. Except in the presence of localized pathology such as uterine fibroids and polyps, drugs are the first line of treatment for menorrhagia. If that proves ineffective or unbearable, a hormone-releasing intra-uterine system may be inserted, particularly when the childbearing function needs to be preserved; however, others may opt for endometrial ablation after completing their family. Hysterectomy is commonly used as a last resort but can be performed earlier if the woman wishes to have a guaranteed permanent cure of her menstrual problems.

Drug therapy

Ideal drug therapy for menorrhagia should be effective, safe, and acceptable over the long term; unfortunately, none of the wide variety of drugs available has all these properties[11,12] (Table 25.1). The acceptability of any treatment depends on the balance between effectiveness and side effects. There is uncertainty about the effectiveness of many drug therapies. As the purpose of the treatment of menorrhagia is to improve the quality of life rather than to save life, the side effects are more likely to make an effective drug unacceptable.[11,12]

Efficacy

Mefenamic acid, the most commonly used prostaglandin synthetase inhibitor, reduces menstrual loss by 20–40%, although the response may be greater, reaching up to an 80% reduction, which is proportional to a larger pretreatment loss.[13–18] It is effective for both ovulatory and anovulatory dysfunctional uterine bleeding (DUB), as well as menorrhagia associated with adenomyosis, intra-uterine contraceptive devices (IUCDs) and coagulopathy.[13,19] The antifibrinolytic agent tranexamic acid is also effective in reducing menstrual loss by 45–55% in those with DUB and menorrhagia due to the IUCD.[18,20–24] The drugs are effective for as long as they are taken, with no demonstrable residual effect into the placebo or no-treatment periods;[13,25] however, if the pre-therapy menstrual loss is over 200 ml, neither of these therapies would reduce it to normal levels (<80 ml).[21] It is as yet unknown whether prostaglandin synthetase inhibitors and antifibrinolytic agents have synergistic effects in reducing menstrual loss.

In women with ovulatory menorrhagia, oral progestogen therapy during the luteal phase is not effective;[24,26] however, when it is given for 21 of the 28 days of the cycle, menstrual loss is reduced by 10–30%, although 67% of these women still remain menorrhagic.[17,27] It is, however, more appropriate for those with anovulatory menorrhagia, in whom menstrual loss is diminished by 50% with 14 days of therapy.[27] The oral contraceptive pill (OCP) is effective for either ovulatory or anovulatory menorrhagia. Earlier studies using the OCP with a higher dose of oestrogen showed reduction in menstrual loss by 53%, although about 20% of the patients did not respond.[20] The contemporary preparations containing a much smaller dose of oestrogen are similarly effective.[28,29] Continuous use of the OCP, especially of one with a high progestogen content, may be beneficial in women with menorrhagia due to endometriosis, adenomyosis and coagulopathy.[29,30]

Danazol is an effective drug which, at moderate to high doses, induces amenorrhoea in the majority; at a low dose it reduces menstrual loss by 60–80%

without any effect on the cycle length.[6,16,31] The gonadotrophin-releasing hormone (GnRH) agonist is another effective type of therapy, resulting in amenorrhoea in over 90% of women.[32] It is also an effective medical treatment of fibroids in the short term; however, the regression of fibroids is rarely complete and usually is not sustained after the therapy has been withdrawn.[33,34] Danazol and GnRH have a carry-over effect, such that 3 months' therapy may have up to 6 months of beneficial effect, but menorrhagia eventually recurs after the treatment is stopped.[16,31,32] For those who are not suitable for surgery, GnRH analogue may be continued with oestrogen–progestogen replacement ('add-back') to minimize the hypo-oestrogenic side effects.[35]

Benefits

Mefenamic acid is effective for associated dysmenorrhoea and menstrual migraine.[15,16,21,25] Tranexamic acid also improves dysmenorrhoea, possibly only by reducing the menstrual loss.[18,21] Progestogens have no effect on dysmenorrhoea but the OCP is one of the most effective treatments available.[28] Both danazol and GnRH agonists are also effective for dysmenorrhoea and the latter is useful for premenstrual syndrome and menstrual migraine.[16] Progestogens and the OCP have additional benefits of reducing the duration of bleeding, making cycles more predictable and eliminating premenstrual spotting.[17,28]

Limitations

Irrespective of the type of medical treatment, the satisfaction and acceptability rates are about 30–40% and only 20% of patients are willing to continue therapy after 3 months.[36] Moreover, none of the drugs can cure menorrhagia, which usually recurs when the treatment is stopped.[5,16] Mefenamic acid and tranexamic acid cause mild to moderate side effects in 20–60% of users.[16–18,20] As these drugs are taken only intermittently during menstruation, the side effects are less of a problem; nevertheless, one-quarter of users stop treatment after 3 months[18] and there is no report of long-term continuation. The side effects of progestogens and the OCP make their use less popular, particularly in those who are at higher risk of cardiovascular disease and thrombo-embolism or who suffer from premenstrual syndrome. Danazol therapy is associated with a most distressing catalogue of side effects, which makes it unsuitable for more than 3–6 months' treatment.[16] The GnRH analogues can not be given long term, owing to the adverse effects of the hypo-oestrogenic state, including bone demineralization.[37]

Relative cost

Mefenamic acid, progestogens and the OCP are the most economic choices, whereas tranexamic acid, danazol and GnRH analogue are relatively more expensive. As the treatment of menorrhagia may need to be continued for a considerable length of time, intermittent therapy with mefenamic acid and tranexamic acid reduces the prescribing costs. The cost of a 6-month course of treatment would be as follows: mefenamic acid (£10), tranexamic acid (£50), the OCP (£5–10), progestogen (£30), danazol (£60) and GnRH analogue (£350).

Intra-uterine system

Medicated intra-uterine systems (IUSs) releasing progesterone (Progestosert) or levonorgestrel (the LNG–IUS), originally developed for contraception, have been shown to reduce blood loss substantially and even lead to amenorrhoea in a significant number of users.[38,39] This seems ideal for those in whom drug therapy is ineffective or intolerable, and who would prefer to avoid surgical treatment.

Efficacy

Progestosert reduces menstrual loss by 40% after a month and by up to 65% after 12 months of insertion.[38] Similarly, the efficacy of the LNG–IUS depends on the duration of use, with the decrease in menstrual loss ranging from 82% after 3 months to 85–88% after 6 months and 96–97% after a year.[22,39] About one-third of women become amenorrhoeic within a year of insertion and the pattern of menstrual loss remains unchanged thereafter.[39,40] The use of the LNG–IUS among those awaiting hysterectomy has been shown to obviate surgery in 64–82% of women.[41–43] Nevertheless, within a year of insertion, 44% of patients opted for hysterectomy, owing to dissatisfaction with the treatment; after an average follow-up of 3 years, less than half were continuing with the treatment.[43] However, this was a selective population waiting for hysterectomy and patients did not necessarily have an open mind towards the treatment.

Benefits

In addition to the use of the LNG–IUS as an effective contraceptive, there are other benefits including the relief of dysmenorrhoea, regression of endometrial hyperplasia and prevention of fibroid growth.[40,42] A possible therapeutic effect on fibroids has also been suggested, as their size actually reduced after 6–18 months of use.[44] It is also not associated with an increase in pelvic inflammatory disease and ectopic pregnancy, as is the case with other coils; rather, it reduces the incidence of these conditions, compared with that in sexually active women not using any contraception.[45] Owing to the minimal systemic absorption of hormones, progestogenic side effects develop in only a small proportion of cases.[39] As the mechanism of action is not by suppressing ovarian function, there is no risk of hypo-oestrogenic side effects such as may occur with danazol and GnRH analogues.

Limitations

The IUS can be slightly difficult to insert, particularly in nulliparous women, and some cervical dilatation may be needed prior to insertion. Other coil-related complications, such as perforation, embedment, expulsion and fragmentation, are all possible. Irregular spotting or intermenstrual bleeding is common, particularly in the early months; although this diminishes gradually in frequency, it is the commonest reason why women discontinue treatment.[22,38–44] Even with the lower and more constant level of progestogen release from the IUS, some women still experience adverse progestogenic side effects due to systemic absorption.[39] Ovarian follicular enlargement or cysts have also been reported to be more common but do not require any treatment.

Relative costs

The cost of the LNG–IUS to the National Health Service is about £100, an initial price that is higher than that of any other medical treatment; however, the system lasts for 3–5 years, during which the cumulative cost of all the other medical treatments would be higher. It is also likely to reduce the number of future surgical treatments — which, if they were reduced even by less than one-quarter, would represent a considerable achievement in making the use of the LNG–IUS cost effective.

Endometrial ablation

Conservation of the uterus is increasingly being demanded, as nearly one-half of all women with menorrhagia have no local pelvic pathology.[3] These patients are eminently suitable for endometrial ablation if they do not wish to preserve their fertility. Complete removal of the endometrium may be accomplished by techniques, including photocoagulation with the Nd:YAG laser, resection with a diathermy wire loop, or electrocoagulation using a diathermy rollerball under direct hysteroscopic guidance or by inserting a thermal coagulation probe into the uterine cavity. The hysteroscopic treatment may also be selective, allowing resectoscopic excision of focal lesions such as polyps and submucous fibroids, particularly in those who wish to retain their fertility.

Efficacy

Endometrial ablation is not always successful in reducing menstrual loss and the effectiveness appears to diminish with time over the first 3 years, although not thereafter.[46–49] There is very little variation in the overall success rates between the different methods. Long-term follow-up studies have reported amenorrhoea in about 25–30% of women and a significant decrease in menstrual loss in a further 45–60%, giving a satisfaction rate of approximately 75–80%.[46–54] The accompanying dysmenorrhoea is relieved in 60–80% of women, with some improvement in PMS, but atypical pelvic pain is not cured. Postoperative cyclical pain due to haematometra may sometimes develop and the prevalence of pain increases with time after endometrial ablation.[55,56] After the initial ablation, 6–23% of women have needed reoperation, including a repeat ablation in 8–16%, and subsequent hysterectomy in 4–16% of patients.[46–54] The probability of requiring a hysterectomy following repeat ablation is 40%.[57] The outcome of endometrial ablation depends on correct patient selection, as there is a significantly high failure rate in younger women (<35 years), in those with an enlarged uterus (>12 weeks), and in the presence of fibroids and adenomyosis.[46–48,50,58]

Benefits

The procedure can be accomplished on an outpatient basis with a minimum of discomfort, inconvenience and cost. It is helpful in patients at high risk for general anaesthesia as it can also be performed with sedation and local anaesthesia. As there is no need for pelvic exploration, the incidence of postoperative complications is lower; nevertheless, serious problems do occur.[59] In comparison to hysterectomy, women require a shorter hospital stay, use less analgesia, have a quicker recovery and resume normal activities earlier after endometrial resection.[60–63] Many also appreciate the option of losing their symptoms while retaining their uterus in the absence of gross pathology. Similarly, there is no alteration in ovarian function after the treatment, unlike that noted in one-quarter of women after hysterectomy. Endometrial ablation also has a beneficial effect on depression, sexuality and general health;[61,62] however, the initial improvement in health-related quality of life at 1 month is offset by a subsequent fall as early as 4 months after operation.[64]

Limitations

The most significant complications after endometrial ablation are (a) haemorrhage, (b) uterine perforation, and (c) fluid absorption leading to hyponatraemia, neurological symptoms, haemolysis and death. In a large series, endometrial resection was abandoned in 5% of women and the uterus was perforated in 2%. The complication rate was higher when resection was combined with hysteroscopic myomectomy.[48] The largest survey published to date on the outcome of endometrial ablation in England and Wales reported a complication rate of 4.4% and the need to perform additional surgery in 1.2% of cases as a result, even though 60% of the operators had very little experience.[59] All women need to use contraception, as any subsequent pregnancy is likely to be complicated, with the risk of foetal growth retardation and placental adhesion. As complete removal of the endometrium is not guaranteed after endometrial ablation, perimenopausal women require progestogen together with oestrogen replacement therapy to prevent endometrial neoplasia. This reduces the compliance to hormone replacement therapy (HRT), owing to progestogenic side effects and the possibility of recurrent and/or heavy withdrawal bleeding.

Relative costs

With endometrial resection the hospital costs are about one-half those with hysterectomy and greater savings are made if the reduced morbidity and sickness leave are taken into consideration: total health service costs are about £500 for endometrial ablation and over £1000 for hysterectomy.[64] The financial savings are twofold: first, there is a small reduction in the operative cost; the second (and more substantial) benefit is the saving in ward costs. Thus, the capital cost of instruments can easily be recouped from the savings of the first 100 cases.[65] However, the need for re-treatment in nearly one-quarter of women within 2 years after endometrial ablation offsets its cost advantage and the cumulative hospital cost amounts to 71% of that for hysterectomy.[54] In addition, there are cost implications for the patient, her family and community, during a much longer total convalescence period after more than one surgical operation.

Hysterectomy

Hysterectomy is the most effective treatment for both menorrhagia and dysmenorrhoea, resulting in the highest level of satisfaction:[5,54,66,67] it is the only treatment that can guarantee a 100% cure rate. Thus, despite considerable debate about the appropriate use of major surgery for a condition that is not life threatening, it is still the most commonly performed surgical intervention in women during the reproductive period.[68]

Route of hysterectomy

The superiority of hysterectomy by the vaginal route is undisputed, with a better cosmetic result, less discomfort, fewer complications, shorter hospital stay, quicker recovery and earlier return to normal activity than that with abdominal hysterectomy.[69-71] However, the abdominal route is commonly preferred when dealing with unexpected pathologies such as endometriosis, pelvic inflammatory disease and ovarian cysts.[8] The vaginal approach has also been thought to be difficult, particularly in nulliparous women, in the presence of an enlarged uterus, or if simultaneous oöphorectomy is to be performed. These limitations have led to the development of laparoscopically assisted vaginal hysterectomy (LAVH), because with this technique it is possible to divide adhesions, secure uterine and ovarian vessels, and separate the uterus from surrounding structures prior to its vaginal removal.[72] Thus, LAVH converts an abdominal to a vaginal procedure and has all the benefits of vaginal hysterectomy. If the conversion from the laparoscopic to the vaginal route takes place early in the operation, the operating time and incidence of complications are lowered.[73] The duration of hospital stay and convalescence period are similar after LAVH and vaginal hysterectomy, but are relatively higher after abdominal hysterectomy.[74,75]

Since the advent of LAVH, it has become apparent that most of the traditional contraindications of vaginal hysterectomy — such as previous pelvic surgery, mild endometriosis, history of pelvic sepsis, uterine fibroids and the need for oöphorectomy — are not valid. At least two prospective randomized controlled trials have failed to show that LAVH has any advantage over vaginal hysterectomy. This includes the need for oöphorectomy, which can be accomplished vaginally in the vast majority of women.[72,73] Thus, LAVH does seem to be a waste of time for most women, except in those with gross pelvic diseases (such as extensive pelvic adhesions, severe endometriosis and adnexal pathology) and when vaginal access is considerably reduced due to a narrow subpubic arch and/or a moderately enlarged uterus (>14–16 weeks). In these circumstances, a vaginal procedure would be difficult, if not impossible; LAVH will obviate a laparotomy and the associated increased postoperative pain and longer recovery period.

Total or subtotal hysterectomy

Subtotal hysterectomy is a safer technique, with less chance of damage to the bladder, ureter and rectum. The operating time is shorter, as removal of the cervix can be the most difficult and time-consuming part of hysterectomy, be it via laparotomy or laparoscopy. As the topography of the pelvic floor is maintained, such a technique is associated with a lower incidence of pelvic haematoma, vault infection and prolapse.[76] With a laparoscopic supracervical approach, the benefits of shorter operating time, lower morbidity and more rapid recovery time than LAVH are more relevant;[77,78] however, subtotal hysterectomy can be accomplished also through the vaginal route. It has also been claimed that sexual function is better preserved after subtotal hysterectomy, although this is, as yet, unsubstantiated.[76]

Benefits

Hysterectomy is prophylactic against not only uterine and cervical cancer but also ovarian cancer, if combined with oöphorectomy.[79] It definitely cures dysmenorrhoea and PMS when bilateral oöphorectomy is also performed. HRT is more acceptable after hysterectomy, owing to the absence of bleeding and progestogenic side effects.[80] All prospective studies on the psychological outcome of hysterectomy have shown a relatively higher incidence of preoperative depression, which improves in the majority of patients after hysterectomy.[81,82] The evidence is more varied for sexual functioning, with some patients expressing dissatisfaction but others reporting either no change or an improvement.[81,83,84] If adequate HRT is given to correct any associated ovarian failure, psychosexual function improves even more after hysterectomy.[85]

Limitations

After hysterectomy, the need for postoperative analgesia is greater, the risk of complication is higher and the convalescence period is longer than after endometrial ablation.[54,60–62,64] This is particularly the case after abdominal hysterectomy. Immediate postoperative complications include haemorrhage, wound infection, urinary retention and infection, and vaginal discharge.[67] In a review of nine papers comparing different types of hysterectomy, the rates of both major and minor complications were very similar (2.3–7.8% and 0.9–4.5%, respectively) and the total complication rates were 6.8–8.7%.[86] However, a meta-analysis of 29 studies showed an overall complication rate of 15.6% for LAVH, compared with 24.5% for vaginal hysterectomy and 42.8% for abdominal hysterectomy.[87] Many experienced gynaecologists would question the high rates; however, such enormous variation between different reports is due to different clinical practices — such as the use of prophylactic antibiotics, which reduces the incidence of postoperative infection from 21% to 9%.[88] Although the psychosexual sequel of hysterectomy is generally beneficial, this may not be the case in the absence of adequate HRT, as in one-quarter of these patients there is premature ovarian failure, resulting in a greater risk of cardiovascular disease and osteoporosis.[89] There have also been reports of residual ovarian pain, prolapse, and urinary and bowel dysfunction, although these facts are not universally accepted.[57]

Relative costs

Hysterectomy is more expensive than other treatments for menorrhagia, but the use of the vaginal route reduces the cost gap relative to endometrial ablation.[69,71] Proponents of LAVH have suggested that its overall cost would be less, in that it facilitates early discharge from the hospital and a rapid return to productive employment. Ironically, the economic impact of prolonged operating time and expensive disposable devices has been a target of the critics, as these costs far outweigh the savings accruing from a shorter hospital stay: the costs of LAVH are twice those of abdominal hysterectomy, thrice those of vaginal hysterectomy and five times those of transcervical resection of the endometrium (TCRE).[72,74,90] However, others have shown that, despite the higher operative cost, the total cost of treatment is less because of the shorter hospital stay after LAVH.[91] LAVH will definitely become less expensive in the future, as laparoscopic instruments become cheaper and operating time is reduced with increasing experience.[72]

Treatment selection

Menorrhagia is rarely a life-threatening situation and its management is therefore seen as a means to achieving a better quality of life. It is, therefore, appropriate that

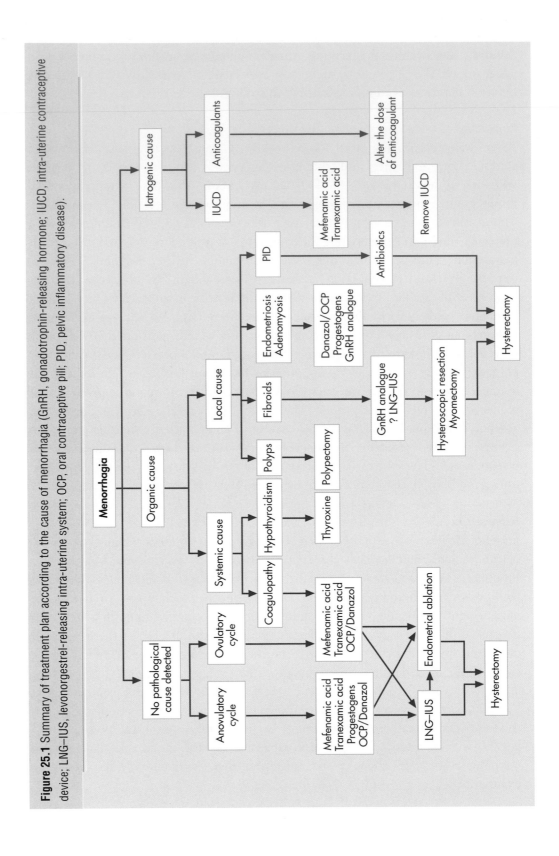

Figure 25.1 Summary of treatment plan according to the cause of menorrhagia (GnRH, gonadotrophin-releasing hormone; IUCD, intra-uterine contraceptive device; LNG–IUS, levonorgestrel-releasing intra-uterine system; OCP, oral contraceptive pill; PID, pelvic inflammatory disease).

women themselves should participate in the decision-making process, which aims for a correct balance between efficacy and side effects in a particular individual. The choice of treatment should take into account the woman's age, need for contraception and desire to retain her uterus, together with the nature and severity of the complaint, the presence of any pelvic pathology and the outcome of any previous treatment. The economic impact of the health-care decision — including the cost of the treatment, bed occupancy, or time away from work — has also become increasingly significant.

In the absence of local uterine pathology and iatrogenic problems, or after correcting the systemic illness, medical treatment should be considered first (Fig. 25.1). Mefenamic acid and tranexamic acid are the drugs of choice as they are effective when taken intermittently (only during menstruation) and would therefore be more tolerable. The OCP may be used as a first line of treatment in younger women, for whom it is acceptable as a long-term remedy since they require contraception and have the added benefit of good cycle control. It is, however, unsuitable for most menorrhagic women, who are commonly in their 40s and who, if sterilized, are usually reluctant to continue with something they consider to be a contraceptive agent. Progestogens may be used if the primary drug fails but should be limited to cases of anovulatory menorrhagia and to those patients with irregular cycles. Similarly, danazol and GnRH analogues are the second-line drugs for menorrhagia; because of their side effects they are used for only a short time (3–6 months), perhaps while waiting for surgery. GnRH analogues are a useful adjunct to myomectomy in reducing the fibroid volume and blood flow. For those who are not suitable for surgery, a GnRH analogue with 'add-back' oestrogen–progestogen replacement may be used in carefully selected patients.

If drug therapy fails or cannot be tolerated, owing to side effects, other therapies for menorrhagia should be given (Table 25.2). The LNG-releasing IUS is the first true alternative to surgical treatment, and is particularly suitable for those young women who wish to preserve their fertility or who disfavour endometrial ablation owing to a higher failure rate. When the LNG–IUS is used in perimenopausal women, the progestogenic effect on the endometrium is adequate for them to start oestrogen replacement therapy. The continuation rate is higher if such patients are counselled about the possibility of breakthrough bleeding, with the assurance of spontaneous recovery within 6 months. It may be useful to supplement cyclical oral progestogens or tranexamic acid for the first 3 months to avoid any heavy and erratic bleeding.

Surgical treatment is required for those who have not responded or who prefer not to have an LNG–IUS, those with pelvic pathology and those who are absolutely determined that they do not want to experience further menstruation. For women in the last category, hysterectomy is the treatment of choice. Endometrial ablation is suitable only for women who have completed their families, who would prefer to avoid hysterectomy and who are happy to accept a reduction in menstrual loss rather than amenorrhoea (which cannot be guaranteed). It is also appropriate when laparotomy for hysterectomy is dangerous or impossible because of dense pelvic adhesions or an ileal conduit, and in women for whom general anaesthesia is to be avoided. Endometrial ablation should be limited to women over 35 years of age, with a uterus less than 12 weeks in size, or a submucous fibroid less than 5 cm in diameter, and in the absence of adenomyosis and endometrial

Table 25.2 Comparison of factors influencing the choice of non-medical therapy for menorrhagia

Factor	Intra-uterine system	Endometrial ablation	Hysterectomy
Efficacy	Reduction in menstrual loss by 96% after 1 year but only 50% of women continue after 3 years	Hypomenorrhoea in 45–60%, amenorrhoea in 25–30% and satisfaction in 75% of women	Amenorrhoea guaranteed in every woman and highest rate of long-term satisfaction
Benefits	• Effective contraceptive • Reduced risk of ectopic pregnancy and PID • Relieves dysmenorrhoea • Regression of fibroid and endometrial hyperplasia • Ovarian function unaltered	• Relieves dysmenorrhoea and PMS in some women • Can avoid general anaesthesia • Short hospital stay, minimum postoperative pain, and earlier return to normal activities • Retains ovarian function	• Removes any pelvic pathology • Cures dysmenorrhoea and PMS with bilateral oöphorectomy • Protects from the future risk of uterine pathology including cancer • HRT more acceptable without bleeding and progestogenic side effects
Limitations	• Irregular bleeding or spotting • Coil-related complications: expulsion, fragmentation, embedment and perforation • Unsuitable with enlarged and distorted uterine cavity	• Continued contraceptive need • Uterine bleeding, perforation and excess fluid absorption • Higher failure in <35 years, large uterus >12 weeks size, with fibroid and adenomyosis • Uterine pain and haematometra	• Postoperative complications: haemorrhage, wound infection, urinary tract infection, vaginal discharge and vault prolapse • Prolonged recovery period • Premature ovarian failure • Urinary and bowel dysfunction
Relative cost	£100	£500	£1000

HRT, hormone-replacement therapy; PID, pelvic inflammatory disease; PMS, premenstrual syndrome.

hyperplasia. If menstrual symptoms persist or recur after endometrial resection, a repeat ablation may be suitable in the absence of dysmenorrhoea.

Hysterectomy is often regarded as the last resort when all other treatment for menorrhagia has failed. However, many clinicians (and their patients) feel that it is appropriate to opt for hysterectomy in the first place rather than to prolong suffering through failure of several other treatments, none of which can guarantee a cure. The route of hysterectomy should be decided in relation to the patient's weight, uterine size, degree of uterine mobility, pubic arch angle, past surgical history, any pelvic pathology, whether ovaries are to be removed and (finally) the preference of the surgeon. The decision on whether the cervix and ovaries should be removed should rest with the patient, after she has been thoroughly counselled about the advantages and disadvantages of this procedure.

Conclusions

Treatment of menorrhagia aims to improve the quality of life in women who are unable to cope with excessive menstrual bleeding. Although one treatment may be more effective than another, it may not be suitable for certain individuals. Medical treatment cannot cure menorrhagia and needs to be continued long term to prevent recurrence. The acceptability of such treatment is also low because of its limited efficacy, possibly intolerable side effects or, simply, the unappealing prospect of long-term drug therapy. The LNG–IUS is an effective alternative and has reduced the need for surgical treatment, but it may not be acceptable to those who develop menstrual irregularity and spotting. Endometrial ablation offers the advantages of lower morbidity and rapid recovery after surgery, but menorrhagia persists in about one-quarter of women, who would need further treatment. At present, hysterectomy is the only treatment that can guarantee a cure for menorrhagia. With such a variation in the efficacy, benefits and limitations of different treatments, it is up to the individual woman and her clinician to chose the most suitable option. Some may decide to undergo hysterectomy for permanent relief from the debilitating symptoms, despite the risks of major surgery; others may prefer to accept the uncertain outcome of less-radical treatments for the sake of lower morbidity.

References

1. Coulter A, Peto V, Jenkinson C. Quality of life and patient satisfaction following treatment of menorrhagia. Fam Pract 1994; 11: 394–401

2. Coulter A, McPherson K, Vessey M. Do British women have too many or too few hysterectomies? Soc Sci Med 1988; 27: 987–994

3. Fraser I S. Hysteroscopy and laparoscopy in women with menorrhagia. Am J Obstet Gynecol 1992; 162: 1264–1269

4. Fraser I S, McCarron G, Markham R. A preliminary study of factors influencing perception of menstrual blood loss volume. Am J Obstet Gynecol 1984; 149: 788–793

5. Studd J W W. Hysterectomy and menorrhagia. Baillieres Clin Obstet Gynaecol 1989; 3: 415–424

6. Shaw R W. Assessment of medical treatment for menorrhagia. Br J Obstet Gynaecol 1994; 101 (suppl 11): 15–18

7. Coulter A Kelland J, Peto V, Rees M C. Treating menorrhagia in primary care. An overview of drug trials and survey of prescribing practice. Int J Technol Assess Health Care 1995; 11: 456–471

8. Vessey M P, Villard-Mackintosh L, McPherson K et al. The epidemiology of hysterectomy: finding in a large cohort study. Br J Obstet Gynaecol 1992; 99: 402–407

9. Studd J W W. Shifting the indications for hysterectomy. Lancet 1996; 345: 388–389

10. Bridgeman S A. Increasing operative rates for dysfunctional uterine bleeding after endometrial ablation. Lancet 1994; 344: 893

11. Consumer's Association. Drugs for menorrhagia: often disappointing. Drug Ther Bull 1990; 28: 17–19

12. Higham J, Shaw R. Risk–benefit assessment of drugs used for the treatment of menstrual disorders. Drug Safety 1991; 6: 183–191

13. Anderson A B M, Hynes P J, Guillebaud J, Turnbull A C. Reduction of menstrual blood loss by prostaglandin-synthetase inhibitors. Lancet 1976; i: 774–776

14. Hall P, Maclachlan N, Thorn N et al. Control of menorrhagia with cyclo-oxygenase inhibitor naproxane sodium and mefenamic acid. Br J Obstet Gynaecol 1987; 94: 554–558

15. Fraser I S, Pearse C, Shearman R P et al. Efficacy of mefenamic acid in patients with a complaint of menorrhagia. Obstet Gynecol 1981; 58: 543–551

16. Dockeray C J, Sheppard B L, Bonnar J. Comparison between mefenamic acid and danazol in the treatment of established menorrhagia. Br J Obstet Gynaecol 1989; 96: 840–844

17. Cameron I T, Haining R, Lumsden M A et al. The effect of mefenamic acid and norethisterone on measured menstrual blood loss. Obstet Gynecol 1990; 76: 85–88

18. Bonnar J, Sheppard B L. Treatment of menorrhagia during menstruation: randomised controlled trial of ethamsylate, mefenamic acid, and tranexamic acid. Br Med J 1996; 313: 579–582

19. Fraser I S, McCarron G, Markham R et al. Measured menstrual blood loss in women with menorrhagia associated with pelvic disease and coagulation disorder. Obstet Gynecol 1986; 68: 630–633

20. Nilsson L, Rybo G. Treatment of menorrhagia. Am J Obstet Gynecol 1971; 110: 713–720

21. Andersch B, Milsom I, Rybo G. An objective evaluation of flurbiprofen and tranexamic acid in the treatment of idiopathic menorrhagia. Acta Obstet Gynecol Scand 1988; 67: 645–648

22. Milsom I, Anderson K, Andersch B, Rybo G. A comparison of flurbiprofen, tranexamic acid and levonorgestrel-releasing intrauterine contraceptive device in the treatment of idiopathic menorrhagia. Am J Obstet Gynecol 1991; 164: 879–883

23. Rybo G. Tranexamic acid therapy is effective treatment in heavy menstrual bleeding. Clin Update Safety Ther Adv 1991; 4: 1–8

24. Preston J T, Cameron I T, Adams E J, Smith S K. Comparative study of tranexamic acid and norethisterone in the treatment of ovulatory menorrhagia. Br J Obstet Gynaecol 1995; 102: 401–406

25. Vargyas J M, Campeau J D, Mishell D R Jr. Treatment of menorrhagia with meclofenamate sodium. Am J Obstet Gynecol 1987; 157: 944–950

26. Cameron I T, Leusk R, Kelly R W, Baird D T. The effect of danazol, mefenamic acid, norethisterone and a progesterone impregnated coil on endometrial prostaglandin levels in women with menorrhagia. Prostaglandins 1988; 34: 99–110

27. Fraser I S. Treatment of ovulatory and anovulatory dysfunctional uterine bleeding with oral progestogens. Aust N Z J Obstet Gynaecol 1990; 30: 353–356

28. Ekstrom P, Juchnicka E, Laudanski T, Akerlund M. Effect of an oral contraceptive in primary dysmenorrhoea — changes in uterine activity and reactivity to agonists. Contraception 1989; 40: 39–47

29. Fraser I S, McCarron G. Randomised trial of 2 hormonal and 2 prostaglandin-inhibiting agents in women with a complaint of menorrhagia. Aust N Z J Obstet Gynaecol 1991; 31: 66–70

30. Dockeray C J. The medical treatment of menorrhagia. In: Chamberlain G (eds) Contemporary obstetrics and gynaecology. London: Butterworths, 1988: 299–314

31. Fraser I S. Treatment of dysfunctional uterine bleeding with danazol. Aust N Z J Obstet Gynaecol 1985; 25: 224–226

32. Shaw R W, Fraser H M. Use of a superactive luteinizing hormone-releasing hormone (LHRH) agonist in the treatment of menorrhagia. Br J Obstet Gynaecol 1984; 91: 913–916

33. Friedman A J, Barbieri R L, Benacerraf B R, Schiff I. Treatment of leiomyomata with intranasal or subcutaneous leuprolide, a gonadotrophin-releasing hormone agonist. Fertil Steril 1987; 48: 560–564

34. Maheux R, Lemay A, Merat P. Use of intranasal luteinizing hormone-releasing hormone agonist in uterine leiomyomas. Fertil Steril 1987; 47: 229–233

35. Thomas E J, Okuda K J, Thomas N M. The combination of a depot gonadotrophin releasing hormone agonist and cyclical hormone replacement therapy for dysfunctional uterine bleeding. Br J Obstet Gynaecol 1991; 98: 1155–1159

36. Cooper K G, Parkin D E, Garratt A M, Grant A M. A randomised comparison of medical and hysteroscopic management in women consulting a gynaecologist for treatment of heavy menstrual loss. Br J Obstet Gynaecol 1997; 104: 1360–1366

37. Studd J W W, Leather A T. The need for add-back therapy with gonadotrophin-releasing hormone agonist therapy. Br J Obstet Gynaecol 1996; 103(suppl 14): 1–4

38. Bergqvist A, Rybo G. Treatment of menorrhagia with intrauterine release of progesterone. Br J Obstet Gynaecol 1983; 90: 255–258

39. Andersson K, Rybo G. Levonorgestrel-releasing intrauterine device in the treatment of menorrhagia. Br J Obstet Gynaecol 1990; 97: 690–694

40. Sivin I, Stern J. Health during prolonged use of levonorgestrel 20 mg/d and the Copper T Cu 380 Ag intrauterine contraceptive devices: a multicentre study. Fertil Steril 1994; 61: 70–77

41. Puolakka J, Nilsson C, Haukkamaa M et al. Conservative treatment of excessive uterine bleeding and dysmenorrhoea with levonorgestrel intrauterine system as an alternative to hysterectomy. Acta Obstet Gynaecol Scand 1996; 75(suppl): 82

42. Barrington J W, Bowen-Simpkins P. The levonorgestrel intrauterine system in the treatment of menorrhagia. Br J Obstet Gynaecol 1997; 104: 614–616

43. Lahteenmaki P, Haukkamaa M, Puolakka J et al. Open randomised study of use of levonorgestrel releasing intrauterine system as alternative to hysterectomy. Br Med J 1998; 316: 1122–1126

44. Sturridge F, Guillebaud J. Gynaecological aspects of levonorgestrel-releasing intrauterine system. Br J Obstet Gynaecol 1997; 104: 285–289

45. Cheng Chi I. An evaluation of the levonorgestrel-releasing IUD: its advantages and disadvantages when compared to the copper releasing IUDs. Contraception 1991; 4: 573–587

46. Garry R, Shelley-Jones D, Mooney P, Phillips G. Six hundred endometrial laser ablations. Obstet Gynecol 1995; 85: 24–29

47. Derman S G, Rehnstrom J, Neuwirth R S. The long term effectiveness of hysteroscopic treatment of menorrhagia and leiomyoma. Obstet Gynecol 1991; 77: 591–594

48. O'Connor H, Magos A L. Endometrial resection for the treatment of menorrhagia. N Engl J Med 1996; 335: 151–156

49. Chullapram T, Song J Y, Fraser I S. Medium-term follow-up of women with menorrhagia treated by rollerball endometrial ablation. Obstet Gynecol 1996; 88: 71–76

50. Magos A L, Baumann R, Lockwood G M, Turnbull A C. Experience with the first 250 endometrial resections for menorrhagia. Lancet 1991; 337: 1074–1078

51. Baggish M S, Sze E H M. Endometrial ablation: a series of 568 patients treated over an 11-year period. Am J Obstet Gynecol 1996; 174: 908–913

52. Scottish Hysteroscopy Audit Group. A Scottish audit of hysteroscopic surgery for menorrhagia: complications and follow-up. Br J Obstet Gynaecol 1995; 102: 249–254

53. Thijssen R F A. Radiofrequency induced endometrial ablation: an update. Br J Obstet Gynaecol 1997; 104: 608–613

54. Sculpher M J, Dwyer N, Byford S, Stirrat G M. Randomised trial comparing hysterectomy and transcervical endometrial resection: effect on health related quality of life and costs two years after surgery. Br J Obstet Gynaecol 1996; 103: 142–149

55. Fraser I S, Angsuwathana S, Mahmoud F, Yezerski S. Short and medium-term outcomes after rollerball endometrial ablation for menorrhagia. Med J Aust 1993; 158: 454–457

56. Jacobs S, Blumenthal N. Endometrial resection follow-up: late onset of pain and the effect of depot medroxyprogesterone acetate. Br J Obstet Gynaecol 1994; 101: 605–609

57. The management of menorrhagia. Effective Health Care Bull 9. University of Leeds. London: Churchill Livingstone, 1995

58. Daniell J, Kurtz B R, Ke R W. Hysteroscopic endometrial ablation using the roller ball electrode. Obstet Gynecol 1992; 80: 329–332

59. Overton C, Hargreaves J, Maresh M. A national survey of the complications of endometrial destruction for menstrual disorders. The MISTLETOE study. Br J Obstet Gynaecol 1997; 104: 1351–1359

60. Gannon M J, Holt E M, Fairbank J et al. A randomised controlled trial comparing endometrial resection and abdominal hysterectomy for the surgical treatment of menorrhagia. Br Med J 1991; 303: 1362–1364

61. Dwyer N, Hutton J, Stirrat G M. Randomised controlled trial comparing endometrial resection with abdominal hysterectomy for the surgical treatment of menorrhagia. Br J Obstet Gynaecol 1991; 100: 237–243

62. Pinion S B, Parkin D E, Abramovich D R et al. Randomised trial of hysterectomy, endometrial laser ablation and transcervical endometrial resection for dysfunctional uterine bleeding. Br Med J 1994; 309: 979–983

63. O'Connor H, Broadbent J A M, Magos A L, McPherson K. The Medical Research Council randomised trial of endometrial resection versus hysterectomy in the management of menorrhagia. Lancet 1997; 349: 897–901

64. Sculpher M J, Bryan S, Dwyer N et al. An economic evaluation of transcervical endometrial resection versus abdominal hysterectomy for the treatment of menorrhagia. Br J Obstet Gynaecol 1993; 100: 244–252

65. Rutherford A J, Glass M R. Management of menorrhagia. Br Med J 1990; 301: 290–291

66. Carlson K J, Miller B A, Fowler F J. The Maine women's health study: I Outcomes of hysterectomy. Obstet Gynecol 1994; 83: 556–565

67. Clarke A, Black N, Rowe P et al. Indications for and outcome of total hysterectomy for benign disease: a prospective cohort study. Br J Obstet Gynaecol 1995; 102: 611–620

68. Coulter A, McPherson K. The hysterectomy debate. Q J Soc Affairs 1986; 2: 379–396

69. Kovac S R, Christie S J, Bindbeutel G A. Abdominal versus vaginal hysterectomy: a statistical model for determining physicians' decision making and patient outcome. Med Decis Making 1991; 11: 19–28

70. Sheth S S. Vaginal hysterectomy. In: Studd J W W (ed) Progress in obstetrics and gynaecology, Vol 10. London: Churchill Livingstone, 1993: 317–340

71. Power T, Goodno J, Harris V. The outpatient vaginal hysterectomy. Am J Obstet Gynecol 1993; 168: 1875–1880

72. Summitt R L, Stovall T G, Lipscomb G H et al. Randomised comparison of laparoscopy-assisted vaginal hysterectomy with standard vaginal hysterectomy in an outpatients setting. Obstet Gynecol 1992; 80: 895–901

73. Richardson R E, Bournas N, Magos A L. Is laparoscopic hysterectomy a waste of time? Lancet 1995; 345: 36–41

74. Nezhat C, Bess O, Admon D et al Hospital cost comparison between abdominal, vaginal and laparoscopy-assisted vaginal hysterectomies. Obstet Gynecol 1994; 83: 713–716

75. Dorsey J H, Holtz P M, Griffiths R I et al. Cost and charges associated with three alternative techniques of hysterectomy. N Engl J Med 1996; 335: 476–482

76. Drife J. Conserving the cervix at hysterectomy. Br J Obstet Gynaecol 1994; 101: 563–564

77. Ewen S P, Sutton C J G. Initial experience with supracervical hysterectomy and removal of the cervical transformation zone. Br J Obstet Gynaecol 1994; 101: 225–228

78. Schwartz R O. Laparoscopic hysterectomy: supracervical vs. assisted vaginal. J Reprod Med 1994; 39: 625–630

79. Studd J W W. Prophylactic oophorectomy. Br J Obstet Gynaecol 1989; 96: 506–509

80. Khastgir G, Studd J W W. Hysterectomy, ovarian failure and depression. Menopause 1998; 5: 113–122

81. Gath D, Cooper P, Day A. Hysterectomy and psychiatric disorder: I. Levels of psychiatric morbidity before and after hysterectomy. Br J Psychol 1982; 140: 335–342

82. Ryan M M, Dennerstein L, Pepperell R. Psychological aspects of hysterectomy: a prospective study. Br J Psychol 1989; 154: 516–522

83. Dennerstein L, Wood C. Sexual response following hysterectomy and oophorectomy. Obstet Gynecol 1977; 49: 92–96

84. Helstrom L, Lundberg P O, Sorbom D, Backstrom T. Sexuality after hysterectomy: a factor analysis of women's sexual lives before and after hysterectomy. Obstet Gynecol 1993; 81: 357–362

85. Khastgir G, Studd J W W. Hysterectomy and depression. In: Studd J W W, Edwards L (eds) Hysterectomy and HRT. London: RCOG Press, 1997: 98–116

86. Munro M G, Deprest J. Laparoscopic hysterectomy: does it work? A bicontinental review of the literature and clinical commentary. Clin Obstet Gynecol 1995; 38: 401–425

87. Garry R, Phillips G. How safe is the laparoscopic approach to hysterectomy? Gynaecol Endosc 1995; 4: 77–79

88. Mittendrof R, Aronson M, Berry R et al. Avoiding serious infections associated with abdominal hysterectomy: a meta-analysis of antibiotic prophylaxis. Am J Obstet Gynecol 1993; 169: 1119–1124

89. Siddle N, Sarrel P, Whitehead M I. The effect of hysterectomy on the age at ovarian failure: identification of a subgroup of women with premature loss of ovarian function and literature review. Fertil Steril 1987; 47: 94–100

90. East M. Comparative cost of laparoscopically assisted vaginal hysterectomy. N Z Med J 1994; 107: 371–374

91. Raju K S, Auld B J. A randomised prospective study of laparoscopic vaginal hysterectomy versus abdominal hysterectomy each with bilateral salpingo-oophorectomy. Br J Obstet Gynaecol 1994; 101: 1068–1071

CHAPTER 26

Endometrial balloon ablation

R. W. Dover

Introduction

Menorrhagia sufficient to affect daily activities may occur in up to 25% of middle-aged women.[1] However, this widespread problem, which has been responsible for an increasing number of hysterectomies over the last two decades,[2] is associated with abnormal pathology in only 50% of patients.[3,4] This, in addition to a complication rate of up to 42.8% associated with abdominal hysterectomy,[5] and coupled with a steadily rising number of women who wish to retain their uterus, has led to the development of endometrial ablation as an alternative treatment for abnormal uterine bleeding.

Published figures concerning techniques in common usage at the moment show that both hysteroscopic endometrial laser ablation (ELA) and transcervical resection of the endometrium (TCRE) are capable of achieving high levels of patient satisfaction when performed by experienced clinicians.[6–8] The outcome is highly dependent on the ability and technique of the surgeon, with more skill and experience giving both better results and, more importantly, fewer complications.[9–11]

Until recently, the long-term efficacy of endometrial ablation (EA) has been unclear. However, recent data have suggested that, in experienced hands, 90% of women undergoing TCRE did not have a hysterectomy, and 80% no further gynaecological surgery during the first 5 postoperative years.[7] Unfortunately, although EA has been shown to have long-term benefits and avoids the high rates of morbidity associated with abdominal hysterectomy, it does have a morbidity and complication rate of its own. Uterine perforation, fluid overload from the uterine irrigant, and haemorrhage have been estimated to occur in 1% of patients undergoing ELA,[8] while perforation at the time of TCRE may vary between 1 and 3.7%.[9,12] It is of some interest that the incidence of perforation is related to the expertise of the surgeon, with one series reporting that 52% occurred during the first five cases of each individual's experience.[13]

The established therapeutic benefits of EA have led to many attempts to develop alternative, locally ablative techniques. These aspire to equal or exceed the efficacy of those currently available, while simultaneously aiming to eliminate the previously described complications. The intention is for them to be suitable for use by general gynaecologists, who will not have undergone the lengthy periods of training necessary in order to achieve good outcomes with low complication rates with ELA and TCRE. Indeed, the only skills needed for successful use of one of these new techniques, are those required to fit an intra-uterine device.[14] This is in stark contrast to TCRE, where the benefits of further surgical experience may still be apparent until at least 200 patients have been treated.[10]

Three of these new therapies are discussed below, but it is important to appreciate that these procedures are comparatively recent innovations and that they do not have the wealth of published literature associated with ELA/TCRE, the techniques they are seeking to supersede. It is also important to be aware that the interpretation of patient outcomes following EA therapy is a confusing area: many authors use differing terminology and this hinders direct comparisons between alternative therapies. In addition, many of the endpoints chosen are highly subjective and, therefore, difficult to assess accurately. An objective outcome measure is therefore desirable, the most pertinent being the need for a second procedure or a hysterectomy. As mentioned earlier, a recent paper[7] has published results in this format. If it is accepted that objective endpoints are more reliable, then papers not published in this style should, perhaps, be viewed with some degree of caution.

The second issue of importance is that therapeutic failures can occur up to 36 months postoperatively, at which point a plateau is reached,[7] and that almost one-half of those seeking further treatment do so 12 months after their original surgery.[10] This implies that follow-up data for any period less than this are likely to show a higher success rate than those obtainable in the long term; once again, some caution must be used in interpreting these results.

The balloon systems

Three balloon system techniques are considered here. Although they are all variations on the basic idea of an inflatable balloon that conforms to the shape of the endometrial cavity, there are important differences between them. Whereas the Vesta DUB (Valleylab, Boulder, CO, USA) balloon utilizes radiofrequency energy delivered to the endometrium via monopolar electrodes, both the Cavaterm (Wallsten Medical SA, Morges, Switzerland) and the ThermaChoice Uterine Balloon Therapy system (Gynecare Inc, Menlo Park, CA, USA) are reliant on heated fluid to cause endometrial destruction.

Whatever differences may exist with regard to the mode of action, the preoperative assessment is common to all three procedures. In essence, the aim is to select a group of patients with menorrhagia that have structurally normal uteri and who have no desire for further children or to undergo a hysterectomy. Cervical smears and endometrial biopsy should exclude cellular abnormalities; structural anomalies of the uterus, such as leiomyomas or excessive cavity length, will be detected by ultrasound. As with EA, the procedures are not contraceptive and counselling needs to be given in this area. Patients about to undergo ELA/TCRE usually have their endometrium thinned by the administration of either danazol or one of the gonadatrophin-releasing hormone analogues (GnRHa) in order to aid the surgical procedure. However, pharmacological endometrial suppression adds to the cost of the procedure and causes well-documented (although transient) side effects. The balloon modalities deal with this aspect somewhat differently, as mentioned in the relevant section on each.

The other issue common to all three therapies is the use of heat, although, as mentioned earlier, the source is different. All three modalities have undergone

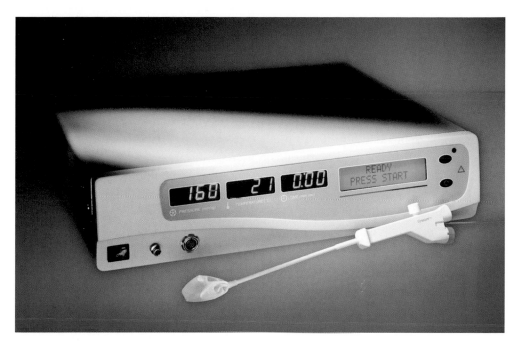

Figure 26.1 The ThermaChoice Uterine Balloon Therapy system. (Reproduced by permission of Gynecare Inc., Menlo Park, CA, USA.)

similar trials whereby their ability to destroy the endometrium has been assessed. The extent of thermal spread has also been investigated, both in vitro and in vivo, with none of the balloon systems causing a significant degree of thermal spread to adjacent viscera.

The ThermaChoice Uterine Balloon Therapy system

The first of these new procedures to be considered is the ThermaChoice Uterine Balloon Therapy system, shown in Figure 26.1. This consists of a plastic catheter 16 cm long by 4.5 mm diameter with a latex balloon attached to the distal end that houses a heating element and thermistor. The proximal end, which allows for inflation of the balloon, connects to a unit that monitors and controls preset intraballoon temperature, pressure and length of treatment.

Prior to insertion, the system is tested for leaks and the uterine cavity is assessed hysteroscopically. The device is then inserted transcervically to reach the fundus. A solution of 5% dextrose is used to distend the balloon incrementally until a stable pressure is obtained. Initial work suggested that this occurred at 70–80 mmHg,[15] but subsequently it has been suggested that 160–170 mmHg is optimal.[14] Indeed, in this later study, the first 15 patients were treated with pressures between 80 and 140 mmHg, whereas the final 15 experienced pressures of 150–180 mmHg. When discussing their results, the authors suggest that this may be a factor related to a poor outcome, as their seven failures were all among the initial 15 patients.

Once a stable intra-uterine pressure has been achieved, the heater is activated and maintains the intraballoon solution at a temperature of 87 ± 5 °C. Earlier work has suggested a treatment length of 8 minutes.[15,16]

The patients treated more recently[14] have been subjected to hysteroscopy immediately postoperatively. Uniform blanching has been noted over the fundus and anterior and side walls, with pink unblanched areas being seen near the ostia (especially if the uterus was arcuate), and on the posterior uterine wall. The authors conjectured that this incomplete blanching was a result of uneven energy distribution within the balloon and that, perhaps, it could be rectified by continual agitation of the balloon in order to improve the circulation (unlike the Cavaterm, there is no mechanism to circulate the fluid automatically within the ThermaChoice). The authors also pointed out that the immediate post-treatment hysteroscopic appearances were not predictive of the patient's eventual outcome.

The first published data describing the therapeutic usage of the ThermaChoice were in relation to a multicentre trial involving 18 patients.[16] The follow-up ranges from 6 to 34 (mean 17.5) months, during which seven of 18 patients (39%) reported light bleeding, and eight (44%) reported spotting or amenorrhoea. A success rate of 83% is claimed, although it is notable that three patients underwent a second procedure (two hysterectomy and one TCRE), during this comparatively short follow-up. Of the failures, one had no identifiable endometrium at histological assessment, whereas the other two had varying degrees of normal endometrial tissue still present within the cavity.

The other published data relating to the initial experience with this device is also comparatively disappointing,[14] even though the follow-up extends only to 12–18 months. Of the 30 patients undergoing the procedure, seven (23%) were deemed to have experienced no improvement; these all underwent TCRE or hysterectomy. In addition, a further six patients, all of whom had improved to some degree, underwent further surgery. In total, therefore, 13/30 (43%) underwent a second procedure by 18 months. It is possible, as suggested earlier, that inadequate balloon distension may have been responsible for these poor outcomes, as the results of later studies all using the higher pressure reveal much-improved outcomes.

Studies are also in progress to assess the impact of endometrial preparation. In the more recent study, nine women took a short course of danazol preoperatively, with the other procedures occurring at all times of the cycle. The results of the danazol-treated group are not given separately. This has significant implications, as it is known that endometrial glandular elements may be present deep within the myometrium and that, in order to destroy these areas, resection or ablation should include the endometrium and up to 3 mm of myometrium.[17] The thermal balloon is capable of penetrating up to 5 mm into the myometrium,[15] but this does not take account of the varying depth of the endometrium, which may be up to 7 mm deep in the secretory phase.[17] Endometrial suppression reduces the depth to 1.5–2.0 mm[18] and it is therefore probable that some degree of endometrial preparation may improve the outcome. This suggestion has been supported by recent evidence showing that the postoperative outcome was, in fact, improved by the preoperative administration of GnRHa.[19]

The largest series of any of the balloon systems has just been presented and confirms the improved outcomes achieved by using the higher balloon inflation pressures.[20] This series involved 408 patients, of whom 296 had been followed for 6 months and 150 for 12 months. At 12 months, 32% experienced amenorrhoea or spotting, with a further 31% classified as hypomenorrhoeic. In 12% of patients the menstrual loss was unchanged. It is worth noting that 36% of these women underwent the procedure using local anaesthesia, with or without sedation.

As mentioned earlier, the standard methods used to achieve endometrial ablation at present are TCRE and ELA. A retrospective study has sought to compare the outcomes achieved by these in the hands of an experienced single operator with the results achieved with the ThermaChoice.[21] Success, defined as amenorrhoea or hypomenorrhoea, was achieved in 83% of the Nd:YAG patients (follow-up 38–130 months), in 81% of the TCRE patients (follow-up 6–73 months) and in 82% of the balloon patients (follow-up 6–15 months). It is possible that longer follow-up will lead to some decline in the success rate for the balloon patients, but, interestingly, other workers have found that the results attained not only with the ThermaChoice[19] but also with the Vesta DUB Treatment system appear to be very durable.[22,23] The retrospective nature of this study may concern some clinicians, but its results are supported by a recent prospective, randomized study comparing the balloon systems with standard ablation procedures.[24] The patients received either rollerball ablation (n = 125) or the ThermaChoice (n = 130). No hormonal endometrial preparation was used, the surgeons relying on mechanical curettage. At 6 months' review the mean reduction in menstrual diary scores was 83.6% for the balloon patients and 88.5% for the rollerball group. Although there is some small difference between these groups, two points need to be appreciated: first, this difference was not statistically significant ($p>0.05$); secondly, it must be remembered that the outcomes from traditional ablations can deteriorate up to 36 months postoperatively, whereas the outcome following a balloon ablation appears to be slightly more durable. The other point of note is that 75.2% of the balloon procedures were completed in less than 30 minutes, whereas the figure for rollerball ablation was only 31.0%. In these times of ever-increasing operating theatre costs, this difference (provided that the outcomes are equivalent) is highly significant. The last area to highlight is that of safety: there were no adverse intra-operative events in the balloon group, compared with one uterine perforation, two cases of fluid overload and one cervical laceration in the rollerball group.

Whatever the current concerns regarding the long-term efficacy of this procedure, there is one aspect that is of major significance: the diameter of the system is only 4.5 mm, and this has obvious implications with regard to the ease of insertion. Use of the Cavaterm and Vesta DUB Treatment system necessitates cervical dilatation to Hegar 9 and 10 respectively, and this difference does tend to favour the ThermaChoice when the ideal device for use in an outpatient setting is being considered. The 8-minute treatment cycle also compares favourably with the 15 minutes currently used by the Cavaterm, although it is longer than the 4 minutes needed by Vesta. This technique has also been performed without general anaesthesia, 21 of the 30 procedures in one of the trials[14] and 36% in a different study[20] being performed under neuroleptic anaesthesia.

The Cavaterm system

The Cavaterm system, shown in Figure 26.2, also utilizes heated fluid to destroy the endometrium, but does differ significantly from the ThermaChoice. It consists of two major components — a silicone balloon catheter and heating element, and a central unit that houses the power source and the pump to ensure continual circulation of the heated fluid.

There are three important points to note with regard to this system. The first is that the silicone balloon is adjustable and thus can be altered according to the

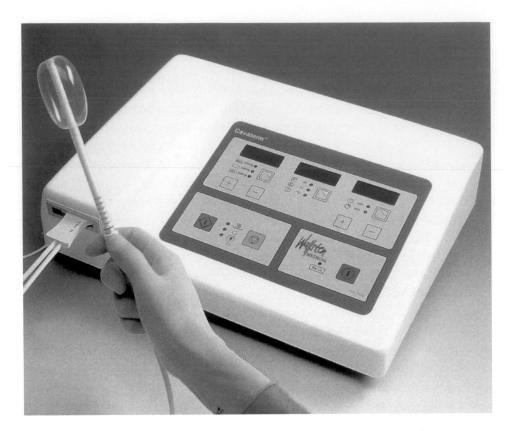

Figure 26.2 The Cavaterm system. (Reproduced by permission of Wallsten Medical SA, Morges, Switzerland.)

length of cavity about to be treated. The second feature follows from the first: ensuring an optimal fit of the balloon to the cavity reduces the chances of heat affecting the cervix (which may lead to stenosis), or damage to the underlying major vessels. The shaft of the catheter is insulated in an attempt to eliminate the occurrence of high temperatures in the vagina and cervical canal, which have led to problems in the past with other ablative techniques.[25] Finally, an oscillating pump causes the liquid to vibrate, consequently activating a backvalve system within the catheter tip, which forces the liquid to circulate vigorously inside the balloon. The hot circulating liquid is thus maintained within the balloon. Adequate circulation ensures constant temperatures within the balloon and on its surface, and therefore a uniform degree of thermal damage. In the absence of circulation, temperature differences of up to 18 °C within the balloon have been noted,[26] and other workers have suggested that this may be a cause of unequal energy distribution within their systems.[14]

One further difference with the Cavaterm system is that the patient inclusion criteria differ slightly from those of the other balloon therapies, which aim to exclude any degree of structural uterine abnormality. In contrast, the Cavaterm protocol allows the inclusion of women with myomas, as long as these are less than 50 mm in diameter. This has major implications, as it will markedly increase the number of potential patients for this device.

Prior to the procedure being performed, the cervix is dilated to Hegar 9 in order to accept the 8 mm diameter catheter. Of the initial series of 44 patients, 29 had their procedure under general and 15 under spinal anaesthesia.[26] After sounding the cavity to determine the balloon length, curettage is performed. This mechanically prepares the endometrium, meaning that hormonal pretreatment is not required, and the procedure can be performed at any phase of the menstrual cycle. In addition, a further histological specimen is obtained.

After the balloon length has been adjusted to the sounded length, the Cavaterm catheter is introduced to reach the fundus, and the balloon is filled with glycine until a pressure of 180–200 mmHg is obtained. This level of pressure is thought to be important for two reasons: the first is that it ensures adequate contact between the balloon and endometrium; the second reason is that, at this level of pressure, in excess of systolic blood pressure, a marked diminution in endometrial perfusion is obtained and consequently there is a reduction in heat loss from the system. This means that the therapeutic temperature can be reached more quickly and maintained using less power, allowing for a better depth and more uniform degree of penetration.

Once the system is activated, the therapeutic balloon surface temperature of 75 °C is quickly reached and then maintained for 15 minutes, after which the fluid is removed and the balloon withdrawn.

During manufacture, the heating element is preset to a working temperature of 80 °C, which yields a balloon surface temperature of 75 °C. The element has a large surface area, minimizing the need for a high temperature. This temperature cannot be altered, thereby eliminating the possibility of boiling that might lead to balloon expansion and possible rupture.

Apart from the initial heating studies in vivo and in vitro,[27] this device has thus far been trialled in over 1000 patients, although published data are available only in relation to 44.[26] During this study the treatment time was set at 30 minutes, this being based on previous experience of hyperthermia in malignant tumours. The follow-up time in this series was only 12 months, but the initial results were encouraging: of the 44 patients, 38 had an improvement in their menstrual loss, with 12 being amenorrhoeic and 11 having minimal loss only. None were postmenopausal on biochemical assessment. Three patients had not noticed any improvement and three had undergone hysterectomy.

After this first series, the treatment time was reduced to 15 minutes. At the time of initial presentation the follow-up on this group of 30 patients was very short, with only 14 having been followed for 6 months or longer.[28]

Combined data concerning the first group of patients treated for 30 minutes and all the subsequent patients treated for only 15 minutes have recently been presented.[29] These data relate to 130 patients, 60 of whom have been followed for more than 12 months, with 36 of these having follow-up ranging from 20 to 37 months. Of the initial 60 patients, seven have undergone hysterectomy, leaving 53 with more than 12 months' follow-up. Of these 37 are currently experiencing either amenorrhoea or spotting, with a further 12 having a normal menstrual loss, although this is a marked improvement on their preoperative menstrual bleeding. All 53 of these patients rate their level of satisfaction with the procedure as either good or excellent. It is of some interest to consider the reason for hysterectomy in the seven patients undergoing this operation. One patient was found to have atypical hyperplasia on preoperative curettage and underwent hysterectomy 5 weeks later; histological assessment revealed that the endometrium had been completely destroyed by the balloon ablation. Two patients continued to bleed heavily and underwent surgery at 4 and 16 months post-treatment. Examination of the resected uteri revealed pedunculated myoma, although the area accessible to the balloon had been completely destroyed. A further patient was found to have a uterine septum that would have prevented adequate balloon contact. The authors have made the point that all of these patients should have been excluded from the trial as, in keeping with the other balloon systems, cellular or major uterine abnormalities are contraindications to inclusion in these trials. Of the other three patients undergoing hysterectomy, two were diagnosed as suffering from postablation sterilization syndrome; and one woman (who bled less than preoperatively, but more than she found satisfactory) was found to have adenomyosis on examination of the resected specimen.

At present, Cavaterm patients are treated on an arbitrary day of their menstrual cycle; they receive no prior endometrial suppression, relying instead on pretreatment curettage to prepare the endometrium mechanically. This protocol appears to produce good results, but a recently presented series has suggested that these results could be improved still further.[30] These workers used a single GnRH injection 1 month prior to using the Cavaterm system. No curettage was performed at the time of surgery; consequently, all patients had previously undergone hysteroscopy and endometrial biopsy. This series contains only 12 patients and the follow-up is limited to 9–15 months, but the results are, none the less, impressive: eight of the patients are currently completely amenorrhoeic; three have oligomenorrhoea, while one has gained no discernible benefit. The first eight patients had their procedure performed under general anaesthesia; in the last four it was performed under paracervical block and intravenous sedation. The small numbers and short follow-up mean that these results must be viewed with some degree of caution, but this may represent a simple refinement to the treatment protocol that results in a major improvement in outcome.

The Vesta DUB Treatment system

The final procedure to be considered is the Vesta DUB Treatment system, shown in Figure 26.3. In common with the previous devices, it is based on the concept of an inflatable balloon; however, in this instance, rather than being a container for heated fluid it acts as a carrier for monopolar electrodes.

The system comprises two components, one of which is the electrode balloon constructed from an expandable polymer that allows the balloon, as it is inflated, to conform to the shape of the uterine cavity. The other is a hardware control component that connects to a standard electrosurgical generator, and controls the application of radiofrequency energy to the 12 monopolar electrodes located on the balloon. Six electrodes are applied to each uterine surface, each containing its own thermistor which is continually checked by the control unit so that energy levels can be altered to maintain the desired temperature level.

Preclinical studies, in common with the previously described devices, did not reveal thermal spread to adjacent organs, and demonstrated consistent thermal injury extending into the myometrium to a depth of 3 ± 1 mm when the treatment protocol of temperature and time (75 °C and 4 min, respectively) was used.[31]

Although long periods of endometrial suppression are not required with the Vesta DUB System, it is the only balloon system to use pharmacological methods routinely to prepare the endometrium. Unless surgery can be scheduled for the early follicular phase, a withdrawal bleed is procured just before treatment by the use of

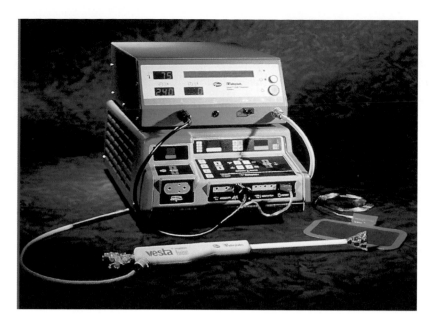

Figure 26.3 The Vesta DUB Treatment system. (Reproduced by permission of Valleylab Inc., Boulder, CO, USA.)

a short course of either a progestogen or a combined contraceptive pill.

The cervix is dilated to Hegar 10 and the treatment device slowly inserted until the distal end is in contact with the fundus. In an effort to reduce the risk of perforation, the Vesta DUB inserter has been designed with an atraumatic blunt-nosed sheath. Once this is adjacent to the fundus, the distal end is retracted to reveal the electrode balloon. The lumen of the instrument is patent, and used to test for unrecognized perforations before the electrodes are heated. A small volume (3–5 ml) of normal saline is injected through the lumen into the uterine cavity. Absence of resistance to this influx of fluid means that the uterine cavity must be carefully inspected to exclude a perforation. The balloon is then maximally distended by the use of an air-filled syringe connected to the inflation port. The volume of air required is usually between 7 and 10 cm³ and a constant degree of pressure is maintained manually. In contrast to the other systems, the exact intra-uterine pressure is not measured during the Vesta procedure.

Temperature and time of therapy are set at 75 °C and 4 min, respectively, and the system is then activated. A warm-up period of 40–60 s is needed in order to reach the target tissue temperature, at which point the therapeutic phase begins. During this, the thermistors sense the temperature at each electrode so that local energy levels can be adjusted to ensure that the temperature remains within a narrow range. At the end of 4 minutes, the system automatically shuts off and the balloon can be removed.

This system is currently being trialled in an international therapeutic study; although the data have yet to be published, they have recently been presented.[22,23] To date, 206 patients have been treated, with 79 of these having been followed up for 12 months or longer. According to their status at most recent review, 81.3% are either amenorrhoeic or have had a marked diminution in their menstrual loss.

There have been 12 documented treatment failures so far; where factors have been identified, they appear similar to those noted by other workers utilizing balloon systems, notably, distortion of the uterine cavity by a submucous leiomyoma and development of a haematometra. Interestingly, all patients developing problems did so before 15 months of follow-up. At present, no problems have become apparent after this period of follow-up has been passed, suggesting a good degree of durability for the treatment outcomes.

The need for the use of concrete endpoints in the presentation of results has been discussed earlier. Of the balloon systems, in only the Vesta DUB group have the data been presented in an actuarial format. Comparison of these results with those dealing with the 5-year follow-up of TCRE patients[7] reveals that they are on the same course. It must, however, be noted that the limit of review of the Vesta DUB Treatment system patients is just over 24 months, but that the TCRE data have shown that treatment failures may occur until 36 months. Caution must, therefore, be exercised when reviewing these initially promising results.

Conclusions

It does appear that, in some cases, good short-term therapeutic results can be achieved with the use of the balloon systems, but their long-term durability is as yet unproven. The numbers involved in the published and presented trials are small, and the length of follow-up too short, to demonstrate whether the results obtainable are equivalent to those achieved by TCRE/ELA.

The ease of use and apparent safety are encouraging aspects of these new modalities. All the devices have been designed with simplicity in mind, and their use requires only basic skills that are well within the remit of all practising gynaecologists. If the long-term outcomes are found to be satisfactory, then this ease of use may well be the pivotal factor in enabling many more women to gain access to this proven therapy.

There are some areas where improvements do need to be made, and these adjustments will become obvious as clinical experience with the therapies increases. The final treatment protocols have not yet been established in all cases, and changes here — such as the routine use of pretreatment of the endometrium — may well improve the efficacy still further, as has already been discussed.

The one area where all modalities need to improve is patient selection. The mode of action of all these devices is thermal damage to the adjacent endometrium. Any distortion of the cavity, whether from a leiomyoma or uterine septum, will reduce the extent of balloon contact and leave a varying proportion of endometrium untreated. Identification and exclusion of patients with irregular endometrial cavities — an established cause of failure across all the modalities — will mean that the therapies will not be performed on patients who may well be expected to do badly and who would, in all likelihood, benefit more from an alternative treatment. This may be helped if all potential patients undergo pretreatment hysteroscopy in an attempt to exclude structural uterine anomalies, as the use of ultrasound alone (as in some protocols) appears to be insufficient for this purpose.

On the basis of initial experience, few serious complications appear to develop following these new procedures. It should, however, be remembered that these complications occur infrequently and the numbers of patients that have received these therapies is small; perhaps these initially encouraging results, therefore, are a reflection both of the numbers involved and of the skill of the clinicians trialling these devices.

Undoubtedly, there will be some clinicians who will be alarmed by the presence of atypical hyperplasia on one of the pretreatment specimens and cite this, coupled with the lack of an operative histological specimen, as a reason not to use these techniques. The exception here is the Cavaterm system, where the preoperative curettage provides a histological sample. It should, however, be remembered that, of the currently used procedures, only TCRE produces tissue for histological assessment, with both ELA and rollerball coagulation destroying the endometrium in situ. This does, however, serve as a timely reminder of the need to obtain a good preoperative endometrial sample, which is as true for the present techniques as it is for balloon therapy.

Although the numbers and length of follow-up are small, it does seem that some conclusions can be drawn from the published trials with regard to the future. Further work with longer follow-up is undoubtedly necessary before the true benefits of these procedures are known, but on initial inspection they all appear to have some merit. As such, it seems likely that ablative therapy based on an inflatable balloon system will be a treatment option for many women in the near future. This does not, however, mean the end of the currently practised techniques; there are limitations to the balloon therapies that are unlikely to be overcome. Leiomyomas are common, and many women with menorrhagia will have a distorted uterine cavity and thus be unsuitable for balloon therapy. These limitations have been recognized by the manufacturers, with cavity irregularities being contraindications to inclusion in their trials and also responsible for some of their treatment failures. At present it would seem that TCRE and ELA are the only ablative options for these women and, consequently, will be in demand for the foreseeable future.

References

1. Gath D, Osborn M, Bungay G et al. Psychiatric disorder and gynaecological symptoms in middle-aged women: a community survey. Br Med J (Clin Res) 1987; 294: 213–218

2. Coulter A, Bradlow J, Agass M et al. Outcomes of referrals to gynaecology outpatient clinics for menstrual problems: an audit of general practice records. Br J Obstet Gynaecol 1991; 98: 789–796

3. Rees M C P. Heavy painful periods. In: Drife J O (ed) Dysfunctional uterine bleeding and menorrhagia. Ballieres Clin Obstet Gynaecol 1989; 3: 341–356

4. Office of Population Censuses and Surveys. Hospital Inpatient Enquiry. HMSO, London, 1985

5. Dicker R C, Greenspan J R, Strauss L T et al. Complications of abdominal and vaginal hysterectomy among women of reproductive age in the United States. Am J Obstet Gynecol 1982; 144: 841–848

6. Magos A L, Baumann R, Lockwood G M, Turnbull A C. Experience with the first 250 endometrial resections for menorrhagia. Lancet 1991; 337: 1074–1078

7. O'Connor H, Magos A. Endometrial resection for the treatment of menorrhagia. N Engl J Med 1996; 335: 151–156

8. Garry R, Erian J, Grochmal S A. A multi-centre collaborative study into the treatment of menorrhagia by Nd-YAG laser ablation of the endometrium. Br J Obstet Gynaecol 1991; 98: 357–362

9. Pyper R J D, Haeri A D. A review of 80 endometrial resections for menorrhagia. Br J Obstet Gynaecol 1991; 98: 1049–1054

10. Holt E M, Gilmer M D G. Endometrial resection. In: Gordon A G (ed) Endometrial ablation. Ballieres Clin Obstet Gynaecol 1995; 9(2): 279–297

11. Davis J A. Hysteroscopic endometrial ablation with the Nd-YAG laser. Br J Obstet Gynaecol 1989; 96: 928–932

12. Maher P J, Hill D J. Transcervical endometrial resection for abnormal uterine bleeding — report of 100 cases and review of the literature. Aust N Z J Obstet Gynaecol 1990; 30(4): 357–360

13. Macdonald R, Phipps J. Endometrial ablation: a safe procedure. Gynaecol Endosc 1992; 1(1): 7–9

14. Vilos G A, Vilos E C, Pendley L. Endometrial ablation with a thermal balloon for the treatment of menorrhagia. J Am Assoc Gynecol Laparosc 1996; 3(3): 383–387

15. Neuwirth R S, Duran A A, Singer A et al. The endometrial ablator: a new instrument. Obstet Gynecol 1994; 83: 792–796

16. Singer A, Almanza R, Gutierrez A et al. Preliminary clinical experience with a thermal balloon endometrial ablation method to treat menorrhagia. Obstet Gynecol 1994; 83: 733–735

17. Reid P C, Sharp F. Hysteroscopic Nd-YAG endometrial ablation: an in-vitro and in-vivo laser tissue interaction study (abstr) III European Congress on Hysteroscopy and Endoscopic Surgery, Amsterdam, 1992

18. Sutton C J G, Ewen S P. Thinning the endometrium prior to ablation: is it worthwhile? Br J Obstet Gynaecol 1994; 101: 10–12

19. Stabinsky S. Personal communication. California: Stanford University, 1997

20. Maher P. Four hundred patients treated for menorrhagia with a uterine thermal balloon (abstr). 6th Annual Congress of the International Society for Gynecologic Endoscopy, Singapore, 1997

21. Loffer F. A comparison of endometrial ablation results obtained by a single investigator using the Nd:YAG laser, the resectoscope and the ThermaChoice balloon system, (abstr). 6th Annual Congress of the International Society for Gynecologic Endoscopy, Singapore, 1997

22. Dover R. Thermoregulated radiofrequency endometrial ablation (abstr). British Society for Gynaecological Endoscopy, London, 1996

23. Dover R. The Vesta DUB treatment system for endometrial ablation (abstr). 6th Annual Congress of the International Society for Gynecologic Endoscopy, Singapore, 1997

24. Walsh B. Endometrial ablation for menorrhagia: a comparative clinical trial of thermal balloon therapy versus rollerball (abstr). 45th Annual Clinical Meeting, The American College of Obstetricians and Gynecologists, Las Vegas, 1997

25. Phipps J H, Lewis B V, Roberts T et al. Treatment of functional menorrhagia with radiofrequency endometrial ablation. Lancet 1990; 335: 374–376

26. Friberg B, Wallsten H, Henriksson P et al. A new simple, safe and efficient device for the treatment of menorrhagia. J Gynecol Tech 1996; 2: 103–108

27. Friberg B, Persson B, Willen R, Ahlgren M. Endometrial destruction by hyperthermia — a possible treatment of menorrhagia. Acta Obstet Gynecol Scand 1996; 75: 330–335

28. Friberg B. Cavaterm — a new technique for endometrial ablation by thermal coagulation (abstr). World Congress of Hysteroscopy, Miami, 1996

29. Friberg B. Cavaterm, endometrial ablation by thermal coagulation, results at 2–3 years follow-up (abstr). 6th Annual Congress of the International Society for Gynecologic Endoscopy, Singapore, 1997

30. Phillips G. Endometrial ablation with a thermal balloon catheter (abstr). 6th Annual Congress of the International Society for Gynecologic Endoscopy, Singapore, 1997

31. Soderstrom R, Brooks P, Corson S. Endometrial ablation using a distensible multielectrode balloon. J Am Assoc Gynecol Laparosc 1996; 3(3): 403–407

Laparovaginal approach to fibroids: laparoscopically-assisted vaginal myomectomy (LAVM)

S. Nair

Introduction

Myomectomy, an operation evolved to remove uterine leiomyomata with preservation of the uterus, had its origins in 1840 when Amussta of Paris excised a prolapsed submucous tumour transvaginally;[1] subsequently, Washington Atlee removed a pedunculated subserous myoma transabdominally in 1844.[2]

At this time, the pioneers of gynaecological surgery were accustomed to procuring the pedicles of ovarian cysts and hence myomectomies were confined to pedunculated fibroids. Hysterectomy became the most popular operation as it required only severance of the uterus from the cervix or vagina, involving the familiar concept of pedicle surgery for removal of adnexal masses.

The fundamental principles that govern the modern operation of myomectomy were attributed to William Alexander in 1898.[3] The problems of haemorrhage and sepsis plagued this technically more complex operation, involving the removal of tumours embedded in the uterine wall. Hence, it did not gain popularity until championed during the 1920s by Bonney in England[3] and by Kelly and Noble,[4] Mayo[5] and Rubin[6] in the United States.

The encouraging results produced by these surgeons served to stimulate interest in myomectomy. In fact, Victor Bonney had reported in 1931 over 800 of these operations.[7] Bonney had a high regard for reconstructive surgery preserving the reproductive organs. He was instrumental in increasing the awareness among gynaecologists of the more conservative myomectomy as the operation of choice for young women with myomatous uteri, rather than the more radical operation — the hysterectomy.

Nevertheless, hysterectomy continued to be the primary operation for the treatment of dysfunctional bleeding and anatomical uterine abnormalities. Improved surgical morbidity and mortality and ineffective medical therapy were responsible for the trend towards more radical surgery.

In recent years, however, social changes have made it important to conserve the uterus and the reproductive potential of women who are tending to delay marriage and/or child bearing. This is especially so with the advent of effective contraception. The propensity for the occurrence of myomata in later reproductive years has thus made the prospect of the conservative myomectomy more attractive to the patient and her gynaecologist than ever before.

There was no dramatic evolution in the technique of surgical extirpation of myomata until recently, with the advent of minimal-access operative laparoscopic surgery. The earliest description of laparoscopic myomectomy had been from one of the fathers of laparoscopic surgery, Professor Kurt Semm;[8] and in later years, the laparoscopically-assisted minilaparotomy approach was proposed by Nezhat et al.[9] There has been a resurgence in the totally laparoscopic approach, even for those women wishing to increase their fertility.[10] However, controversy still abounds regarding the integrity of the laparoscopic repair of the myomectomy defect and the risk of scar dehiscence.[11–13]

To this end, the need for meticulous reconstruction of uterine defects to ensure the integrity of the repair is critical to reproductive function. There are reports in the literature of uterine dehiscence occurring during a pregnancy following laparoscopic myomectomy.[11–13] There are distinct shortcomings in laparoscopic suture reconstruction of the post-myomectomy uterus, whether intra- or extracorporeal, that even the most dexterous and skilful endoscopist will acknowledge. Especially in large and multiple myomata, recommendation of a purely laparoscopic approach where subsequent fertility is a consideration is generally still not accepted by the majority of the fraternity.[9,12]

To achieve meticulous and expeditious repair of uterine defects after myomectomy, two major routes have been used in conjunction with the laparoscopic initiation and subsequent completion of the myomectomy. These include a suprapubic transverse minilaparotomy, i.e. laparoscopically-assisted minilaparotomy myomectomy (LAMM),[9] or a transvaginal approach utilizing a colpotomy, i.e. laparoscopically-assisted vaginal or laparovaginal myomectomy (LAVM). The utility of this approach for only fundal and posterior fibroids has been described by Pelosi and Pelosi,[14] whereas with anterior intramural fibroids the LAMM was performed.

The laparoscopic phase of these two approaches retains the advantages of minimal-access surgery in minimizing the size of the abdominal incision. It also allows the surgeon to survey the entire peritoneal cavity and to handle any concomitant pathology or perform associated surgery such as adhesiolysis, adnexal surgery or appendicectomy. It also enables appropriate siting of the uterine incision, application of vasoconstrictor agents, and initiation and completion of the process of myomectomy — which would be hindered and difficult if performed through a small minilaparotomy incision or via the vagina.

The major disadvantage of the wholly laparoscopic approach is that laborious and time-consuming morcellation is required for extirpation of large myomata. As mentioned earlier, laparoscopic suture repair of uterine defects is less than ideal:[9,12] it is technically demanding to perform adequate and acceptable suturing of deep defects from a two-dimensional video image using instruments a long way from the operative site, with the inherent loss of fine dexterity. Although a minilaparotomy can overcome these problems, it still results in a sizeable abdominal incision.

The laparovaginal approach, however, avoids the need for a painful abdominal incision. In women, an excellent portal of access exists in the way of a colpotomy for removal of large tissue masses, either wholly or after limited laparoscopic or vaginal morcellation. The uterus can then be everted through the colpotomy and the uterine defect, however deep and extensive, repaired in layers in much the same way as would be done via a laparotomy, without compromising the integrity of the repair. Furthermore, the entire uterus can readily be palpated to detect and remove any further intramural fibroids.

Technique of laparovaginal myomectomy

In order to master this technique, the surgeon should have acceptable experience of operative laparoscopy and be proficient in vaginal surgery — i.e. in techniques of vaginal hysterectomy and, if possible, vaginal myomectomy for posteriorly placed myomata.

Selection of patients for LAVM depends on the availability of the standard laparoscopic and vaginal surgical equipment and on patient factors such as size and multiplicity of the fibroids, vaginal capacity, accessibility of the uterus through the vagina and the presence of adhesive disease of the pelvis. It would be prudent in the early learning phase of this procedure to select a patient who has a single fibroid, preferably situated posteriorly or at the fundus and generally not larger than 6–8 cm. The vaginal aspect of surgery would be easier if the patient were multiparous and had a capacious vagina and a mobile uterus. Dense pelvic adhesions from previous surgery, inflammation or endometriosis could prove frustrating for the surgeon in his initial foray into this type of surgery.

In the laparoscopic phase of this procedure, a 10 mm trocar is inserted either directly or after preliminary establishment of carbon dioxide pneumoperitoneum by passage of the Verres needle intra-umbilically. In instances where the myomatous uterus extends to or beyond the umblicus, an open laparoscopy[15] or insertion of the Verres needle and a 5 mm trocar at the left upper quadrant of the abdomen, 3–4 cm below the subcostal margin and along the midclavicular line, would be necessary to avoid injury to the uterus. In the left hypochondrium insertion, splenomegaly must be excluded and a nasogastric tube is necessary to deflate the stomach to prevent an inadvertent gastrostomy.

Laparoscopic phase

Positioning of the accessory ports depends very much on the size of the myomatous uterus. To provide better accessibility and leverage of instruments from the fixed points of access through the abdomen, the lateral ports are best placed high and lateral along the abdomen for large myomatous uteri. A suprapubic port is often useful as it allows the surgeon to use further graspers or dissectors to facilitate the myomectomy. After preliminary infiltration of the myoma site with vasopressin

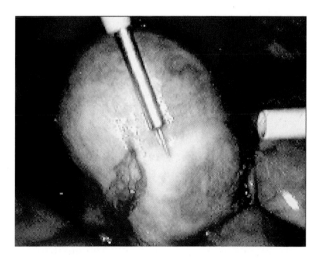

Figure 27.1 Infiltration of vasopressin into the myoma site using a 5 mm aspiration needle.

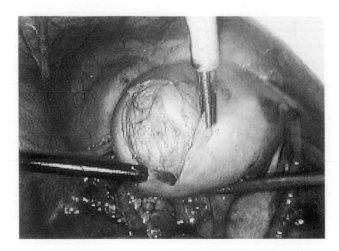

Figure 27.2 The uterine incision.

(0.2 units/ml), a vertical incision is made over the uterus through the suprapubic port using a monopolar spatula electrode (Figs. 27.1 and 27.2).

In removing large myomata, a 10 mm myoma screw (Fig. 27.3) can be passed through the 10–11 mm umbilical port to anchor, and/or to apply traction to, the myoma. Application of cephalad traction together with visualization via a 5 mm laparoscope through one of the lateral ports can expedite the myomectomy and provide the necessary visualization.

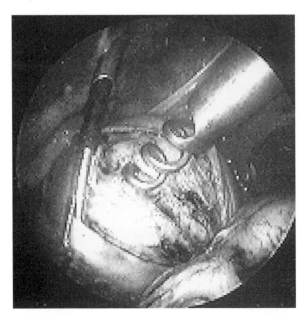

Figure 27.3 Traction via a 10 mm myoma screw through an umbilical port.

By a combination of 5 mm graspers and the 5 mm bipolar forceps insinuated between the pseudocapsule and the fibroid, meticulous and haemostatic enucleation of the fibroid is accomplished (Fig. 27.4). Traction and counter-traction is applied, using instruments through the three ports, gradually delivering the myoma from its uterine bed.

It is important to use the bipolar coagulating forceps to desiccate the fibrous interconnecting bands that sometimes carry the vessels feeding the myoma, in order

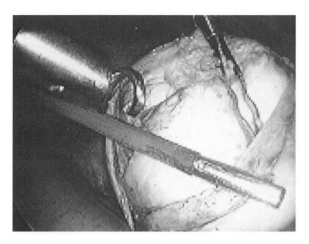

Figure 27.4 Enucleation using myoma screw traction and dissection with bipolar coagulating forceps.

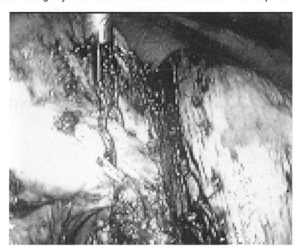

Figure 27.5 Bipolar dessication of vascular bridges between fibroid and myoma 'bed'.

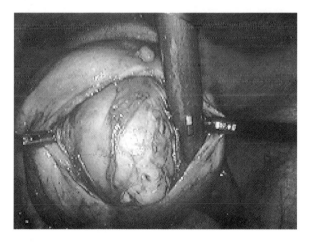

Figure 27.6 Myoma enucleation using 10 mm spoon forceps.

to prevent bleeding (Fig. 27.5). Haemorrhage from the uterine defect can be difficult to control laparoscopically, especially when the vessels retract into the depths of the myometrium. During laparoscopy, it is also difficult to apply haemostatic sutures rapidly as readily as at laparotomy.

Another energy modality, the harmonic ultrasonic scalpel (US Surgical Corp., Norwalk, NJ, USA: Ethicon Endoscopy, Cincinnati, OH, USA) has been shown to assist in blunt dissection and morcellation of myomata while minimizing tissue trauma and blood loss.[10] However, this device is expensive and not as universally available as the bipolar coagulating forceps. All the author's cases were performed using electrosurgery.

Remote palpation of the uterus using a spoon forceps (Fig. 27.6) via the umbilicus can often help in the detection of large intramural fibroids, which are best enucleated to reduce the bulk of the uterus and hence facilitate its delivery through the colpotomy incision.

If the myoma is deeply embedded in the myometrium, the author has, on occasion, introduced the index finger (Fig. 27.7) by enlarging the suprapubic incision. Introduction of the finger and dissecting and enucleating the fibroid is extremely rewarding, even in posteriorly placed fibroids, as it enables the surgeon to exert significant yet controlled palpation pressure to enucleate the myoma. This approach also enables the surgeon to palpate for other fibroids. Once again, care must be taken to secure any major vessels before finger-dissecting through the tissue bridges.

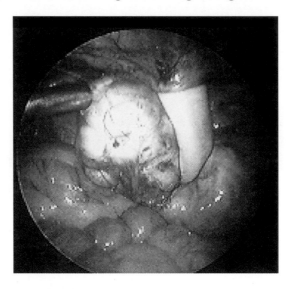

Figure 27.7 Myoma enucleation using finger dissection.

As a precautionary manoeuvre, the author anchors large myomata that have been removed with a laparoscopic stitch upon the fibroid with the suture drawn through the lateral port site peripheral to the trocar (Fig. 27.8). There have been instances where an entire uterus has been 'lost' in the upper reaches of the abdomen, requiring a laparotomy to retrieve it![16]

It is important to have myomata anchored via the laparoscopic myoma screw, claw forceps or vulsellum (Fig. 27.9) for introduction into the cul-de-sac and eventual removal through the colpotomy.

On occasion, the author has found that some myomata are too large to fit into the depths of the cul-de-sac for easy vaginal access. It must be remembered that the pelvic canal progresses downwards and forwards, and large myomata may not be delivered beyond the level of the ischial spines. Hence, limited laparoscopic morcellation sufficient to allow vaginal delivery of large fibroids may sometimes be required (Fig. 27.10).

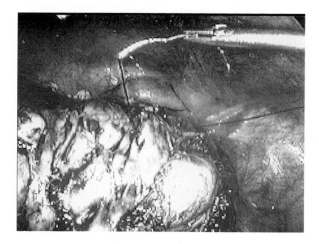

Figure 27.8 Securing enucleated fibroids by sutures via lateral ports prior to removal.

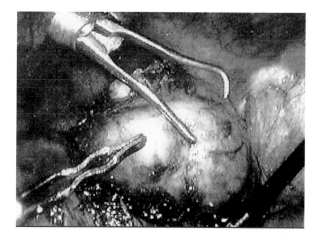

Figure 27.9 A 10 mm vulsellum is used to grasp the myoma.

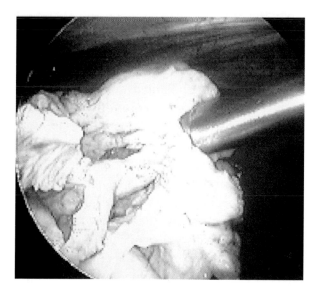

Figure 27.10 Laparoscopic morcellation of the fibroid.

There are a variety of ways in which the large myomata can be anchored or grasped vaginally through the colpotomy. The laparoscopic vulsellum is a very useful device to grasp the myoma, but this must be done under laparoscopic surveillance to avoid inadvertent rectosigmoid injury.

The colpotomy can be made either vaginally or laparoscopically. The vaginal incision is made as in a vaginal hysterectomy. The cervix is lifted anteriorly using a tenaculum. After prior vasoconstrictor infiltration, a fold of vaginal mucosa is lifted using the Bonney's forceps and an incision made transversely. The incision is carried through the mucosa and the peritoneum until the pouch of Douglas is entered. Loss of pneumoperitoneum can be slowed if the myoma is used to plug the cul-de-sac. A 10–12 mm trocar with a laparoscopic claw forceps or vulsellum can be introduced through a small colpotomy incision to grasp the fibroid under laparoscopic guidance. Alternatively, if vaginal access is difficult, the colpotomy can be made laparoscopically, delineating the posterior fornix by introducing a wet swab carried on the sponge forceps and tenting the posterior fornix. A spatula electrode is used to perform the colpotomy laparoscopically, using the 'cut wave' form of current. This is possibly the method to be preferred if there is endometriosis involving the rectovaginal septum. Prior laparoscopic enterolysis of the rectosigmoid colon from the posterior vagina can be accomplished to prepare for the colpotomy. In either case, great care must be taken to retract the rectosigmoid colon out of harm's way during the delivery of myomata through the colpotomy using atraumatic laparoscopic bowel graspers or retractors. Long-bladed Briesky–Navratil retractors introduced vaginally (Aesculap A.G., Tuttlingen, Germany) are used to protect the rectum and also provide leverage to negotiate the fibroid and evert the uterus through the colpotomy (Figs. 27.11–27.13).

By removing the largest myoma the bulk of the uterus is reduced. This facilitates negotiation of the myoma along the pelvic canal out through the colpotomy. Pelosi and Pelosi[14] have preferred to keep the myoma partially tethered to the uterus at its base in order to facilitate subsequent transvaginal uterine exteriorization by traction on the myomata. This method is easier in women with a very capacious pelvis and smaller myomata. An alternative method used by the author, especially when there are constraints in space and large multiple myomata are present, is to enucleate laparoscopically as many of the larger myomata as possible. The myomata are removed in turn, either intact or with limited morcellation, through the colpotomy. With the recent advent of electronic motor-driven laparoscopic morcellators, myoma morcellation can be expedited. This phase of the procedure is less cumbersome after reduction of the uterine volume, so that it occupies less space in the anterior pelvis.

Once the uterus has been 'debulked' and reduced in volume after prior laparoscopic myomectomy, it can be delivered through the colpotomy by a combination of blunt pressure from the spoon forceps laparoscopically and concomitant traction transvaginally via atraumatic sponge forceps applied over the edges of the uterine defect. Occasionally this is difficult if the uterus is fairly large or the uterine defect is anterior or anterofundal. Hence, application of the long vulsellum or claw forceps into the uterine defect or the posterior aspect of the uterus is necessary for gentle constant traction in order to prevent trauma to the uterus. Pelosi and Pelosi[14] describe application of traction sutures in the midline of the posterior uterine wall. However, the same effect could be accomplished by using a

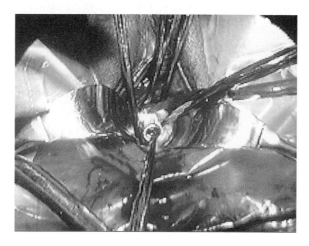

Figure 27.11 Vaginal morcellation of the fibroid held by myoma screw.

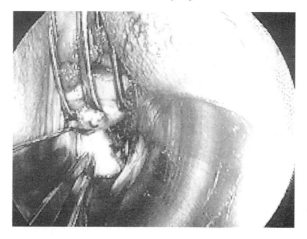

Figure 27.12 Upward traction of the posterior lip of the cervix to gain access to the fibroid in the pouch of Douglas through colpotomy.

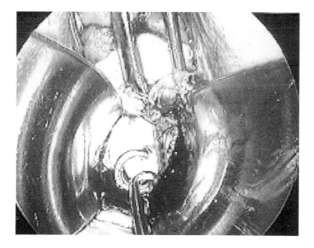

Figure 27.13 Delivery of the fibroid through colpotomy using myoma screw.

fine-toothed tenaculum, which provides a quicker, less cumbersome and more controlled traction than application of sutures. In nullipara, if the vaginal capacity is inadequate, a midline episiotomy can develop sufficient 'give' round the introitus for delivery of fibroids or the uterus for repair of the defect.

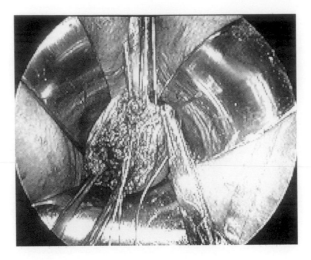

Figure 27.14 Meticulous layered transvaginal repair of a uterine defect.

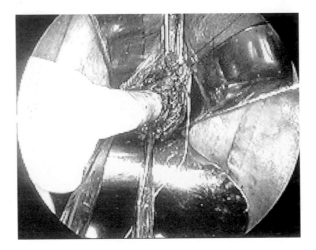

Figure 27.15 Meticulous layered transvaginal repair of a uterine defect.

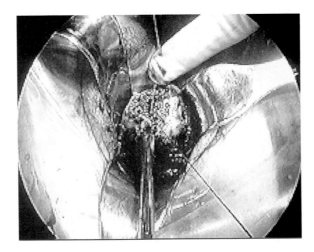

Figure 27.16 Transvaginal meticulous and secure layered suture repair of an uterine myoma defect.

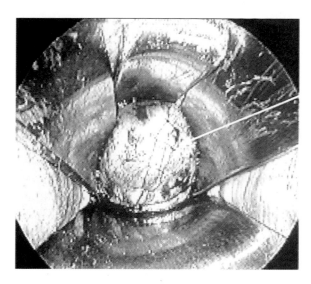

Figure 27.17 Completed repair.

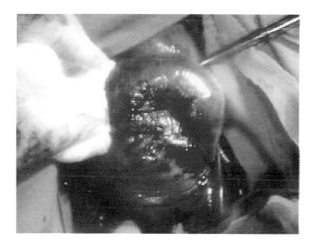

Figure 27.18 Completed transvaginal repair (inversion technique, see text).

Once the uterus has been delivered out through the introitus, even the deepest defect and/or multiple defects can be suture-repaired as meticulously as can be achieved via a laparotomy (Figs. 27.14–27.18). The author uses Monocryl (Ethicon, Edinburgh, UK) absorbable sutures because they are akin to monofilament sutures in that they pass through the tissues smoothly and atraumatically and have very high tensile strength. This is important to ensure good haemostasis and firm apposition of surrounding myometrium in order to minimize the formation of dead space and haematoma. If the uterine cavity is entered, the myometrium over and adjacent to it is repaired via continuous fine 4/0 Vicryl or Monocryl sutures without involving the endometrium. The serosa of the uterine defect is apposed using fine continuous running sutures. A technique used by the author to close the uterine defect involves burial of the surrounding myometrium and serosa in the depths of the uterine defect, using purse-string sutures. In this way, the large cavity left in the uterus is further reduced and obliterated, hence reducing the eventual size of the incision line. There is, therefore, less scarred surface on which adhesions might occur, and the serosal surfaces are in apposition without any myometrium appearing.

Fundal and posterior fibroids are technically more accessible by the laparovaginal method; however, anteriorly placed myomata can also be removed and repaired in a similar manner (Fig. 27.19). Despite being anterior in position, the uterus can be everted through the posterior colpotomy (Fig. 27.20) and introitus by delivering the fundus as described earlier and thrusting the cervix cephalad in very much the same fashion as that involved in Doderlein's hysterectomy. To progress further inferiorly to the apex of the anterior uterine defect (i.e. nearer to the cervix), a series of anchoring sutures, applied progressively towards the cervix while repairing the defect stepwise, will eventually enable the entire defect to be repaired securely. Alternatively, if application of sutures is not feasible, then long sponge forceps or single-tooth tenaculi can be used to grasp the edges of the anterior uterine defect to draw down the defect gently for repair at the introitus. If this is not possible, a suprapubic minilaparotomy could be used to repair this defect (and, of course, any other defects present over the entire uterus).[9,14]

Cautious and controlled but adequate traction upon the uterus to deliver it out through the introitus is critical if tearing or rupture of vessels (especially within the infundibulopelvic ligaments) is to be prevented. Jerky and hurried excessive

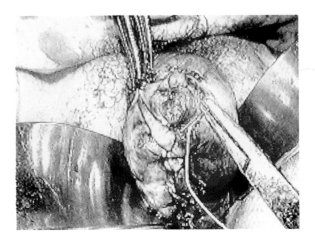

Figure 27.19 Transvaginal repair of an anterior myomectomy defect.

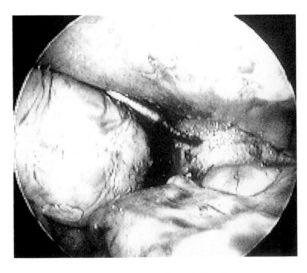

Figure 27.20 Posterior colpotomy to remove the enucleated fibroids.

traction forces could potentially result in disastrous consequences, such as haematomata dissecting up the retroperitoneal space from ruptured infundibulopelvic vessels.

After repair of the myomectomy site, the uterus is reintroduced into the abdomen via the colpotomy. During the whole procedure the uterus is kept moist with saline. Meticulous haemostasis is maintained by a combination of sutures and electrodiathermy. The colpotomy is carefully repaired using absorbable running sutures, taking care to secure the angles of the colpotomy incision to prevent postoperative haemorrhage.

A large Redivac or Jackson–Pratt drain is introduced via the abdominal port sites to drain the pelvis. The author initially used to drain the pelvis transabdominally; however, in one case a vault haematoma occurred, which was subsequently drained transvaginally under ultrasound guidance. Very often the Redivac or Jackson–Pratt sump drains, upon vacuum suction, become obstructed. Thereafter, drains were left to pass out through the colpotomy, using gravity to drain off the most dependent area in the pelvis, i.e. the cul-de-sac. A T-tube drain has since been used and this has been found to be more effective (Figs. 27. 21–27.23). Drains are left only when

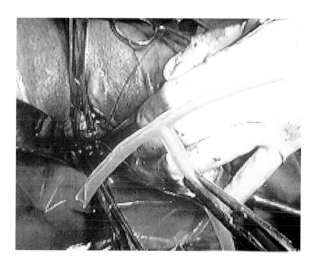

Figure 27.21 Using a T-tube to drain the pelvis — introduction at repair of colpotomy.

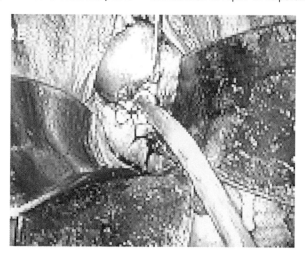

Figure 27.22 Drainage of the pelvis with the T-tube drain out through the posterior colpotomy.

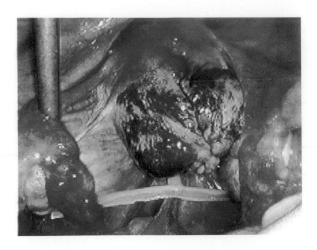

Figure 27.23 Using a T-tube to drain the pelvis — intra-abdominal view at check laparoscopy.

very large uterine defects have been repaired or absolute haemostasis has been difficult to achieve.

Copious lavage and further pinpoint haemostasis using bipolar coagulation is accomplished laparoscopically (Fig. 27.24). The whole abdomen is again inspected, taking care to lavage the subdiaphagmatic areas as some blood and fluid can collect in these recesses, owing to the steep Trendelenburg position of the patient that is sometimes necessary in order to perform the laparoscopic myomectomy.

The rectus sheath defect at the umbilical incision is repaired in layers using a C-shaped needle (Polysorb O, US Surgical Corp.) in order to prevent any acute herniation of the omentum or intestine. About 20 ml Marcaine (bupivacaine 1%) is infiltrated into the umbilicus and the accessory trocar sites to minimize postoperative pain. The skin edges at the 5 mm accessory trocar sites are apposed using 'Steri-strips'. If required, subcuticular Vicryl sutures are used to appose the skin edges.

Experience with LAVM

A total of 57 LAVM procedures were attempted by the author between June 1995 and October 1997. The age, weight and parity distribution of the patients are shown in Table 27.1.

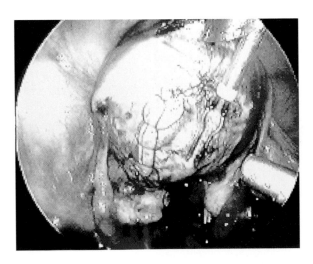

Figure 27.24 Meticulous bipolar pinpoint haemostasis at final laparoscopy.

Table 27.1 Age, weight and parity of 57 patients undergoing laparoscopically-assisted vaginal myomectomy (LAVM)

Patient features	No. of patients
Age (years)	
<25	8
25–34	12
35–44	27
>45	10
Weight (kg)	
>49	13
50–59	27
60–69	11
>70	6
Parity	
0	11
1	7
2	23
≥3	16

The most frequent indication for myomectomy was menorrhagia (19 cases) followed by dysmenorrhoea and abdominal pain (10 cases) including two of acute pain and febrile morbidity due to degeneration of the fibroid. A total of 14 cases were operated on as part of their treatment for subfertility. An abdominopelvic mass was the presentation in another eight cases. In six cases, the patients were asymptomatic and were discovered to have a pelvi-abdominal mass on routine health screening.

With regard to previous major abdominal surgery, in 14 cases patients previously had undergone caesarean section (CS) (1 CS, six; 2 CS, three; 3 CS, five patients). Eleven patients had previously undergone myomectomy, all performed abdominally; laparoscopic adnexal surgery (e.g. oöphorectomy, cystectomy, tubal surgery) had previously been performed in five cases. Appendicectomies had been the history in three cases. In only two cases had transcervical resection of the endometrium been performed and one patient had undergone abdominal surgery other than gynaecological surgery (i.e. open cholecystectomy). All patients were carefully counselled about the need for surgery and the exact nature of the surgery, and were told that the traditional approach (i.e. the laparotomy) was still an option and might be embarked upon should technical difficulties or complications arise during the LAVM. A detailed informed consent form was signed by each patient, with the full knowledge that this procedure was a new approach to performing the same surgery as would be done via a laparotomy. Preoperative preparation involved mechanical bowel preparation, one day before surgery. (The colonic lavage solution comprised sodium chlorite, bicarbonate and sulphate [anhydrous]; potassium chloride; and Macrogel [Delta West, Western Australia], 1.5–2.0 litres).

Prophylactic antibiotics (usually either ampicillin, gentamicin and flagyl or a cephalosporin and flagyl) were given at induction of anaesthesia and for 48 hours thereafter. In febrile patients, a full course of antibiotics was administered (i.e. for at least 7–10 days). Gonadotrophin-releasing hormone analogues (GnRHa) were used only in cases of significant anaemia (i.e. haemoglobin < 10.0 g/dl) for 3 months, together with iron supplements to improve haemoglobin levels. The use of GnRHa did pose some technical problems, such as difficulty in enucleation of the fibroid due to a lack of a definite dissection plane between the myoma and the pseudocapsule.

In five cases of very large myomata (>10 cm), preoperative bilateral embolization of the uterine arteries was performed under fluoroscopic guidance in order to reduce intra-operative bleeding. Although this was successful in reducing blood loss, it added significantly to the overall cost of surgery and hence was not continued for the remainder of the LAVM procedures.

In selecting patients for LAVM, care was taken to ensure that the patients were fit to withstand anaesthesia and laparoscopy for a prolonged period. In addition, the pelvic and vaginal capacity (especially in nullipara and virgins) was cautiously assessed in relation to the total mass of fibroids to be extirpated. The assessments were carried out during examination per vaginam and/or per rectum in the clinic setting, as well as before embarking on surgery when the patient had been anaesthetized in the operating theatre. In only two cases was a totally laparoscopic myomectomy (TLM) preferred over the LAVM. In the first case a large anterior pedunculated fibroid was transected at its narrow base and removed piecemeal through gradual morcellation via the umbilicus; the site of attachment to the uterus did not require any repair as there was no defect. In the other instance, a large multilobulated broad-ligament fibroid was dissected out and removed by morcellation via the umbilicus. In this case, the myoma was attached to the right lateral mid-body of the uterus via a narrow pedicle and did not require repair of the uterus; only the defect in the broad ligament was closed laparoscopically.

In two other cases, a minilaparotomy myomectomy was performed instead of the LAVM. In the first case, the lesion turned out to be an adenomyoma associated with dense pouch of Douglas obliteration by endometriosis. The adenomyoma was difficult to dissect and 'enucleate' laparoscopically as there were no distinct planes of cleavage as expected; instead, the adenomyoma was excised and the defect repaired through a minilaparotomy incision. In the second case, the patient was a virgin and, although she had consented to the LAVM, at anaesthesia the pelvis and vagina were found to be too restrictive to allow the 15 cm myoma to be removed expeditiously. Hence, the myomectomy was performed laparoscopically as described earlier, followed by suture repair via a 4 cm minilaparotomy over the suprapubic area.

Thus, discussion of the surgical outcome takes into account only the remaining 53 cases where LAVM was completed.

Surgical outcome

Of the LAVM procedures performed, in 18 the dominant fibroid was an anteriorly placed myoma, the remainder comprising primarily fundal and/or posterior fibroids. Although anterior in site, myomata that were significantly large were first removed laparoscopically and the uterus then everted so that the anterior myoma defect became accessible via the introitus for layered suture repair. The laparoscopic

Table 27.2 Characteristics of the myomata removed

Characteristics	Mean (range)
Size of dominant myomata (cm)	8.5 (5–18)
Weight of myomata (g)	333.0 (180–852)
Number of myomata removed	3.4 (1–13)

vulsellum was employed to assist in delivery of the uterus, as described earlier. Conversely, a low posterior cervical myoma defect was repaired after prior transvaginal myomectomy. The intravaginal repair was performed after replacement of the uterus intra-abdominally because only then was it possible to access the posterior cervical myomectomy site vaginally. Prior 'debulking' of the uterus allowed easier delivery of the uterus, such that even anterior cervico-isthmic myomectomy defects were accessible vaginally. Small anterior fibroids (i.e. <2 cm) were extirpated entirely transvaginally after laparoscopic myomectomy of adjacent fundal or posterior fibroids.

A total of 96 myomata were removed. The myomata ranged in size from less than 1 cm to the largest single myoma measuring 18 cm in diameter (Table 27.2). The maximum weight of myomatous tissue removed from a single patient was 852 g, and the largest number of myomata removed from one patient was 13: in this case, the four largest fibroids were removed laparoscopically, allowing sufficient reduction of uterine volume to enable delivery of the uterus transvaginally, where the rest of the palpable fibroids were subsequently removed vaginally followed by suture repair of the defects.

In two cases the myomata had undergone degeneration and liquefaction. However, in both instances it was possible to enucleate the solid segments of the fibroid completely. A frozen section was taken in one 43-year-old patient, but there was no histological evidence of a leiomyosarcoma.

In 37 cases, limited morcellation was required before the fibroid could be reduced to a size that allowed delivery via the colpotomy. The author found that it was not so much the actual size of the myoma that impeded delivery but rather whether it was hard and 'gritty', requiring morcellation to a manageable size. Some fibroids were more compressible and pliable in consistency, or were large but lobulated and thus could be delivered via the colpotomy intact or with limited morcellation.

Morcellation was sometimes accomplished transvaginally, especially where the myoma could be delivered low enough into the pelvis to make it accessible to anchorage via myoma screws or claw forceps introduced vaginally. In four (nulliparous) patients a small midline episiotomy was required to facilitate removal of the fibroids. Nevertheless, in two patients (one nulliparous and one who had two previous births by caesarean section), an extension of the colpotomy was sustained. Thus far, there have not been any instances of dyspareunia due to painful scarring of the episiotomy or colpotomy in those women who were sexually active. Concomitant laparoscopic procedures included pelvic adhesiolysis involving the adnexae (12 cases) and pouch of Douglas enterolysis (four cases). In eight patients who had undergone previous surgery, anterior abdominal wall enterolysis and/or omentolysis had to be performed to facilitate myomectomy. In addition to the myomectomy, three patients had cystectomies and one patient an oöphorectomy for a benign cystic teratoma. In two cases, incidental appendicectomy was carried out at the patient's request. A total of eight patients had simultaneous tubal sterilization. One patient underwent concomitant hysteroscopic resection of a submucous myoma. The mean overall operating time of the LAVM procedures was 170 (range 152–300) min and the mean estimated blood loss was 480 (range 50–1800) ml. The operating time was generally 1½ hrs longer than the average operating time for abdominal myomectomies in the author's institution. The most time-consuming cases often involved instances where adhesiolysis was required for dense pelvic adhesions or when there were large and multiple myomata requiring laborious morcellation. However, this was less time consuming than performance of a totally laparoscopic myomectomy for large myomata.

The mean duration of hospitalization was 3.8 (range 1–13) days. This was far shorter than that for myomectomies performed by laparotomy in the author's institution (7.6 days). In nine cases, surgery was on a day-case basis. In two cases, involving complications, prolonged hospitalization was necessary.

In the first case involving prolonged hospitalization, the patient stayed in hospital for 9 days. She had developed tense abdominal distension, ileus and a swinging fever, and appeared ill and dehydrated, on the third postoperative day, after being well and consuming a normal diet for the first two days. A bowel injury was suspected and exploratory laparotomy was conducted with the general surgeon in attendance. However, fortunately, no bowel trauma was discovered: the peritoneal cavity was clear of any blood, or faeculent or exudative materials; nevertheless, the abdomen was lavaged and swabs were taken for culture. After the laparotomy, the patient's symptoms and fever promptly subsided. She was taking food orally one day after the laparotomy and was discharged 4 days later. There was no overt cause for the ileus and bowel distension (such as acute bowel obstruction from a volvulus or adhesion bands) nor was there any electrolyte imbalance. The symptoms were attributed to peritonitis from a possible intra-abdominal transmission of vaginal organisms, although blood, urine and vaginal cultures were negative for pathogens.

In the second case, the patient stayed in hospital for 13 days. There was 'spiking' fever from postoperative day 4 and a haematoma was discovered on transvaginal scan in the pouch of Douglas on postoperative day 6. Despite broad-spectrum antibiotics, the fever did not subside; transvaginal ultrasound-guided drainage of the haematoma was therefore performed on day 8. This resulted in resolution of the fever, granulocytosis and pelvic pain within 4 days, when the patient was discharged well from hospital. On review of the operative notes it was apparent that this patient had sustained an extension of the colpotomy due to removal of large myomata (13 cm) and, despite laparoscopic visualization to check on haemostasis, it was very likely that a bleeding point had resulted in a pelvic haematoma.

These were two major complications in this series of LAVMs. Other minor problems included 11 cases of fever, which all resolved by postoperative days 4 and 5 with the use of broad-spectrum antibiotics.

In the 11 nulliparous women who underwent LAVM procedures, six wished to become pregnant and did so within 3–18 months of the procedure. Although patients were advised to defer plans for pregnancy for at least 6 months, two became pregnant before this time. Of the six patients who were hoping for pregnancy, four were on concurrent fertility treatments (one in vitro fertilization [IVF], one superovulation with gonadotrophins and intra-uterine insemination [SO-IUI] and two on ovulation induction with clomiphene). There have thus far been five normal vaginal deliveries and one on-going pregnancy.

Of the multiparous patients, eight were contemplating further child bearing. A total of five patients were on fertility programmes — one IVF and four on ovulation induction with clomiphene.

To date, among all the multipara, there have been three successful pregnancies. Two patients were delivered vaginally, while one with an ongoing pregnancy has been scheduled for caesarean section because of a previous caesarean section for cephalopelvic disproportion. This time the baby was estimated to be too large (abdominal circumference far above the 97th centile) for a safe trial of the scar and not because of any suspicion of the integrity of the LAVM scar. There were two first-trimester miscarriages among the multipara.

Of those patients who did not wish to become pregnant, two had spontaneously conceived; both patients opted for termination of their pregnancy and one underwent concurrent laparoscopic tubal sterilization.

In the author's institution, second-look laparoscopies are not routine. In this series of LAVM procedures, repeat laparoscopies took place in four cases. One was for tubal sterilization, as described earlier; here, no adhesion barrier was used and a loop of small bowel was densely adherent to the fundal myomectomy site. There were also filmy adhesions over the site of colpotomy in the pouch of Douglas, but the fallopian tubes were free and not involved in adhesions. In two other cases, recurrent pelvic pain and dysmenorrhoea prompted an exploratory second laparoscopy. Here again there were omental and bowel adhesions to the fundal myomectomy site, but these were not densely adherent and were easily lysed laparoscopically. In both these cases, Interceed (TC7, Ethicon, Sommerville, NJ, USA) was used as an adhesion barrier and probably had helped to reduce the severity of the adhesions (Fig. 27.26). In the fourth case, a repeat laparoscopy was done to evaluate fertility potential after 13 months of ovulation induction with clomiphene. This patient was subsequently referred for IVF, as she was 36 years old and had endometriosis and there was severe teratospermia in her husband's seminal assay. The endometriosis in this case was largely confined to the pelvic side-walls and the pouch of Douglas, causing partial obliteration of the cul-de-sac. There were also dense bowel adhesions to the myomectomy site, involving the rectosigmoid, despite prior use of the Interceed adhesion barrier. Whether the bowel adhesions were due primarily to the endometriosis rather than the myomectomy scar was difficult to ascertain. By the time of the 'second-look' laparoscopy, the fallopian tubes had been distorted by progressive endometriosis. The patient is currently on her second thaw cycle of IVF.

With regard to postoperative pain, patients who had undergone LAVM had low pain scores similar to those of the patients who underwent total laparoscopic myomectomies in the author's institution. Even patients who had an episiotomy did not experience significant perineal pain: only oral analgesia was required, and only for the first 24 hours. All the patients were ambulant and taking a full diet by the first postoperative day.

In contrast, patients undergoing LAMM, performed by the author and other

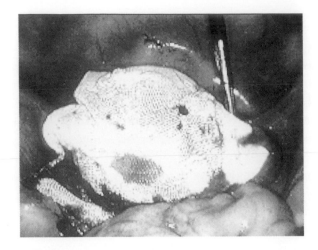

Figure 27.25 Placing an adhesion barrier over the myomectomy site.

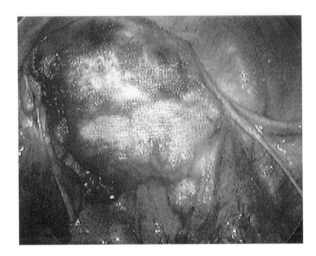

Figure 27.26 The adhesion barrier over the myomectomy site.

surgeons in the same institution, required parenteral analgesia in the form of pethidine injections or morphine infusion for at least 24–48 h postoperatively. The duration of hospitalization for the LAMM patients was, however, similar to that for those undergoing LAVM, but the mean pain scores of the former were higher, and the period before return to normal activity was three times longer (LAVM, 5 days; LAMM, 17 days). Patients who underwent open myomectomy in the author's institution had the highest pain scores and longest duration of analgesia requirements (parenteral, 24–36 h, oral, 5–22 days); most of these women were not able to return fully to their routine activities until about a month later. These patients stayed longer in hospital and became fully ambulant only on postoperative days 5 or 6.

Controversial aspects of laparoscopic myomectomy

Much controversy surrounds laparoscopic myomectomy. The most important debating point is the question of the integrity of repair of the myomectomy repair. Scar dehiscence of myomectomy defects repaired via a laparotomy is almost unheard of, whereas there have been a few case reports of uterine rupture following laparoscopic myomectomy.[11–13]

Laparoscopic suture repair of myomectomy defects, although having its protagonists,[10] has not yet achieved universal acceptance. This is primarily because of the increased manual dexterity and prolonged operating time required to perform securely a layered repair of deep defects. The two approaches available to the gynaecological endoscopist for the repair of myoma defects using conventional techniques and instruments are minilaparotomy or colpotomy. Minilaparotomy still results in a sizeable abdominal incision. For large myomatous uteri, a clinically significant reduction in size of the abdominal incision can be achieved by concurrent laparoscopy that allows good visualization of the myomata and instrumentation to facilitate and complete the myomectomy. Upon 'debulking' the uterus, an incision that gives sufficient access to suture repair the myomectomy defect is all that is needed. Similarly, if large abdominal incisions are to be avoided altogether, selected patients could undergo the laparovaginal approach (LAVM) as described.

A potential disadvantage of the LAVM procedure, however, is the possibility of sepsis due to the exposure of the pelvic organs to the exterior via the vagina. Furthermore, the close proximity of the surgical field to the perineum and anal region, and thus the potential for infection, is an important consideration. Aseptic technique, using barrier drapes across the perineal region such that only the introitus is accessible, plus adequate pelvic drainage, careful and meticulous haemostasis afforded by laparoscopy and broad-spectrum antibiotics can help to negate or minimize this shortcoming of the procedure.

Indeed, in this series, one patient developed a vault haematoma, which the author suspects was due to persistent bleeding from the vaginal incision, not adequately secured during colpotomy closure. The patient who underwent the laparotomy may possibly have had some degree of peritoneal irritation from sepsis that could have been treated conservatively by broad-spectrum antibiotics; however, the author thought it prudent to perform an exploratory laparotomy, as faecal peritonitis from large bowel perforation (which was the provisional diagnosis) can result in significant morbidity and mortality.

The majority of the patients, however, recovered far more quickly from surgery in comparison to those following open myomectomy (3.8 days vs 7.6 days). This was reflected in a significant reduction in morbidity, with earlier return to normal routine activity. Furthermore, the improved cost-effectiveness of the procedure, due to reduction in hospital stay and the ability of the patients to return to work earlier, far outweighed the increased cost due to longer operating times.

Whether the laparoscopic approach had reduced the propensity for pelvic adhesions was not conclusively studied in this series. There is a paucity of published data on this aspect of laparoscopic myomectomy; however, one recent study, comparing open myomectomy with the laparoscopic approach, showed a reduction in adhesion scores on second-look laparoscopy for the latter group.[17] The putative explanation for this could be the more meticulous haemostasis and lavage afforded by check laparoscopy using physiological irrigant and precise bipolar coagulation. The Interceed adhesion barrier used in this series mandated a blood-free surgical site for maximum efficacy, which was achieved via laparoscopy.

Conclusions

LAVM is proposed as an efficient method for the surgical extirpation of clinically significant myomata. It allows organ-preserving myomectomies to be performed with minimum morbidity, using newer minimal-access techniques and established vaginal manoeuvres to facilitate and expedite tissue reduction. It also enables resilient suture repair of the myomectomy defects to ensure the proper integrity of the uterine scar in women planning further child bearing.

References

1. Kelly H A. Myomectomy–hysteromyomectomy. In: Kelly H A (ed) Operative gynaecology, Vol. II. New York: Appleton & Co., 1898: 338–402

2. Atlee W L. Case of successful extirpation of a fibrous tumour of the peritoneal surface of the uterus by large peritoneal section. Am J Med Sci 1845; 9: 309

3. Bonney V. The techniques and results of myomectomy. Lancet 1931; 220: 171–177

4. Kelly N A, Noble C P. Gynaecology and abdominal surgery. Philadelphia: Saunders, 1908

5. Mayo W J. Myomectomy. Surg Gynecol Obstet 1922; 34: 548

6. Rubin I C. Progress in myomectomy. Am J Obstet Gynecol 1942; 44: 196

7. Bonney V. The technical minutiae of extended myomectomy and ovarian cystectomy. London. Hoeber, 1946

8. Semm K. New methods of pelviscopy (gynaecologic laparoscopic) for myomectomy, ovariectomy, tubectomy and adnectomy. Endoscopy 1979; 2: 85–93

9. Nezhat C, Nezhat F, Bess O et al. Laparoscopic assisted myomectomy: a report of a new technique in 57 cases. Int J Fertil 1994; 39: 39–44

10. Miller C E, Johnston M, Rundell L M. Laparoscopic myomectomy in the infertile woman. J Am Assoc Gynecol Laparosc 1996; 3: 525–532

11. Harris W J. Uterine dehiscence following laparoscopic myomectomy. Obstet Gynecol 1992; 80: 545–546

12. Dubuisson J B, Chavet X, Chapron C et al. Uterine rupture during pregnancy after laparoscopic myomectomy. Hum Reprod 1995; 10(6): 1475–1477

13. Friedmann W, Maier R F, Lutt Kus A et al. Uterine rupture after laparoscopic myomectomy. Acta Obstet Gynecol Scand 1996; 75(7): 683–684

14. Pelosi M A III, Pelosi M A. Laparoscopic-assisted transvaginal myomectomy. J Am Assoc Gynecol Laparosc 1997; 4: 241–246

15. Hasson H M. A modified instrument and method for laparoscopy. Am J Obstet Gynecol 1971, 110: 886

16. Semm K. Professor and Head of Dept, Dept of Obstetrics & Gynaecology, University of Kiel, Kiel, Germany. Personal communication, 1992

17. Bulletti C, Polli V, Negrini V et al. Adhesion formation after laparoscopic myomectomy. J Am Assoc Gynecol Laparosc 1996; 3: 533–536

Note: vs indicates the differentiation of conditions. Abbreviations used: AUB/DUB, abnormal/dysfunctional uterine bleeding; IU(C)D/IUS, intrauterine (contraceptive) device/intrauterine system; PDT, photodynamic therapy.